AF344323

TOPICS IN PUBLIC HEALTH

Edited by **David Claborn**

Topics in Public Health

http://dx.doi.org/10.5772/58484
Edited by David Claborn

Contributors

Suélia De Siqueira Rodrigues Fleury Rosa, Mário Fabrício Fleury Rosa, Diego Colón, Célia A. Reis, José M. Balthazar, Maria Do Carmo Reis, Denise Zak, Francisca Carvajal, Jose Manuel Lerma-Cabrera, Charles Ntungwen Fokunang, Maria De Lourdes Pereira, Elsa Dias, Fernando Garcia E Costa, Simone Morais, Lauren Ramsay, Christopher Charles, Hajime Sato, Satomi Noguchi, Stephen C. Edberg, David Claborn, Christie Oestreich, Muhiuddin Haider

CBS, Edition **2017**

Published by InTech

Janeza Trdine 9, 51000 Rijeka, Croatia

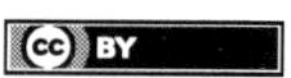

Notice

Publishing Process Manager Iva Simcic

Technical Editor InTech DTP Team

Cover Designer InTech Design Team

Additional hard copies can be obtained from orders@intechopen.com

Topics in Public Health, Edited by David Claborn
p. cm.
ISBN 978-953-51-2132-9

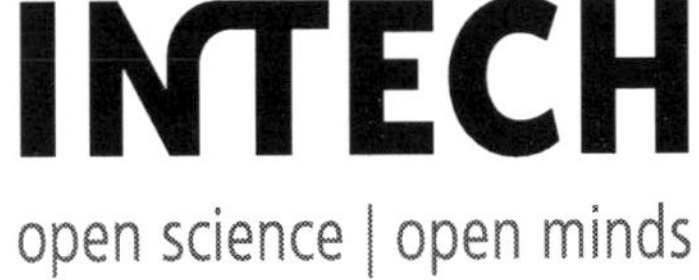

Contents

Preface

The American Centers for Disease Control and Prevention (CDC) define public health as "the science of protecting and improving the health of families and communities through promotion of health lifestyles, research for disease and injury prevention, and detection and control of infectious diseases." The focus of this definition is the population, and this is important in most other definitions of public health. Nevertheless, definitions do vary, especially in societies where clinical medicine is provided as part of a national system and is funded primarily through the national coffers. Understandably, the public often sees public health as the provision of clinical care through publicly-funded facilities. Historically, however, public health was what communities did to address infectious disease. Classic examples include John Snow's successful attempt to link cholera transmission to specific water sources, the control of malaria during the construction of the Panama Canal, and the control of yellow fever in Cuba. Perhaps the most successful of all public health initiatives is the elimination of smallpox through the use of systematic immunization.

As the successes in control of infectious diseases accumulated, the role of public health workers evolved to address other types of health threats. One notable example is the identification of pellagra as a disease due to a nutritional deficiency. This work by the U.S. Public Health Service led to dietary recommendations that ended a decades-long epidemic of pellagra in the American South. Such work led to more applications of the public health discipline to addressing the health of populations. Today, public health is broadly defined, reflecting efforts that include more aspects of the health and healthcare professions. Some authorities have postulated 10 essential health services that any public health agency should provide. These include:

(1) Monitoring the health status of supported populations;

(2) Diagnosing and investigating health problems and hazards in the community;

(3) Educating and empowering people to address health issues;

(4) Mobilizing community partnerships to address health problems;

(5) Developing and implementing policies that address health issues, both at the community and individual levels;

(6) Enforcing laws and regulations that protect human health and safety;

(7) Facilitating linkages between people and personal health services to ensure access to healthcare when it would be unavailable otherwise;

(8) Providing a competent workforce of health workers;

(9) Evaluating effectiveness, accessibility and quality of health services;

(10) Researching new solutions to existing health problems.

In light of this newer, broader definition of public health, this book presents chapters on a wide range of public health topics, including new technologies for testing potable water, the role of the news media in communicating health risks to the public, and specific health issues associated with migrant or displaced populations. The purpose of this book is not to provide an introduction to public health, but rather to provide a forum for updates on new technologies and new analysis of current issues in the field.

David Claborn, DrPH
CDR USN (ret.)
USA

Emerging Issues in Global Public Health

An Overview of The Public Health Global Perspective on the Grand Challenges of Non-Communicable and Chronic Diseases Within the Framework for Developing new Drugs

Estella Tembe-Fokunang, Charles Fokunang,
Zacharia Sando, Barbara Atogho Tiedeu,
Frederick Kechia, Valentine Ndikum,
Marceline Ngounoue Djuidje, Jerome Ateudjieu,
Raymond Langsi, John Fomnboh Dobgima,
Joseph Fokam, Luc Gwum, Obama Abena,
Tazoacha Asonganyii, Jeanne Ngongang,
Vincent K. Titanji and Lazare Kaptue

Additional information is available at the end of the chapter

http://dx.doi.org/10.5772/59070

1. Introduction

Non-communicable diseases (NCDs) known to cause more than half of all deaths in sub Saharan Africa over the past two decades has shown a steady increase to become a public health concern,. [1-4]. More than 30% of these deaths are recorded before the age of 60 in the resource poor countries. The mortality and morbidity caused by the NCDs is globally on the increase. However, the greatest impact has been recorded in sub Saharan Africa where healthcare facilities and medical awareness is low. In the developing countries NCDs is on the rise at the same proportion with infectious diseases that has led to an increasing disease burden, [2].

Other studies in sub-Saharan Africa has indicated that women within the ages of 15–49 are dying from NCDs faster than the women living in high-income countries [3-4]. The burden of

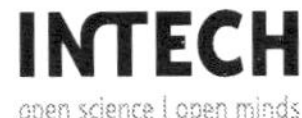

early mortality and disability poses a serious problem to socio economic and human development [3]. In countries where the public health systems are not well developed, payment for health care service for the poor is difficult and creates more financial burden to the poor subsistent population. The assess to treatment for metabolic disease such as diabetes has been shown to cost a patient in some developing economies like India about 15-25% of their household earnings [5-6]. Studies conducted by the World Bank showed that cardiovascular disease can lead to high expenditure for about 25 % of India families and also creates poverty to about 10 % of low income families [5-7]. The socio economic implication of population living with NCDs ranges from time off work usually unpaid, high unemployment rate and also early retirement from work. [6-8]. the world economic forum (WEF) based on socio economic situation in developing economies attempts to place the NCDs among the top global concern to economic empowerment [6-8].

Well-structured and coordinated primary prevention with elaborate health care disease surveillance can potentially help reduce in developing countries like Africa [8].Base on the good health care policy implementation strategies there has been a concerted effort by health actors to develop and formulation of effective health programmes for the prevention and potential control strategies for NCDs that was initiated during the World Health Assembly that took place 2000. Some great initiatives has been implemented by WHO member countries towards the control of tobacco consumption, an unregulated excessive alcohol intake, and the global control of diet and nutrition, physical activity and health. A lot of effort has been taken to reduce potential NCDs as indicated report in the action plan of WHO of 2008-2013 [8-10]. In the sub Saharan Africa regions the reduction of NCDs is not view as a technical resource issue, but it is a highly political problem which in most cases does not create an enabling health working environment. The health sectors and the policy-makers in most sub Saharan African countries are aware of the burden of NCDs, and also the existence of cost-effective interventions for implementation, unfortunately health intervention policy is not priority [10-12]. So far, some donors and the international development community have been slow to respond, in part because NCDs are not among the Millennium Development Goals [11]. So far with all the repeated donor mobilization and commitments as demonstrated by the Paris Declaration on Aid Effectiveness and the Accra Agenda for Action, NCDs still receive below 3 % of the development assistance for health across most countries in sub-Saharan Africa despite the fact that NCDs are known to cause more than of all premature deaths in these regions [11-14].

The WHO's Action Plan for the Global Strategy for the Prevention and Control of NCDs has put in place a strategic health development platform for change and since its adoption in 2008, a global movement promoted by leaders from developing countries to develop a common partnership operational platform is effective to some extend [14-16[.The Some partnership global initiative has led to important decisions like that taken at Doha which led to some resolution and declarations made on NCDs and different injuries advocating consideration for integrating the NCD prevention and control into the health management framework [16]. Deliberations at the United Nations Economic and Social Council meeting in July 2009 led to a United Nations General Assembly Resolution in May 2010, requesting the United Nations to convene an important meeting in September 2011 inviting the participation of heads of state and government [17-18]. Drawing inspiration from the HIV/AIDS crucial meeting in 2001 that was the turning point in unlocking the HIV epidemic, this meeting also provided an opportunity to raise awareness and shift in paradigm in research towards the NCDs within the framework of the global health development agenda [19-21].

The distribution of the burden f NCDs has shown a big disease gap between the high income earning countries where the health service is very developed and organized and the low income countries where the health system is not well organized and less accessible to the poor subsistence population as shown in Figure 1. There disease burden is more severe with the highly active population within the age range of 15-59 years recording between 48 %-56 %.

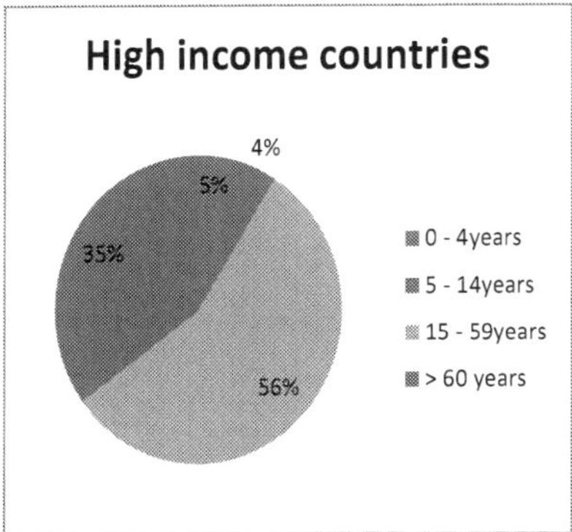

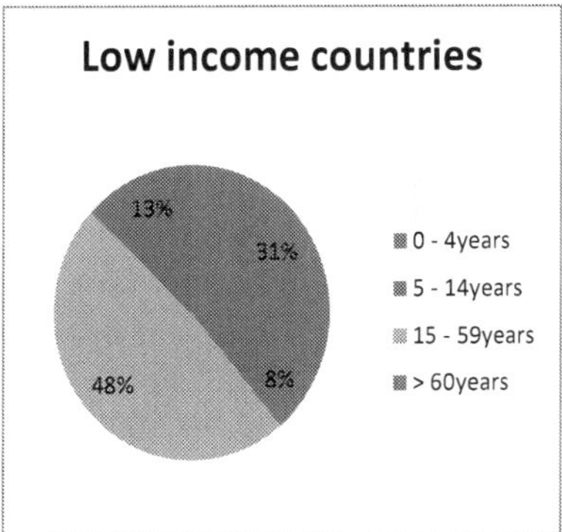

Figure 1. Disease burden distribution in high income and low income countries (Data source-WHO 2013) [26]

Many efforts have been made to organize important workshops, conferences on NCBs through the support of Global Health, and stakeholders in health within the WHO mapped sectors, and in Africa coordinated by the new partnership for Africa (NEPAD), Africa Union support programmes.

Workshops and consultation forums have contributed towards the production of vital support documents that serve in the promotion of awareness on NCDs and also important end of meeting resolution are made through national declaration by the health sector stakeholders that helps in identifying and targeting strategic areas for possible control intervention. In some developing countries efforts have been made towards the creation the health actors' national programmes to deal with NCDs through national consultations and coordination that requires a high level of commitments from the health stakeholders. There is effort made toward putting in place a well-developed health monitoring system for sector action evaluation, accountability and participation potential of the NGOs and other affiliated nonpublic health actors, the public health partnership sectors and to a greater extend efforts made to enhance the strategies promoting the action plan of established by WHO [22-24]. Resolutions and declarations form organized symposiums and many organized conferences helps in setting priorities by policy makers within the WHO member states and a roadmap to put in place sustainable implementation strategies. There is the need for the promotion of the awareness and sensitization of NCDs through the outcome of a consultation frame work organized by the health sectors in the WHO members states, at the level of research institutions, research groups focused on developing and establishing effective policy and legislation that supports NCDs portfolios [25].

To develop good control strategies for NCDs there is the need for total participation of the entire public health sectors, actors in health research institutions. The holistic approach involving the total participation of all stakeholders has shown to be more effective for a sustainable NCDs in Africa and also support resource poor countries to implement good control programmes, and channel public health policies towards the intensification of the prevention action and capacity strengthening for NCDs control and management systems [24-26]. In the WHO member states where there is well organized structures to support and promote health professionals leadership and the efforts to promote NCDs management initiatives, are known to play a significant role in shaping study of the epidemics and managing the cases of premature deaths in Africa [4, 7, 27]..Some of the main indicators of diseases that are used such as disease incidence and prevalence, do not give a clear indication when considering the disease burden involving an individual in a community in poor resource economy

The unit measure for that is applied to express an indication of the disease burden is known as the DALY and one DALY which represents the loss of the equivalent of one year of full health [27]. By using the DALYs, measurement the disease burden involve in early deaths and little disability such as measles or drowning, could be compared to other diseases that cannot cause death but has potential to cause disability as the case of cataract that causes blindness [1, 2, 28-29] NCDs is known to cause about half of the disease burden in the low-and middle-income countries [22-24], and about one half of the disease burden involves non-communicable diseases. Among the NCDs Ischaemic heart disease and stroke constitutes the biggest sources of this disease burden and the cardiovascular diseases account for more than one quarter of the total disease burden. Currently, injuries have been shown to account for about 17% of the disease burden in adults aged 15–59 years, within the low- and middle income economies in Europe, USA and the Eastern Mediterranean Regions, where more than 30% of the entire disease and injury burden are recorded among men aged between 15–44 years. [29-30].

1.1. Leading causes of burden of disease

Recent studies have shown that the four non-fatal conditions are found in the 20 leading causes of burden of disease, while the two leading causes of death such as ischaemic heart disease and cerebrovascular disease, and are among the top six causes of burden of disease as indicated in table 1. The four primarily non-fatal conditions are also shown to be among the 20 leading causes of burden of disease; such as hearing loss, alcohol use disorders, and unipolar depressive disorders to name but a few.. To assess the main causes of loss of health in any populations it is very relevant to take into consideration the non-fatal conditions as well as deaths. The income levels are also known to be linked with major differences in burden of disease [3-5]. The two leading causes of burden of disease in the world are infectious diseases such as lower respiratory infections and diarrheal diseases. HIV/AIDS is known to be the fifth cause of burden of disease globally, and three other infectious diseases follows on the top 15 causes as shown in Table 1.The leading causes of burden of disease in developing nations are very similar to those recorded globally, with the exception of the statistics for malaria and tuberculosis (TB). As indicated in Table 1, out of the top ten causes of death, eight belongs to the Group I, however the leading causes in developed nations are all NCDs, with the exception of road traffic accidents which is the tenth leading cause of death [29-30].

1.2. The disease and injury burden for women

In a broader perspective depression is now known to be among the leading cause of disease burden among young adult women with mental disorders that are known as the main source of lost years of healthy life for women of aged 15–44 years [23].Mental disorders make up three of the ten leading causes of disease burden in developing countries, and four of the leading ten in developed countries. Case of self-inflicted injuries have been reported to be among the leading ten causes for the developing economies [3, 11, and 30]. Injuries have also been shown to be important for boys beyond infancy, however, the causes of burden of disease are broadly similar for boys and girls but with, a marked sex differences that is seen between the age range of 15–59 years. The burden of reproductive problems is generally restricted to developing nations, and this is vital such that the maternal conditions make up two out of the ten leading causes of disease burden in women of age groups 15–44 years [29-30]. The HIV/AIDS, and other maternal conditions are among the main factors contributing to the high disease burden for women in developing countries with respect to developed countries. In sub Saharan African and in the South-East Asia regions, the disease burden from maternal conditions is responsible for about eight percent of the total global disease burden shown in women between the aged groups of 15–59 year [32-34]. In developing countries great contribution can be made towards reducing the burden of disease by developing strategies aim at reducing loss of healthy years that can be enhanced by putting in place better facilities to implement proper care for pregnant women, promote antenatal and neonatal care, years loss Almost all of this loss of healthy years of life is avoidable.in low-income countries, better care for women in pregnancy and childbirth could make a great. The Millennium Development Goal provides an opportunity for women to have access to a skilled birth attendant during childbirth. This opportunity where available has reduced to a greater extent the disease burden through the prevention maternal and neonatal deaths. [9, 35].

1.3. Causes of non-communicable disease

The burden of NCDs are derived from various past and cumulative risks; and the future burden are now determined by current population exposures to risk factors. Studies have shown that the major risk factors for NCDs epidemics are more complex than those for infectious disease and are well known to be responsible for most of such risk factors. [2-6]. Many populations are exposed to the most common groups of NCDs. There are some modification of these NCDs within individuals and location but generally the mode of action is the same worldwide [9-12]. Some determinants on NCD epidemics involves the increase in aging population, low fertility and the decreasing child survival potential

The increase in NCDs globally has been caused by a significant change in lifestyle of the population especially in developing economies. Current trends indicates that more people spend longer period out of their homes working and eating fast food containing high cholesterol level which is a predisposing factor to metabolic diseases, with obvious implication linked to problems such as low fertility and sexual dysfunction [32-34].

World trade and marketing developments concepts is to orientate the nutrition and food strategies transition towards diets formulation with a high proportion of saturated fat and sugars with high cholesterol. The consumption of high cholesterol diet, drug abuse, and common tobacco use with little or no physical activity can lead to worldwide predisposition of NCDs [15-17]. In developed countries, seven of the ten leading risk factors contributing to the burden of disease are for non-communicable disease, compared with six and three of ten in developing countries with low and high rates of mortality, respectively

1.3.1. Non-communicable disease risk

The NCD risks are higher in developing countries and dominate the disease burden of most developed countries, to the extent that they are considered as a health priority in the developed countries [11, 35].The developed countries have well-structured health programmes to manage the NCD risks which generally increase with age. It is therefore important to develop control measures of the different age distributions of populations through age-standardization of DALY rates, to reduce the apparent NCDs risks. Report on the age-standardized DALY rates, are higher in developing countries than in developed nations [35-37]. This disparity is due mostly to cardiovascular diseases, such as the heart disease and stroke, with age standardized burden are significantly higher in developing nations than in developed countries. Other disease burden under the group of sense disorders, vision impairment and ocular anomaly like hearing loss, is more common in developing economies than in the developed countries [35-37].

1.3.2. The Global unequal burden of disease injury

Other reports show that one sixth of the disease burden in adults caused by injuries accounts for 17% of the disease burden in adults aged between 15–59 years [35-37]. In developing countries about 30 % of the main disease and injury burden recorded in men between the ages of 15–44 years are known to result from injuries. In general considering both sexes, road traffic accidents are the third leading cause of burden in the 15-44 age group that is followed by HIV/AIDS and unipolar depression. Due to economic decline and poor road infrastructural development there is a rapid increase in road traffic accidents most especially in the developing countries [12, 38].The relative importance of intentional injuries varies from regions to regions and these category of injuries includes aspects like self-inflicted injuries, suicide, violence and war [37-39]. This type of injury contributes to the increasing rate of the burden, mainly in economically oriented young adults. In most developed nations, suicides top the cause of intentional injury burden, while low income economies aspects of violence and war leading the massive displaced and migratory population are the main cause. Highly politically unstable regions involve in unrest, civil wars like in the Central Africa sub regions, have rates of injury, death and disability among males that are similar to other developing countries [5, 30, and 39]. The death rate resulting from the effect of poisoning is significantly high developing countries than in any other region of the world. Consumption of excess and deaths is also a main cause in developing countries where the unemployment rate is very high and provokes frustration among the youth. Record of the potential death rate resulting from injuries cause by fire is significantly higher for women population in the South-East Asia regions than for the women or men population globally [40].

1.3.3. Global Projection of the burden of disease in 2035

The global forecast for the disease burden per capita is projected to potentially show a decrease in the global DALYs from 1.53 billion in 2014 to about 1.36 billion in the year 2035, given a general decrease of approximately 10 % [40-42]. There is also a projection of increase in population of over 25% during the same time span, which represents a big decrease in the general per capita disease burden worldwide. The DALY rate general have been shown to decrease faster than the global death rate due to a potential shift in the chronic NCDs that has not only occurred in the last decade but has become an economic health issue, that has attained an epidemic magnitude globally [11, 43-45].

Within the coming years the burden of chronic NCDs is anticipated to be on the increase particularly in sub Saharan Africa. This projection raises a concern of the potential death of about 388 million people in the population in the next decade from one or more forms of CNCDs. This health concern has provoked many states to put in place some action plans towards reducing a significant number of premature deaths. [21, 46]. There is the possibility that poor feeding and excessive smoking are two important factors that contribute to the millions of preventable deaths that occur each year.The CNCDs have a significant negative economic impact such that looking at the next 1o years, south east Asia, the UK and India are listed to lose billions in combating the CNCDs.[47-49], Within the framework of globalization, the increasing interconnection of countries and the openness of borders to ideas, people, commerce, and financial capital, has beneficial and harmful effects on the health of populations [2, 14, 50]. The effect of the present current era of globalization on health has to be debated and reconsidered in a wider perspective [5, 52]. Greater emphasis and interest is now focused on the control strategies on the infectious diseases and the threats to world security, the supply of generic drugs and international trade partnership [41, 52].

1.4. The global burden of non-communicable disease and disease injury distribution

Health forecasts projection shows that there are about 56 million deaths globally, of which about 60 % die as a result of NCDs [53]. 16 million deaths are recorded from cardiovascular disease (CVD), especially the coronary heart disease (CHD) and stroke; 7 million from cancer; 3 5 million from chronic respiratory disease; and almost 1 million from diabetes [41, 52]. Mental health problems are known to be the leading cause of disease burden in most countries irrespective of its state of development and this contribute in many ways to the incidence and severity of many NCDs such as the cardiovascular disease and cancer [1, 53]. The disease injury distribution has been grouped into world disease regions of Africa, the Americas, and the

Eastern Mediterranean and European regions. This distribution are well illustrated in Table 1, showing the disease injury categories and the DALY. It is observed that there is major variation between these world disease regions.

Disease incidence or injury	DALYs (millions)	Percent of total DALYs		Disease or injury	DALYs (millions)	Percent of total DALYs
The African sub Regions				**The Region of the Americas**		
1	HIV/AIDS diseases	46.7	12.4	1	Unipolar depressive disorders	10.8	7.5
2	Lower respiratory tract infections	42.2	11.2	2	Violence abuse	6.6	4.6
3	Diarrheal (gastroenterological issues	32.2	8.6	3	cardiovascular disease problems	6.5	4.6
4	Malaria infections-PRD.	30.9	8.2	4	Alcohol abuse disorders	4.8	3.4
5	Neonatal and antenatal infections and other	13.4	3.6	5	Unstained Road traffic accidents	4.6	3.2
6	Birth asphyxia and birth trauma	13.4	3.6	6	Diabetes mellitus	4.1	2.9
7	Premature and low birth weight	11.3	3.0	7	Cerebrovascular disease	4.0	2.8
8	Tuberculosis problems-PRD	10.8	2.9	8	Lower respiratory infections	3.6	2.5
9	Road traffic accidents	7.2	1.9	9	Chronic obstructive pulmonary disorder COPD	3.1	2.2
10	Protein-energy malnutrition	7.1	1.9	10	Congenital malformation anomalies	2.9	2.1

The Eastern Mediterranean sub Regions				**The European sub Regions**		
1	Lower respiratory infection	12.1	8.5	1	Cardiovacular heart disease	16.8	11.1
2	Diarrheal diseases	8.3	5.9	2	Cerebrovascular disease	9.5	6.3
3	Ischaemic heart disease	6.2	4.3	3	Unipolar depressive disorders	8.4	5.6
4	Neonatal infections and other	6.1	4.3	4	Alcohol use disorders	5.0	3.3
5	Cot death and birth trauma	5.5	3.9	5	Hearing loss, adult onset	3.9	2.6
6	Premature death and low birth weight	5.3	3.8	6	Road traffic accidents	3.7	2.4

Disease incidence or injury	DALYs (millions)	Percent of total DALYs		Disease or injury	DALYs (millions)	Percent of total DALYs
7	Unipolar depressive disorders	5.2	3.7	7	Trachea, bronchus, lung cancer	3.3	2.2
8	Road traffic accidents	5.1	3.6	8	Osteoarthritis	3.1	2.1
9	War and conflict problems	3.8	2.7	9	Cirrhosis of the liver	3.1	2.0
10	Congenital malformations	3.7	2.6	10	Self-inflicted injuries	3.1	2.0
The South-East Asia sub Regions				**The Western Pacific sub Regions**		
1	Lower respiratory infection	28.3	6.4	1	Cerebrovascular disease	15.8	6.0
2	Diarrheal diseases	23.0	5.2	2	Unipolar depressive disorders	15.2	5.7
3	Ischaemic heart disease	21..6	4.9	3	COPD	11.9	4.5
4	Unipolar depressive disorders	21.1	4.8	4	Refractive errors	10.6	4.0
5	Prematurity and low birth weight	18.3	4.1	5	Road traffic accidents	9.6	3.6
6	Neonatal infections and other	14.3	3.2	6	Alcohol use disorders	8.6	3.2
7	Birth asphyxia and birth trauma	13.9	3.1	7	Ischemic heart disease	7.9	3.0
8	Tuberculosis	12.4	2.8	8	Hearing loss, adult onset	7.0	2.6
9	Road traffic accidents	11.0	2.5	9	Birth asphyxia and trauma	5.7	2.1
10	Cerebrovascular disease	9.6	2.2	10	Tuberculosis	5.6	2.1

COPD, chronic obstructive pulmonary disease PRD-poverty related diseases

Table 1. Global disease injury distribution in the world disease regions of Africa, the Americas, Eastern Mediterranean region and European Region [13, 29].

There are all indications that communicable diseases in Africa cause more deaths than non-communicable diseases. NCDs contribute significantly to adult mortality with the highest rates recorded in central and eastern European sub regions [54]. They increase the problem of health inequalities within and between affected countries, mainly concerning poor populations due largely to the inequalities in the distribution of major risk factors [3, 55-56].

2. The effects of globalization on disease burden

The study on economic and financial globalization and the World Trade Organization (WTO) show that when the national and the international trade is regulated this can lead to improvement of the health status of the population, although this benefit has little impact in developing countries [7]. Many countries have put in a lot of efforts towards the regulation of national and international trade unfortunately, the limited resources and technical knowhow has not helped to promote the programme. WTO promotion of drug development and new chemical entities has enhance the access to many developed pharmaceuticals, but not all countries have same accessibility due to lack of limited resources. [5, 9]. The development of NCD epidemics where there are limited access to medical care has been influence to some extend by globalization [1-3]. The effect of indirect effects of globalization are linked to national economic performance which act through changes in household income, government spending, and the foreign exchange, and prices regulation within the different countries [50]. National income play an important role in health development however in developing countries the resources for health promotion [51-43]. Some of the drawbacks of globalization on health can be exemplified by increase in production and commercialization of unfriendly health products such as alcohol, tobacco and other substances of health abuses readily available to the population. These commodities unfortunately are very accessible to the population especially in the developing countries where trade regulation of these products where there exist are difficult to enforce. [36, 54].

Significant efforts have been made towards the protection of essential local producers in high income economies and this has had an effect on the management of NCD epidemics. For instance the move by the European Union (EU) to subsidize agricultural products is aimed at regulating the competition that may arise from the primary producers. There is little subsidize unfortunately for fresh produce in low income economies and therefore could reduce the national income [55]. The EU also subsidize the production of tobacco which has been generally considered as a policy anomaly because of the negative health effect tobacco has on the population of consumers. [31, 45, 56]. Some attempts have been made through advocacy for the removal of the agricultural subsidies and this was endorsed in Doha and then in Johannesburg during the World Summit on Sustainable Development and most recently the declaration by the EU gave an indication that the process for lifting subsidies linked to production is in progress.

Modern information and communication technologies (ICT) have been shown to have some positive and negative effects on health. It is evident that global commercialization of products like tobacco, alcohol, and other essential household products could be made available to all parts of the country ICT has made it possible for global commercialization shifting market target to the younger population [3, 11]. In the USA for example millions of dollars are put into persuasive marketing that has encourage young people to develop interest in fast food with high cholesterol content, fizzy drinks, alcohol and tobacco. The power of media publicity and advertisements through the use of more sophisticated technology has promoted the persuasive marketing and also exploiting the poor regulatory environment to capture and penetrate the consumer market [21-26].

2.1. Globalization, nutrition and alcohol on disease burden

Nowadays there has been a great substitution of our natural organic traditional food rich in fruit, vegetables and fibers by diets rich in calories from animal fats and low in complex carbohydrates. The impact of this food substitution syndrome has had more impact in developing countries [3. 11, 17]. Such changes has led to an increased rates of many NCDs in countries previously protected by balanced and healthy diets. Sub-Saharan Africa, Asia and some South American countries are undergoing a big shift in consumption patterns, and consumer life style transformation although rates of heart disease are still low compared to developed countries, and stroke rates have also reduced significantly in countries like Singapore and Japan [46]..

Globally there has been a steady increase transformation in farming [45] food processing, distribution [23] transportation [19] shopping practices [3, 55] and the consumption of food outside of the home (*fast food, take away*) [27]. Cooking has changed with the development of microwave, ovens and other techniques and changing lifestyles, especially in the urban cities where people work long hours out of home [14]. Changing patterns of production and consumption underlie the emergence of NCD epidemics and poses a problem to achieving a sustainable development goals [56]. The impact of alcohol consumption in promoting non-communicable disease epidemics has become very complex and a significant correlation has been shown between alcohol consumption and liver cirrhosis, some cancers, and most causes of injuries and violence. Alcohol also enhances and predispose the population to the risk of cardiovascular disease [22, 36].

2.2. Global policies towards non-communicable disease control strategy

2.2.1. Prevention strategy

The progression of non-communicable disease, especially lung cancer in men and CVD, have reduced significantly in many developed countries than in low income economies. For example in lung cancer, the reduction in mortality is linked to the concerted prgramme developed to reduce tobacco consumption by the population [50-52]. There are indications that, in many European countries, and south East Asia lung cancer epidemics is on the increase especially in women. This increase is linked to the rise in smoking habit developed in women and the lack of traditional health promotion programmes to enhance regulation of tobacco marketing strategies oriented towards young women [9]. The cause of reduction in CVD mortality are complex but are linked to improved management in high risk people, in particular in the USA, and in some countries, such as Finland and Sweden, where there are prevention programmes aimed at reducing the risk levels in combination with other environ-mental changes within the population [46].

The application of existing knowledge could play a major, rapid, and cost-effective contribu-tion to the prevention and control of NCD epidemics [18]. The agenda of most international donors is focused on belief that communicable diseases can be prevented or treated before addressing the problems of NCDs [45]. The report made by the Commission on Macroeco-nomics and Health did not consider as a priority to make any emphasis or awareness on the importance of the growing burden of NCDs [7], this is probably because of the misconception that NCDs are still the preserve of wealthy countries and populations. Generally in developing countries the institutional response to disease prevention and control is still based on the infectious disease paradigm [15, 34].and therefore the global and national ability in managing non-communicable disease epidemics is very inadequate and few countries have successfully put in place a workable prevention and control programmes [1, 16].

2.2.2. Global advocacy for non-communicable disease

The sensitization and active advocacy is still at its infancy at the global level for NCD prevention and control [8], and even the control platforms developed in advanced countries are still not well coordinated to highlight the risk-factor or disease specificity [53]. The lack of coordination between evidence and action in the for example in USA can also be applied globally [25]. Many potential advocacy groups have their origins in specialist organizations of health professionals, and are not coordinated to generate a force as powerful promoters of broad prevention and control policies [16, 35]. This lack of advocacy for health promotion is not in line with the expanding commercial and consumer groups who have placed treatment at the centre of health policy debates and funding priorities [31].A powerful widely coordinated health alliances are necessary for main health professional organizations, consumer groups, corporate industries, and research institution to effectively manage the prevention of major risk factors for NCDs [14, 54].All efforts to promote research to address challenges in chronic non communicable diseases prevention, control are being promoted through research initiatives and stake holder funding opportunities. These challenges and the study research needs have been addressed in table 2.

	Major challenges	Study/Research needed to address goals
Goal A Sensitization/ Advocacy	Increase the political priority of NCD Encourage healthy lifestyle and consumers choices through effective sensitization advocacy and public engagement sensitization Assemble valid information for widespread media coverage and sensitization of economic, social and public health programmes	Engaging stakeholders in partnership for disease prevention How to create public forums to raise awareness of issues relating to chronic NCDs Promote research platform for health involving the government some state sectors such as the health eduction and environment, transportation Research the causes for poor sensitization and promoting awareness to chronic disease in the community.
Goal B Advancing economic legal and environmental policies	The effect of poor health on economic output and productivity The effect State spending and taxation on health System to implement local, national and international policies with trade regulation policies on health related consumer products.	Quantify impact of chronic NCDs on local economies Program on the international implication of changes in health related food consumption Assess motivations associated with domestic spending, and changing lifestyle choices study the health effect of agriculture, climate change and policy interventions Research on health and economic effects of developed community-based interventions

	Major challenges	Study/Research needed to address goals
		Setting up population metrics, health indicators program for policy and programme surveillance
		Research on the efficiency of food-labeling legislation and policies
Goal C Programme management of possible risk factors	Knowledge of environmental and cultural factors linked to social behavior changes Enforcement of sustainable programmes to minimize tobacco consumption Promote healthy food intake in the population Develop sustainable physical activity strategic programmes	Study behavioral modifications to reduce risks Study risk factors, and the factors associated or affect risk in chronic NCDs. Study new medical products for the prevention of heart disease and diabetes Study the socio-cultural, ethnic and genetic diversity linked to risk factors that support behavioral interventions Assess personal risk linked to phenotypes, genotypes and multiple risks factors Evaluate genotype by environment interaction of environment of genes in risk factors and the outcomes Research on new biomarkers and diagnostics for risk and early disease diagnosis.
Goal D Participation in community outreach	Application of business models as main tool to sensitize health and preventable disease Develop business ethics and code of conduct for the food ndustries Enhance community resources such as voluntary and NGOs	Study marketing techniques and marketing data resulting from commercial firms on behavioral patterns. Investigate the mechanisms for consumers and the public have a positive influence on the food industry Research the impact of taste, packaging, labeling and advertising on choice and health of consumers. Create and evaluate community-based strategies to promote healthy living Source the method of effective public-private partnerships to support health
Goal E Identification the health impacts on poverty and urbanization	Study and address how poverty increases risk factors Study and address the links between urbanization and chronic NCD	Assess the relationship between poverty and the risk associated to health Examine the influence of poverty on the adoption of high-risk behavior Identify negative effects of economic growth on health Study the importance in town planning to promote the environment on healthy living
Goal F	Strategies to mobilize resources in health systems in function of the disease burden.	Develop strategies that can incorporate a sustainable health-system control/prevention of non-communicable diseases

Major challenges		Study/Research needed to address goals
Reorientation of the health system platforms	Direct capacity building of health professional within prevention management, Increase number and skills of professionals in prevention and controlof chronic non-communicable diseases Built health systems that integrate screening and prevention within health delivery Increase access to medication to prevent complications of chronic non-communicable diseases	Develop partnership work platforms to promote best practices in delivering accessible, cheap health care Research on ways in supporting an organized education on health promotion Put in place roadmap for the promotion of health training and development of courses targeted on chronic non-communicable diseases Provide local technical knowhow to enhance the training of health personnel Evaluate effective methods to promote optimal resources distribution of health care in poor communities Promote and advocate the use of e-health records in disease forecasting Investigate effective means of developing practical health surveillance tools. Implementation of high throughput screening mechanism that group the population according to health disease predisposition risk factors.

Table 2. Global Challenges in chronic NCDs and advocacy tools for research needs [10, 53].

2.3. Partnerships collaboration for addressing disease burden

The challenges of non-communicable disease are so complex that there is a need for many stakeholders to collaborate in developing a control strategy. For improve the quality and regular access to quality healthy food, there is a need for a meaningful partnership collaboration between producers the consumer groups and the multinational food companies [13, 37]. The WHO has effectively developed a working to handle diet and physical activities with respect to the chronic diseases. This collaborative approach has seen the development of food regulatory guidelines, effective consultations process between WHO, the state, consumer groups, and many companies. Many food producing companies have reported the changes that is occurring in product labelling to reduce competition and promote marketing practices; if widely implemented, these changes could lead to significant benefits of globalization support to public health [40]. Other participatory partnership involving WHO involves working in close collaboration with the people and promote safe alcohol consumption.

2.4. Building Capacity and resources platforms for non-communicable disease management

Strengthening capacity for NCDs management is very important and must be promoted especially in low income economies where health information system management are not well developed. [20, 26].Other constraints in building good resource platforms for NCDs is the slow institutional response to capacity strengthening, lack of vision and mission not align epidemiological survey activities. There is a need for creating an enabling environment for important financial commitment in different countries that may vary depending on the strategic planning programme put in place to build capacities that can plan and manage activities towards combating diseases and sustainable health of the population [9]. There are many initiatives at the national and international level to develop policies and working documents for NCDs management within the framework of public health sectorial health development portfolio, to what extend thses policies are effective can only be known when there is marked improvement or continuous increase in the management of patient health within a define country or jurisdiction.[15, 29].There has been a significant progress in building or promoting research partnership or collaboration by researchers at institutional, national and international level, a global advocacy for NCDs that has attracted some funding by potential donors in the health sector [53] There has been a significant progress made by international consortiums to support investment towards tobacco control research by building institutional research platforms in some developing countries and this is also being extended to other aspects of non-communicable diseases.

3. Global norms and standards in the management of chronic non-communicable diseases

In other to achieve success in NCDs management initiatives there must be respect for international standard norms and ethics regulating the health sector.

Each country needs to develop initiative to train health personnel's on international ethical code of conduct guiding or regulating clinical research for diseases affecting the population and the global trade regulatory issue of health related products [5, 53], The respect of ethical norms in the health sectorial research and development is still not a standard practice in the management of NCDs in developing countries.. Despite the creation of ethical committees and institutional review boards to regulate clinical research there are still problems that are linked to nutrition and lack of physical activity that are difficult to address.

Multi stakeholder and other state policies are initiatives geared towards the sensitization and advocacy to regulate the consumption and sales of food and alcohol especially for the younger population [11].

3.1. Reorientation of health services towards management of non-communicable disease

There has been significant increase in premature loss of lives as a result the lack of a sustainable management system for the control and prevention of NCDs. In some developed countries well developed and user-friendly intervention systems are available for CVD management and these are now successfully transferred to some privileged developing countries to support interventions in CVDs [30]. There has been a significant global initiative to develop an effective disease management system for cancer therapy. This system has contributed significant on the ease of diagnostics, the prevention and treatment and methods for procedures for palliative has also improved. [11, 21, 53]. Considering for example NCD like the of breast cancer and cervical cancer, that has also become a serious health concern in sub Saharan African countries, among women of child bearing age, there is no proper sensitization mechanism about the threat of this disease and the health implication for young child bearing women. In addition diagnostic tools and procedures are not well developed, and in most cases diagnostics are made only when severe cases are reported at the late stage of cancer at the hospitals, health districts or integrated health centres. In most countries of the central Africa sub regions the states has made a lot of effort to fight against cancer by creating health committee at the ministry of health, and a society for cancer research. Despite these initiative by the government the impact is not felt at the rural areas. Activities by some NGOs or other operational bodies is focused in the cities. There are many opportunities for coordinated non-communicable disease risk reduction, care, and long-term management.

4. Conclusion

The advancement of globalization of the major risks for non-communicable diseases is on a steady increase especially in resource countries plague with poverty, political and economic instability. On the other hand, the prospects for non-communicable chronic disease diagnosis, prevention and management and control is still generally at its infancy. We can attain a sustainable progress when the governments, stakeholders of international agencies, non-governmental agencies, and civil society create an enabling environment and acknowledge the integration of non-communicable disease as a risk factor in the public health agenda. The challenges are enormous and the fight to promote healthy food consumption and maintenance of a healthy lifestyle towards reducing metabolic diseases or lifestyle diseases, like diabetes, hypertension, CVD will remain slow until the response or taskforce to NCD epidemics is well developed and structured to meet up with their disease burden. The advocacy and the importance of sensitization of the global community on the importance of non-communicable disease as a public health concern is no longer the responsibility of WHO but a global mobilization of nations, donors, stakeholder and greater promotion and encouragement of research funding opportunities. Advocacy for NCDs has gain so much priority of recent in the public health strategic disease prevention and control in most in Africa to the extent that in Cameroon and its Central African states there has been national and sub-regional consortium for the management of NCDs.

Acknowledgements

The authors would like to thank the European & Developing Countries Clinical Trials Partnership (EDCTP) for the grant funding that enable us to realize part of this project. Furthermore we would also like to recognize the financial support of the Ministry of Higher Education (MINESUP) of Cameroon for the allocation of research subvention and modernization financial support Research support of lecturers. Finally, we acknowledged the support of our data mining process system through the access to information sites and those who sent us research materials.

Author details

Estella Tembe-Fokunang[1*], Charles Fokunang[1,2], Zacharia Sando[1], Barbara Atogho Tiedeu[3], Frederick Kechia[1], Valentine Ndikum[1], Marceline Ngounoue Djuidje[3], Jerome Ateudjieu[1], Raymond Langsi[2], John Fomnboh Dobgima[2], Joseph Fokam[1], Luc Gwum[1], Obama Abena[1], Tazoacha Asonganyii[2], Jeanne Ngongang[1], Vincent K. Titanji[5] and Lazare Kaptue[6,7]

*Address all correspondence to: estellafokunang@yahoo.co.uk

1 Faculty of Medicine and Biomedical Sciences, University of Yaoundé, Cameroon

2 Faculty of Health Sciences, University of Bamenda, Cameroon

3 Faculty of Science, University of Yaoundé , Cameroon

Faculty of Science, University of Dschang, Cameroon

4 Faculty of Science, University of Buea, Cameroon

5 Universite des Montages, Cameroon

6 Cameroon National Ethics Committee for Research in Humans (CNERH), Cameroon

References

[1] Beaglehole R, Yach D,. Globalization and the prevention and control of non-communicable disease: the neglected chronic diseases of adults. The Lancet, 2003. 362 issue 9387:903-908.

[2] Wang W, Russell A, Yan Y; Global Health Epidemiology Reference Group (GHERG). Frailty, dependency and mortality predictors in a cohort of Cuban older adults. Frailty, 2003-2011. EPMA J. 2014 Feb 13;5(1):4.

[3] Zhou M, Liu Y, Wang L, Kuang X, Xu X, Kan H. Particulate air pollution and mortality in a cohort of Chinese men, Environ Pollut. 2014 Mar;186:1-6.

[4] Prescott SL, Pawankar R, Allen KJ, Campbell DE, Sinn JKh, Fiocchi A, Ebisawa M, Sampson HA, Beyer K, Lee BW.A global survey of changing patterns of food allergy burden in children. World Allergy Organ J. 2013 Dec 4;6(1):21.

[5] Patel DN, Nossel C, Alexander E, Yach D. Innovative business approaches for incenting health promotion in sub-Saharan Africa: progress and persisting challenges Prog Cardiovasc Dis. 2013 Nov-Dec;56(3):356-62.

[6] Kengne AP, June-Rose McHiza Z, Amoah AG, Mbanya JC.Cardiovascular diseases and diabetes as economic and developmental challenges in Africa. Prog Cardiovasc Dis. 2013 Nov-Dec;56(3):302-13.

[7] Matheka DM, Nderitu J, Vedanthan R, Demaio AR, Murgor M, Kajana K, Loyal P, Alkizim FO, Kishore SP. Young professionals for health development: the Kenyan experience in combating non-communicable diseases. http://www.ncbi.nlm.nih.gov/pubmed/24262308 Glob Health Action. 2013 Nov 20; 6:22461.

[8] Uchendu OJ, Forae GD. Disese mortality patterns in elderly patients: A Nigerian teaching hospital experience in Irrua, Nigeria. Niger Med J. 2013 Jul; 54(4):250-3..

[9] Okpechi IG, Chukwuonye II, Tiffin N, Madukwe OO, Onyeonoro UU, Umeizudike TI, Ogah OS. Blood pressure gradients and cardiovascular risk factors in urban and rural populations in Abia State South Eastern Nigeria, using the WHO Stepwise approach.PLoS One. 2013 Sep 5;8(9):

[10] Kankeu HT, Saksena P, Xu K, Evans DB. The financial burden from non communicable diseases in low-middle-income countries: a literature review. Health Res Policy Syst. 2013 Aug 16; 11:31.

[11] Turk T, Latu N, Cocker-Palu E, Liavaa V, Vivili P, Gloede S, Simons A. Using rapid assessment and response to operationalise physical activity strategic health communication campaigns in Tonga. Health Promot J Austr. 2013 Apr; 24(1):13-9..

[12] Roberts B, Patel P, Dahab M, McKee M. The Arab Spring: confronting the challenge of non-communicable disease. J Public Health Policy. 2013; 34(2):345-52..

[13] Angkurawaranon C, Wattanatchariya N, Doyle P, Nitsch D. Urbanization and non-communicable disease mortality in Thailand: an ecological correlation study. http://www.ncbi.nlm.nih.gov/pubmed/23279597 Trop Med Int Health. 2013; 18(2):130-40.

[14] Robinson HM, Hort K.Non communicable diseases and health systems reform in low and middle income countries. Pac Health Dialog. 2012 18(1):179-90.

[15] Silva-Matos C, Beran D.Non-communicable diseases in Mozambique: risk factors, burden, response and outcomes to date. Global Health. 2012 21; 8:37.

[16] Remais JV, Zeng G, Li G, Tian L, Engelgau MM. Conversion of noncommunicable and infectious diseases in low and middle-income countries. Int J Epidemiol. 2013 42(1):221-7.

[17] Joshi A, Mohan K, Grin G, Perin DM. Burden of healthcare utilization and out of pocket costs among individuals with NCDs in an Indian setting. J Community Health. 2013 Apr; 38(2):320-7.

[18] Crowther NJ, Early determinants of chronic disease in developing countries. Best Pract Res Clin Endocrinol Metab. 2012 Oct; 26(5):655-65.

[19] Jones AC, Geneau R. Assessing research activity on priority interventions for non-communicable disease prevention in low and middle income countries.Glob Health Action. 2012 23; 5:1-13.

[20] Michaelsen KF, Larnkjær A, Mølgaard C.Amount and quality of dietary proteins during the first two years of life in relation to NCD risk in adulthood. Nutr Metab Cardiovasc Dis. 2012; 22(10):781-6.

[21] Lopez, A. D., Mathers, C. D., Ezzati, M., Jamison, D. T. & Murray, C. J. L. (eds) Global Burden of Disease and Risk Factors (Oxford Univ. Press and World Bank, Washington DC, 2006).

[22] World Health Organization Preventing Chronic Diseases: A Vital Investment (WHO, Geneva, 2005).

[23] Adeyi, O., Smith, O. & Robles, S. Public Policy and the Challenge of Chronic Non-communicable Diseases (World Bank, Washington DC, 2007).

[24] Suhrcke, M., Nugent, R. A., Stuckler, D., & Rocco, L. Chronic Disease: An Economic Perspective (Oxford Health Alliance, London, 2006).

[25] Zwi AB, Yach D. International health in the 21st century: trends and challenges. Soc Sci Med 2002; 54: 1615-1620.

[26] WHO. The world health report 2012. Geneva: World Health Organization, 2012.

[27] Stamler J, Stamler R, Neaton JD, et al. Low risk-factor profile and long-term cardio-vascular and non-cardiovascular mortality and life expectancy. Findings for 5 large cohorts of young adult and middle-aged men and women. JAMA 1999; 282: 2012-2018.

[28] Magnus P, Beaglehole R. The real contribution of the major risk factors to the coronary epidemics: time to end the 'only 50%' claim. Ann Int Med 2001; 161: 2657-2660.

[29] United Nations. Conference on trade and development. Least developed countries report 2002: escaping the poverty trap. Geneva: United Nations, 2002.

[30] Bettcher DW, Yach D, Guindon GE. Global trade and health: key linkages and future challenges. Bull World Health Organ 2000; 78: 521-534.

[31] Ong EK, Glantz SA. Constructing "sound science" and good epidemiology": tobacco lawyers and public relations firms. Am J Public Health 2001; 91: 1749-1757?

[32] Yach D, Bialous SA. Junking science to promote tobacco. Am J Public Health 2001; 91: 1745-1748?

[33] Popkin BM. The Bellagio Conference on the Nutrition Transition and its Implications for Health in the Developing World. Bellagio, Italy, Aug 20—24, 2001. Public Health Nutr 2002; 5: 93-280.

[34] Popkin BM. An overview on the nutrition transition and its health implications: the Bellagio meeting. Public Health Nutr 2002; 5: 93-103.

[35] Ebbeling CD, Pawlak DB, Ludwig DS. Childhood obesity: public-health crisis, common sense cure. Lancet 2002; 360: 473-482.

[36] Beaglehole R, Dobson A. The contributions to change: risk factors and the potential for prevention. In: Marmot M, Elliott P, eds. Coronary heart disease epidemiology. Oxford: Oxford University Press, 2003.

[37] Beaglehole R. Global cardiovascular disease prevention: time to get serious. Lancet 2001; 358: 661-663.

[38] Kahn EB, Ramsey L, Brownson RC, The effectiveness of interventions to increase physical activity: a systematic review. Am J Prev Med 2002; 22: 73-107,

[39] McGinnis JM. Does proof matter? Why strong evidence sometimes yields weak action. Am J Health Promot 2001; 15: 391-396.

[40] Yusuf S. Two decades of progress in preventing vascular disease. Lancet 2002; 360: 2-3.

[41] Ala Din Alwan Gauden Galea David Stuckler. Development at risk: addressing non-communicable diseases at the United Nations high-level meeting.*Bulletin of the World Health Organization* 2011; 89:546-546A. doi: 10.2471/BLT.11.091074.

[42] Shoaee S, Ghasemian A, Najafi B, Kasaeian A, Farzadfar F, Hessari H. National and subnational burden of oral diseases in Iran. 1990-2013 study protocol. Arch Iran Med. 2014 Mar; 17(3):159-68.

[43] Ghasemian A, Ataie-Jafari A, Khatibzadeh S, Mirarefin M, Jafari L, Nejatinamini S, Parsaeian M, Peykari N, Jamshidi HR, Ebrahimi M, Etemad K, Moradi-Lakeh M, Farzadfar F.National Arch Iran Med. 2014 ;17(3):146-58.

[44] de Morais C, Oliveira B, Afonso C, Lumbers M, Raats M, de Almeida MD.Nutritional risk of European elderly.Eur J Clin Nutr. 2013 Nov; 67(11):1215-9.

[45] James J, Soyibo AK, Hurlock L, Gordon-Strachan G, Barton EN.The cardiovascular risk factors in an Eastern island prevalence of the non communicable chronic diseases and associated lifestyle risk factors for cardiovascular morbidity and mortality in the British Virgin Islands. West Indian Med J. 2012 Jul; 61(4):429-36.

[46] *Mortality and burden of disease estimates for WHO Member States in 2004*. Geneva: World Health Organization; 2009.

[47] Narayan KM, Ali MK, Koplan JP. Global non-communicable diseases – where worlds meet. *N Engl J Med* 2010; 363: 1196-8

[48] Jha P, Jacob B, Gajalakshmi V, Gupta PC, Dhingra N, Kumar R, et al., et al. A nationally representative case-control study of smoking and death in India. *N Engl J Med* 2008; 358: 1137-1147.

[49] Mahal A, Karan A, Engelgau M. *The economic implications of non-communicable disease for India*. Washington: The World Bank; 2010.

[50] Adeyi O, Smith O, Robles S. *Public policy and the challenge of chronic non-communicable diseases*. Washington: The World Bank; 2007.

[51] Jamison D, Breman JG, Measham AR, Alleyne G, Claeson M, Evans DB, et al. *Disease control priorities in developing countries*. Washington: The World Bank; 2006.

[52] Daar AS, Singer PA, Persad DL, Pramming SK, Matthews DR, Beaglehole R, et al., et al. Grand challenges in chronic non-communicable diseases. *Nature* 2007; 450: 494-6

[53] *Global status report on noncommunicable diseases 2010*. Geneva: World Health Organization; 2011.

[54] Stuckler D. Population causes and consequences of leading chronic diseases: a comparative analysis of prevailing explanations. *Milbank Q* 2008; 86: 273-326

[55] Nugent R, Feigl A. *Scarce donor funding for non-communicable diseases: will it contribute to a health crisis?* Washington: Center for Global Development; 2010.

[56] Alleyne G, Stuckler D, Alwan A. The hope and the promise of the UN Resolution on non-communicable diseases. *Global Health* 2010; 6: 15 -

Chapter 2

Mental Health — An Issue Neglected by European Public Health Systems?

Denise Zak

Additional information is available at the end of the chapter

http://dx.doi.org/10.5772/59138

1. Introduction

Mental disorders comprise a wide spectrum of illnesses that are characterized by tremendous disabilities and impairments. In addition to this loss of quality of life for patients, mental disorders entail high costs for public health systems. In recent years, there has been an increasing amount of literature on the economics of mental disorders. Overall, there seems to be evidence indicating a notable prevalence of mental disorders and a sizeable treatment gap, expressed in a large number of patients suffering from one (or more) mental disorder(s) who have been treated insufficiently. The question arises whether the unmet need is due to a general lack of awareness within (national) health and social care systems and a kind of misallocation of resources (supply-side problem) or if the utilization of services is hindered by stigma or exclusion (demand-side problem).

Epidemiologic data is scarce, which is presumably the reason why the suffering of the patients as well as the significance of the economic burden are underestimated. Reliable estimates of costs and benefits associated with mental disorders are needed to ensure health care planning and financing.

The aim of this chapter is to provide a comprehensive review of literature on this subject. The economics of the most frequent and most burdensome mental disorders are discussed. Therefore only the cost-of-illness studies on affective disorders, generalized anxiety disorder, schizophrenia and alcoholism are taken into consideration. In the light of demographic developments reference is also made to mental disorders of the elderly (i.e. dementias). Mental disorders which begin in childhood and adolescence (i.e. hyperkinetic disorders, autism) are also outlined to point out the importance of prevention. Accordingly, both age cohorts will increasingly challenge health care systems. In this chapter the range of costs and the meth-

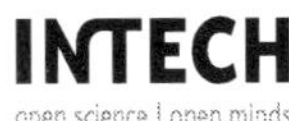

odological constraints of different cost estimates at the European level are discussed in detail as well as the different kinds of challenges for the Austrian health care system.

Only those publications published from 1994-2014 were included because of the changes in diagnostic criteria. Within this timeframe it can be assumed that diagnoses are based on the ICD-10 and DSM-IV criteria respectively, which enhances comparability between the studies analyzed. Regarding the spatial focus, the current 28 member countries of the European Union are part of the analysis, but special attention is paid to the (limited) data available in Austria.

2. Health economics and mental health

In most OECD countries mental health care is insufficiently integrated in the health care system, which is also reflected in the expenditures for mental health [1]. To date, various methods have been developed and introduced to measure the economic impact of ill-health. With a focus on mental health, the cost-of-illness studies have gained interest in the past decades. In general, cost-of-illness studies provide monetary estimates for the economic burden associated with a disease [2]. Thus, information on the allocation of resources and on the relative importance of a disease can be used for further in-depth analyses or (international) comparison.

Generally, the relevant costs are classified into direct, indirect and intangible costs. Direct costs are the expenses for medical goods and services. Often direct costs are subdivided into direct medical and non-medical costs, where the latter refer to all associated services.

Basically, two broad approaches can be distinguished to assess direct costs, i.e. top down and bottom up. Costs in top down analyses are calculated based on aggregated national data and statistics to obtain an estimate of the (health) economic significance of an illness. In contrast, bottom up analyses estimate costs on the basis of resource consumption at the level of the individual patient.

Indirect costs refer to productivity losses owing to a specific illness. There are two approaches to assess indirect costs: the human capital and the friction costs methods. Within the evaluation of mental disorders, the human capital approach is more common and recommended [3]. The core of this method is the assumption that an economy's potential productivity is the sum of the output produced by its population in working age over an expected lifetime. In the case of early retirement or premature death, all productivity losses are projected for the whole life span, resulting in high indirect costs for chronic illnesses. [4]

Suffering, pain and reduced quality of life are also relevant in research on mental health and are summarized as intangible costs. In particular, quantification and monetarization are aggravated by methodological difficulties.

Throughout (mental) health economic studies, the measurement and definition of costs are not consistent. For example, the costs of informal care (i.e. care by members of the family and friends) are often assigned to indirect costs, but can also be assigned to direct non-medical costs. Costs associated with suicide, which are of particular relevance in mental disorders, are hardly taken into account owing to manifold difficulties in valuation.

3. Epidemiology of mental disorders in Europe

The most comprehensive work providing the first epidemiologic and economic data on mental disorders in the European Union is a compilation of recent studies: in a comprehensive review on the costs of disorders of the brain the total costs of 12 selected disorders were estimated at € 386 billion, of which € 240 billion account for mental disorders alone (2004 prices, dementia excluded) [5]. Only those studies including the cost-of-illness data published in the EU-25 member countries and Norway, Switzerland as well as Iceland were selected. In addition, studies based on clinical trials, reviews, quality of life studies and studies dealing with specific treatment forms were excluded. Direct healthcare costs, direct non-medical costs and indirect costs for the following 12 disorders were estimated: affective disorders (depression, bipolar disorders), psychotic disorders (schizophrenia), anxiety disorders (panic disorders, social phobia, special phobias, agoraphobia, generalized anxiety disorder, obsessive compulsive disorder), addiction (illicit drugs, alcohol), dementia, brain tumour, trauma, stroke, epilepsy, multiple sclerosis, Parkinson's disease, migraine and other headaches. The prevalence of these disorders in 2004 amounted to 27% of the total population covered in the study.

Based on this analysis, a follow-up study was initiated. Using a multi-method approach including literature research, the analysis of epidemiologic data and country-specific expert surveys, the 12 month prevalence of the disorders included in the first report [6] as well as 14 new disorders for EU-27 plus Norway, Switzerland und Iceland was estimated [7]. Additionally the age group covered was extended to the major mental disorders for children and adolescents (2-17), adults (18-65) and elderly (65+years). Within this study, substance use disorders (alcohol dependence, opioid dependence, cannabis dependence), psychotic disorders (schizophrenia, other psychotic disorders), mood disorders (bipolar disorders, major depression), anxiety disorders (posttraumatic stress disorder, obsessive-compulsive disorder, generalized anxiety disorder, social phobia, specific phobias, agoraphobia, panic disorder), somatoform disorders, eating disorders (anorexia nervosa, bulimia nervosa), childhood and adolescence disorders (pervasive developmental disorders/autism, hyperkinetic disorders/ ADHD, conduct disorders), personality disorders (dissocial personality disorder, emotionally unstable personality disorder), sleep disorders (non-organic insomnia, hypersomnia, narcolepsy, sleep apnoea), mental retardation and dementias were ascertained.

As a result, it was estimated that each year 38.2% of the EU population would be affected by a mental disorder, whereas the most frequent disorders are anxiety disorders (14%), insomnia (7%) and major depression (6.9%).

In terms of DALY[1], mental disorders rank highest compared to the morbidity burden resulting from all other causes, but at the same time the treatment gap is enormous. The economic estimates were also revised accordingly, resulting in total costs of € 798 billion (2010 prices) of which 40% are indirect costs, 37% direct medical and 23% non-direct medical costs [8][9].

There are also several national cost-of-illness studies available. For instance, the total costs of mental disorders in France were estimated at € 109 billion in 2007 [10]. By using a top down approach, direct health care costs, direct non-medical costs, indirect costs and intangible costs were derived. Within direct health care costs, public psychiatric hospitals had the highest costs of € 6.4 billion while the costs for out-patient care accounted for € 4.7 billion. Direct non-medical costs were estimated at € 6.3 billion, of which € 3 billion were for institutions in the health and social care sector, € 2 billion for allowances, and interestingly also of € 1.3 billion for informal care. In terms of indirect costs, the costs of income compensation accounted for € 4.4 billion and the costs of productivity losses for € 20 billion. Surprisingly, intangible costs, i.e. loss of quality of life, were also assessed, resulting in a loss of 2.2 million QALY[2] and costs of € 65.08 billion.

In a study set out to determine the economic burden of mental disorders in Sweden, annual costs were estimated at € 9.4 billion (2001 values) of which € 1.9 billion were direct costs and € 7.5 billion were indirect costs [11]. From a methodological point of view, these findings are based on prevalence rates of mental disorders, the cost-of-illness approach and a top down perspective.

4. Generalized anxiety disorder

The symptoms of generalized anxiety disorder (GAD) comprise tension, worrying and anxiety symptoms [12][3]. Generalized anxiety disorder is considered to be associated with high individual burden as a consequence of its chronic course [13]. Wittchen [14] found that GAD is the most frequent anxiety disorder treated in primary care settings. In a systematic review, the economic and human burden of this disorder was assessed with the focus on North America and a selection of European countries in the period from 1987 to 2010 [15]. A total of ninety studies met these inclusion criteria. Despite differing diagnostic criteria used in the epidemiologic studies that were analyzed, the effects on productivity, health related quality of life and psychological functioning can be distinguished which lead to burdensome impairments in the sphere of individual functioning and well-being, condensed in high medical costs and the use of health care services. As a further outcome, the health related quality of life impacts are similar to panic disorder or depression. Life time prevalence rates differ among the studies owing to changing diagnostic patterns, but are in the range of 3% to 6%. Estimating

---

1 DALY ("disability adjusted life year") is a health economic measure, expressing a burden of a disease in the number of years lost due to an illness or disability. One DALY equals one year of life in total health. DALYs are calculated as the sum of years of life lost and the years lost to disability.

2 QALY ("quality adjusted life year") measures the quantity and quality of life generated by a health intervention and weights time in different health states.

3 Unless specified differently, all diagnostic criteria used in this chapter refer to ICD-10 guidelines edited by Dilling et al. (8th revision, 2011)

direct and indirect costs associated with generalized anxiety disorder is difficult, but the results suggest that the median medical costs for patients suffering from this disorder are significantly higher than for patients without this disorder. Another aspect under analysis was the treatment rate, limiting the scope of the review only to pharmacologic interventions. Surprisingly, generalized anxiety disorder is still an under-diagnosed and highly untreated disorder, notwithstanding the significant burden of the disease.

Hoffmann et al. [16] analyzed 24 studies and identified the human burden, quantitatively expressed in terms of quality of life and role functioning, as well as the economic burden, defined as health care utilization costs and productivity losses. Only studies based on DSM-III-R, DSM-IV or ICD-10 criteria covering the period from 1990 to 2005 were included, using MEDLINE and PsychLIT database. As a result, the economic consequences and individual burden associated with GAD are considerable and comparable with other mental disorders (i.e. other anxiety disorders, somatoform disorders) as well as somatic problems.

Based on patient survey data from Germany, Spain, Italy, France and the United Kingdom, the economic and human burden of GAD were identified [17]. Cost analyses, as well as bivariate and multivariate approaches, showed that patients suffering from GAD have more co-morbidities, resource use and work impairments and a less health-related quality of life than control groups without GAD.

The costs of anxiety disorders in Europe were assessed by utilizing the mental health supplement of the German National Health Interview and Examination Survey, a community sample (n=4181, age=18-65) conducted in 1998/1999 [18]. The mean costs were derived as excess costs (i.e. compared with individuals without an anxiety disorder) per patient. In the case of GAD, the direct cost per patient amounts t o € 1,230 and the indirect costs to € 399, resulting in a total of € 1,629 (2004 prices).

5. Affective disorders

Affective or mood disorders are characterized by a fundamental change in mood and are accompanied by a change in activity levels. **Bipolar disorders** are marked by a switch of mood, at least two episodes in which the patient's mood and activity levels are significantly disturbed, consisting of an elevation of mood and increased activity (mania or hypomania) and of a lowering of mood and decreased activity (depression). In between the episodes complete remission can be expected. It is interesting to note that more studies on the economics of uni-polar depressions are available than on bipolar type I and II disorders [19]. The co-morbidity of depressive disorders with other mental disorders, as well as somatic illnesses, is high, but studies have neglected the (lifetime) incidence of these major disabling conditions [20]. **Depression** or depressive episodes can vary from being mild, moderate, or severe depending upon the number and severity of the symptoms. Typical symptoms are a lowering of mood, decrease in activity and reduced self confidence accompanied by somatic symptoms such as disturbed sleep and weight loss [12].

5.1. Depression

In 2005, the costs of depression in Sweden from a prevalence based top down perspective amounted to € 3.5 billion, with indirect costs of € 3 billion and direct costs of € 500 million [21]. This study also estimated the intangible costs of suffering based on the QALY losses of patients undergoing treatment (€ 4.1 billion) and for those patients who do not receive any treatment (€ 6.1 billion).

Another study based on a similar methodological approach estimated the total costs for depression at £ 9 billion (2000 values) in England, where direct costs constitute only a minor share of £ 370 million [22]. As part of the "Epidemiology of Mental Disorders (ESEMeD) project", a prevalence based bottom up approach was employed by Friemel et al. to assess the direct costs of depression in Germany, which amounted to € 1.6 billion in 2002 [23].

Berto et al [24] analyzed the costs of depression based on a review of seven studies. According to their findings, depression imposes a remarkable burden on society, which led to direct and indirect costs of $ 43.7 billion in the US as well as of £ 417 million in the UK in 1990. It is interesting that 5 out of 7 studies indicated that in terms of direct costs hospitalization incurs the most costs while medication accounts for only a minor share. The economic burden is high owing to the chronicity, early onset and high prevalence of depression to be found not only among the working population but also in general [25].

5.2. Bipolar disorders

Recently, bipolar disorders in the EU25 and Switzerland, Norway and Island were analyzed. Only studies published after 1980 that were based on DSM-III-R, DSM-IV or ICD-10 criteria were considered. Epidemiologic samples in the clinical population or community, as well as studies using structured or standardized diagnostic interviews, were included in the study [26]. Thus, 14 studies carried out in 10 countries revealed that the 12-month prevalence of these disorders lies within the range of 0.5-1.1%. Another interesting result was that there are only few studies available concerned with the disability and treatment of bipolar disorders. In comparison with other mood disorders, substance use disorders or anxiety disorders, people suffering from bipolar disorders are characterized by a higher level of disability with regard to severity and duration. In addition these patients also have higher productivity losses expressed in absenteeism. The data on treatment and the utilization of health services are scarce. This might be owing to the fact that bipolar disorders are rather rare. However, co-morbidity with other mental disorders, as well as somatic diseases, is high.

The annual societal costs of bipolar disorders in the UK were assessed with the help of health care and statistical databases, and amounted to a total of £ 2.06 billion in 2001/2002 [27]. This estimate includes £ 199 million direct health care costs, £ 86 million direct non-health care costs and £ 1.77 billion indirect costs. In a comparable way, Runge et al analyzed German health insurance data and estimated the annual societal costs of € 5.8 billion (2002 prices) [28]. Indirect costs account for € 5.7 billion, direct costs for € 138 million.

In both studies, bipolar disorders implied a substantial economic burden and the largest share of direct costs was for inpatient treatment (35% in UK; 60% in Germany). In addition, indirect costs exceeded direct costs several times over.

A recent review analyzed systematically 22 cost-of-illness studies [29]. Only studies published since 2000 and meeting 20 elaborated quality criteria were selected with a focus on the cost of illness data for bipolar disorders. Despite the fact that all of the studies reviewed assessed the major costs associated with bipolar disorders, the comparison of estimates was impeded by the plurality of study outcomes on the national and international levels.

Fajutrao et al (2009) [30] carried out a systematic literature review using Medline, Embase and Biosis as well as health technology assessments and treatment guidelines. The analysis of 25 studies dealing with epidemiology, costs and patient related issues (e.g. employment, disability) of bipolar disorders in Europe (i.e. United Kingdom, Sweden, Spain, Germany, France and Italy) emphasises the underestimation of this long-term disorder and high economic burden both in terms of direct and indirect costs.

6. Schizophrenia

Schizophrenia is a chronic and highly disabling mental disorder characterized by thought disorders, hallucinations and delusions (positive symptoms) as well as apathy, incongruity of emotional responses and paucity of speech (negative symptoms) [31]. There is a considerable amount of literature in which the burden of schizophrenia, together with the interrelated dimensions of cognitive functioning, quality of life, stigma and also the burden for caregivers is discussed [32] [33] [34].

There have been some controversial discussions on mortality and associated risk factors [35] [36]. Life expectancy in the light of cardiovascular diseases [37][38] was subject to studies as well as risk factors and suicide rates [39]. To sum up, the causes of mortality in patients with schizophrenia are unnatural deaths, cardiovascular diseases, respiratory diseases and cancer. However, it has been recognized only recently that natural causes are very often the reason for mortality [40].

The costs associated with this disease are high and wide ranging because of the burden on the patients per se, relatives who care for them and society at large [41]. Some analysts [42] have attempted to draw fine distinctions between direct medical and direct non-medical costs, the latter consist of informal care costs. In their prevalence based study on the social costs of schizophrenia in Spain a total of € 1.97 billion (2002 prices) was calculated, of which 53% were direct medical costs (inpatient and outpatient care, medication) accounting for 2.7% of the total public health expenditure.

A notable example of a prevalence based bottom up study provides a differentiated consideration of the costs in 2004/2005 in England [43]: taking into account various populations (private households, residential institutions, prisons, the homeless) the total costs of schizophrenia were £ 6.7 billion. Only £ 2 billion were spent for direct treatment and care costs, but £ 4.7 billion were indirect costs as summarized in the following table.

Lost productivity of patients	3 400
Private expenditures and informal care	615
Benefit payments	570
Lost productivity of carers	32
Administration of benefit payments	14
Criminal justice system	1
Source: table based on [43]	

Table 1. Indirect costs of Schizophrenia in England in 2004 (£ millions)

7. Alcohol

Similarly, studies on alcohol abuse vary considerably in estimating the burden on individuals and society. In the past decade, alcohol and other substance use disorders have gained attention as one of the major public health problems. [44]. Neither prevalence nor costs attributable to addiction are easy to quantify [45]. A specific problem is causality, whether health issues are a consequence of alcohol or some other cause [46]. Whatever the case, co-morbidity with other mental disorders [47] is frequent and there are also causal links to physical problems [48]. Another problem is that the diagnosis and differentiation in the forms of alcohol abuse to be found in studies on the subject range from acute intoxication, harmful use, dependence and withdrawal state [12]. Alongside with increased morbidity and co-morbidity, alcohol is associated with violence [49] and crime [50]. With regard to the prevalence of alcohol abuse disorders, the median 12-month prevalence of alcohol dependence alone in the EU 25 and Norway is 6.1% for the male and 1.1% for the female populations, respectively [51].

Recent evidence suggests that alcohol dependence is even more expensive than alcohol abuse, if health costs per patient are considered [52]. In 2002, a prevalence based Swedish study estimated the societal costs resulting from alcohol consumption at SEK 29.4 billion or 1.3% of GDP [53]. By far the largest share of the total costs were the indirect costs accounting for SEK 18.4 billion. A German study calculated a value of 1.16% of GDP in 2002, based on the concept of attributable fractions and prevalence [54]. This result corresponds to the total costs of € 24.4 billion, including the direct costs of € 8.44 billion and indirect costs of € 15.96 billion. In both studies no specification of alcohol abuse in terms of a mental disorder according to diagnostic manuals is available and the research focus is on alcohol consumption in general. Thus, the potential positive effects (i.e. protective health effects) were discussed too, but presented separately.

8. Dementia and mental health of the elderly

As a consequence of demographic developments the prevalence of mental disorders in old age is assumed to increase [55]. But, so far, little is known about the health care situation of the elderly with mental disorders apart from those with those with dementia and depression [56]. The various forms of dementia are a major health problem for the older generation in Europe. According to ICD-10, various types can be distinguished. Alzheimer's disease is the most frequent form of dementia, but also vascular dementia caused by a stroke (cerebrovascular accident CVA) is very common. With regard to the prevalence of Alzheimer in those who are over 65 years of age, the rate ranges between 5.9% and 9.4%, depending on age, sex and severity [57]. A recent review of 15 cost-of-illness studies based on patient-level data, showed that the median annual costs amounted to € 28,000 (2005 values) which were solely for the care of patients with Alzheimer's disease [58] f. From a societal perspective, the annual baseline costs of dementia in Ireland were estimated at over € 1.69 billion in 2010 [59]. A combination of bottom up and top down approach was adopted. Informal care accounts for 48% of the total costs, residential long-stay care for 43%, while for formal social and health care it is for 9%. For Hungary, the costs of dementia were assessed by a cross-sectional non-population-based study [60], resulting in total annual costs for the demented population of € 846.8 million for 2010. The highest proportion of these costs is attributable to direct costs (55%), followed by informal care (36%) and indirect costs (9%).

The costs for dementia for the EU-27 amounted to € 160 billion in 2008, with a range from € 111 to € 168 billion [61], based on a cost model developed upon 14 cost-of-illness studies reviewed.

9. Child and adolescent mental health

The prevalence of child and adolescent mental disorders has increased [62]. The most common mental disorders in childhood and adolescence are **hyperkinetic disorders** (ICD-10) or **attention-deficit hyperactivity** disorders (ADHD, according to DSM-IV) [63]. The predominant symptoms are ill-regulated, disorganized and excessive activity and lack of persistence in activities requiring cognitive involvement. The children who are affected tend to be impulsive, socially isolated and lack self confidence. The cognitive functions are also frequently impaired. An early onset (usually during the first five years of a child's life) and overlapping difficulties in various aspects of life (education, establishing social ties) continuing until adulthood are distinctive. Symptoms of **conduct disorders** include a persistent pattern of aggressive, dissocial or defiant conduct. A characteristic of this disorder is also the inability to conform with the social expectations appropriate to the child's age. Severe other mental disorders may also exist (e.g. personality disorders). **Autism** is assigned to the group of pervasive developmental disorders and is defined by reciprocal social interaction, abnormalities in patterns of communication, as well as stereotyped behaviour and activities in all areas of the individual's functioning. [12]

The economic burden of mental disorders with onset usually occurring in childhood and adolescence is enormous. The vast majority of literature on ADHD is based on US data, but few European studies are available. From the results of the analysis of German statistical data, medical costs associated with hyperkinetic disorders alone amounted to € 142 million in 2002, which is a first estimate and a rather conservative one [64]. A comparison of children with and without ADHD in Belgium (Flanders) showed that the families and patients are faced with a high (psycho)social and economic burden [65]: based on a questionnaire sent to a non-random sample, the private costs borne by parents amounted to € 533 per year for the parents, and the public costs came to € 779 in 2002. These costs are six and twice as high, respectively, than for children who do not suffer from ADHD. The results of a review of European evidence on ADHD were applied to the case of the Netherlands [66], where the average total costs ranged between € 1,041 and € 1,529 million, depending on the application of high or low level scenarios (2012 prices). The lion's share of the costs at € 648 million was allocated to education including additional school lessons and costs for the services of educational psychologists and other health care professionals. The productivity losses of the members of the family accounted for € 143-€ 339 million, health care costs for the members of the family amount to € 161 million. Patient health care costs ranged from € 84-€ 377 million and social care costs were estimated at € 4.3 million.

Conduct disorders are common too, but prevalence rates vary owing to diagnostic difficulties and to which subjects and/or populations are included in the study [67]. The first German study on the costs of conduct disorders was based on a retrospective analysis of data from a statutory health insurance institution for the period 2006-2009 and resulted in annual mean expenditures of € 2,632, which are 3.8 times higher than those for a matched control group [68]. From a multicentre controlled trial of groups taking over the role of a parent to deal with antisocial behavior in childhood a sample was drawn to estimate the costs of anti-social behaviour in the UK [69]: the annual mean costs of health, voluntary and educational services were estimated to be a £ 1,277, the costs for members of the family, resulting from absence from work, additional repair as well as household tasks were £ 4,637 (2002/2003 prices).

The spectrum of autism disorders was analyzed in two British studies: while Knapp et al. estimated the annual costs, based on prevalence and different data sources for children of different age groups to be £ 2.7 billion and for adults to be £ 25 billion separately (2005/2006 prices) [70], Barett et al undertook a randomized controlled trial of a communication intervention which focussed on autism in children under 5 years of age and used the prevalence rates of the former study. Thus, the estimated service costs for this subgroup amounted to £ 109 million and the wider societal costs at £ 130 million per annum [71].

Based on the British Child and Adolescent Mental Health Surveys, a study on the economic burden of children aged 5-15 with a conduct, hyperactivity or emotional disorder (ICD-10) estimated the national costs for the health, education and social care services at £ 1.47 billion in 2008, the largest share of which was for the education services [72].

10. The Austrian case

The Austrian welfare system can best be described as corporatist and conservative because of the dominance of social insurance and the strong linkage to paid employment [73]. Health, as a dimension of social policy, incurs the second largest proportion of expenditure and is primarily funded by health insurance contributions [74]. In 2012, the total health care expenditures (public and private) amount to € 34,067 million, which corresponds to 11.1% of GDP [75]. A total of 22 social security institutions and the Main Association of Austrian Social Security Institutions (i.e. *Hauptverband der Sozialversicherungsträger*) organize health, accident and pension insurance [76]. There are no specific benefit payments in the case of a mental illness, but the general benefits and other support (e.g. subsidies for education, reintegration programmes, supported employment) are also of high importance for the mentally ill [77].

10.1. Mental health care

In Austria, there is no national mental health care system, but there are reforms and initiatives that are aimed at achieving international targets, such as deinstitutionalization, decentralization of services and equity of mental and somatic illnesses [78]. Because of Austria's federal structure the efforts made by the nine federal provinces in terms of data collection and availability at the level of provinces differ. Thus, the most recent psychiatry report including information on inpatient and outpatient care deals only with the situation in the province of Vorarlberg [79]. Within the last 5 years, besides Vorarlberg, only Styria [80] published up-to-date information on the provision and utilization of services regularly. The last national psychiatry report dates back to 2004 [81], but the Austrian Health Care Structure Plan, as the key planning instrument in the health care sector, includes psychiatric care on all levels of provision [82].

The Main Association of Austrian Social Security Institutions also published a national strategy on mental health [83]. Within this strategy, 25 targets are established that can prevent illness, improve treatment and reduce disability associated with mental disorders. Data on the history of suicide rates and spatial, socio-economic as well as gender patterns is also available [84][85][86]. In addition, a national programme on suicide prevention was adopted recently [87]. A detailed report on alcohol consumption, alcohol related inpatient health service utilization, morbidity and mortality is available for Austria [88].

The federal organisation of health care also necessitates different financing structures of mental health care services [89]. The system of financing psycho-social services is complex. For instance, the model for funding psychotherapy can illustrate the juxtaposition of different possibilities. Psychotherapy can be financed privately, which guarantees the freedom of choice of an adequate psychotherapist. However, based on the principle of benefits in kind, health insurance covers the costs for psychotherapy in total only under specific conditions, but these are limited and waiting lists are long. Finally, a mixed form is the subsidy or co-payment through health insurance [90].

Particularly children and adolescents are a vulnerable but neglected group within the care system [91]. Insufficiencies in the treatment structures are evident in the inpatient and outpatient sectors as well as in the sector of registered doctors, where the respective WHO indicators are not met [92]. Inpatient treatment is predominant, while psychotherapy and specialized ambulatory care practically do not exist without additional costs for those caring for the patient [93].

10.2. The costs of mental disorders in Austria

The costs of mental disorders are huge as the previous sections on selected disorders have shown. Although there have been a few recent studies on this subject, Austrian data is scarce. Based on statutory health insurance data, about 9% of the Austrian population or 900,000 (insured) Austrians made use of the health services to receive treatment for mental illness in 2009 [94].The associated costs in terms of medication, inpatient treatment, psychotherapy, physician services, psychiatric and psychological services, as well as sick pay were estimated at € 790-850 million. This estimate excludes rehabilitation costs as well as disability pensions, where it is important to note that mental disorders are the most common cause for new disability pension claims.

Wancata et al. [95] calculated the costs of 12 mental and neuropsychiatric disorders of the brain as part of the first European cost study [6] [7]. Thus, direct medical costs and direct non-medical costs were derived. Indirect costs were estimated based on the human capital approach. Anxiety disorders, affective disorders (bipolar disorders and depression), addiction (alcohol and illegal drugs), migraine, psychotic disorders, dementia, epilepsy, Parkinson's disease, stroke (cerebrovascular accident), multiple sclerosis, brain tumours and brain trauma were analyzed. With regard to the 12 month prevalence, in 2004 anxiety disorders were the most prevalent disorders (847,622 cases), followed by affective disorders (479,091 cases) and addiction (194,795 cases). In terms of costs per case and per mental disorder, the estimates are based on data from the review on the European level: dementia caused the highest costs at € 13,635 followed by psychotic disorders at € 9,487 and affective disorders at € 5,138 (2004 prices). Taking the Austrian population as a whole, the costs for these 12 disorders amounted to € 8.8 billion, whereas 47% are indirect costs (productivity loss), 37% are direct non-medical costs and 17% are direct medical costs. The authors emphasize that the results must be taken with caution, because the values were extrapolated from averaged and adjusted data taken from other studies owing to the lack of epidemiologic and cost data, respectively. Bearing these limitations in mind, the estimates presented should serve only as a first classification (Table 2).

Costs associated with schizophrenia were analyzed as part of a comprehensive report on this mental disorder in Austria [96]. The most important finding was that there are major gaps in the knowledge and data on this subject. In a short international survey of the studies available, the differences given in the direct and indirect cost estimates on account of the specific characteristics of the underlying health systems and thus of the treatment and care programs, are significant. With regard to the Austrian case, a search in Medline database brought to light one article which dealt with the burden that not only those with this disorder also their families

Mental Disorder	Direct costs	Direct non-health care costs	Indirect costs	Total costs[1]
Affective disorders	617	----	1 845	2 462
Anxiety disorders	427	----	428	856
Dementia	262	833	----	1 094
Addiction	260	40	1 043	1 444
Psychoses	1 095	204	----	1 299

[1] These figures are estimations only. Therefore the sum may not be exact as it is either rounded up or down. Source: estimates extracted from [93]

Table 2. Total costs of selected mental disorders in 2004 (€, millions)

have to bear, respectively. In Austria only few health care service data are recorded directly related to a diagnosis, which is a prerequisite for an appropriate application of cost-of-illness studies. For instance, inpatient care is filed related to the diagnosis, but sick-leaves and prescriptions are not documented according to ICD-10 criteria. Thus, a collection of diagnosis-based data for all health and care services throughout Austria is not feasible, which makes it difficult to obtain statements on the current size and burden of schizophrenia. Despite these limitations, the data from the Main Association of Austrian Social Security Institutions, from the Upper Austrian regional health insurance fund (i.e. *Oberösterreichische Gebietskranken-kasse*), the Austrian Federal Pension Fund and Statistics Austria could be used. As a result, the number of hospital inpatient stays is steadily declining. Not only the number of patients taking sick-leave because of a mental illness, but also the duration of this leave has increased in Austria, but there is no detailed analysis as there is a lack of data. In 2006, the Upper Austrian regional health insurance fund reported 14,010 sick-leave days incurring costs of € 198, 802 for the insured persons with schizophrenia. This comparatively low number might be due to the fact that patients suffering from schizophrenia are likely to prematurely leave the employment market or have difficulties in accessing the employment market. Focusing on pension benefits, it can be said that schizophrenia is one of the most frequent reasons that claims are made. It is an interesting fact that more than 90% of the pension claims made because of schizophrenia are approved, while the refusal rate for claims based on other mental disorders is approx. 39%. The average age of patients with schizophrenia is 40 when they apply for a pension and are thus more than 10 years younger than claimants with other disorders.

A recent cost benefit analysis suggests that alcohol abuse disorders incure high costs for Austria's public health system. As a result, the costs outweigh the "benefits" (i.e. tax revenues) at the rate of 0.25% of GDP (i.e. € 737.9 million, 2011 prices) [97].

At the European level, Austria was also part of the updated review on costs of disorders of the brain in the EU-27 countries [8]. Estimates for selected mental disorders in 2010 are shown below (Table 3). Taking into account that these estimates are highly aggregated and partly based on extrapolation, the results may be classified as first ranges as it is given that primary data in Austria is insufficient.

Mental disorder	Total costs
Addiction	1 282
Anxiety disorders	1 568
Child/ Adolescent mental disorders	425
Dementia	1 451
Mood disorders	2 253
Psychotic disorders	1 961

Source: extracted from [8]

Table 3. Estimates of selected mental disorders in Austria (€PPP million, 2010)

11. Discussion

One may suppose that the blind spots in mental health care research are negligible.. But in view of the limitations in methodologies adopted for the estimates, both with regard to the prevalence of mental disorder and the costs they incur, the conclusiveness of the results may not be given (as indicated by most authors).

When it comes to the economic evaluation of mental disorders, suicidal behaviour and suicide give rise to controversy. On the one hand, it can be argued that suicide must be included in cost analyses in terms of lost productivity owing to premature mortality. On the other hand, suicide attempts result in medical costs. Some authors even discuss the potential savings if a suicide is carried out as treatment is no longer required and pension benefits and care costs are reduced [98]. However, suicide has been excluded or described only qualitatively in most of the recent studies.

Another key aspect is co-morbidity-whether with other mental disorders or somatic illnesses-which can be considered only insufficiently in the studies and approaches available. Multiple co-morbidities are common in patients suffering from mental disorders. Thus, the burden might have been underestimated. A rather sensitive matter is the consideration of criminal justice costs. Establishing a cause-effect link is difficult, but it is a fact that stigmatization and discrimination are interrelated. Stigmatization may also be a reason why patients do not seek any treatment at all. It is assumed, in most of the studies, that a high number of persons with mental disorders remain untreated. This treatment gap also infers that current cost estimates might be too low.

The cost estimates presented show that the burden, both for society and individuals, is tremendous. However, the estimates can be classified as conservative. All of the studies indicate that the indirect costs are an even larger burden than the direct costs incurred by making use of the health services. There are, however, also studies in which only the direct costs for health care systems are estimated. Only one study estimated the intangible costs in monetary terms [21]. Throughout the studies, the costs and cost categories are not applied in a consistent way, since there are no international standards. The comparison of cost estimates, especially in the case of studies utilizing the top-down approach, may be hindered by the presence of heterogeneous public health systems as well. Thus, the different systems of data collection, funding of health and social services, categorizing and grouping of medical and psycho-social services may account for different study outcomes. However, the findings of the cost-of-illness studies are summarized below (Table 4).

Mental Disorder	Reference (year of costs)	Country/ currency	Approach	Direct costs	Direct non health care costs	Indirect Costs	Total costs	% of total public health care expenditure[1]
Depression	[21] (2005)	Sweden €	Prevalence based, top down	500		3 000	3 500	2.4
	[22] (2000)	England £	Prevalence based, top down	370		8 630	9 000	n.a.
	[23] (2002)	Germany €	Prevalence based, bottom up	1 600			1 600	0.9
Bipolar disorders	[27] (2001)	UK £	Health care data, statistics	199	86	1 770	2 060	n.a.
	[28] (2002)	Germany €	Health insurance data, statistics	138		5 700	5 800	0.08
Schizo-phrenia	[42] (2002)	Spain €	Prevalence based	1 044	926		1 970	2.4
	[43] (2004)	England £	Prevalence based, bottom up	2 000		4 700	6 700	n.a.
Alcohol	[53] (2002)	Sweden SEK	Prevalence based	10 987		18 394	29 400	5.8
	[54] (2002)	Germany €	Prevalence based, attributable fractions	7 064	1 377	15 958	24 398	3.9

[1] own calculation based on EUROSTAT [99]. Results include direct costs only. Data of the United Kingdom is not available in Eurostat's

System of National Health Accounts. In the case of Sweden and Germany 2003 values were adopted owing to comparability.

Table 4. Summary of original cost-of-illness studies (millions)

To sum up the cost of illness part of this chapter, the following table presents the total cost estimates converted into Euros (2013 values). As already indicated above, a comparison of single cost estimates is hindered by several factors. However, the scale of the economic burden of selected mental disorders is apparent.

Mental Disorder	Reference (year of costs)	Country	Total costs (millions)	Per capita costs[1]
Depression	[21] (2005)	Sweden	3 948	413
	[22] (2000)	England	15 116	n.a.
	[23] (2002)	Germany	*1 934	24
Bipolar disorders	[27] (2001)	UK	3 434	54
	[28] (2002)	Germany	7 012	85
Schizophrenia	[42] (2002)	Spain	*2 689	58
	[43] (2004)	England	10 733	n.a.
Alcohol	[53] (2002)	Sweden	3 816	399
	[54] (2002)	Germany	29 496	360

*only direct costs

[1] own calculation based on EUROSTAT [100]. Total costs (direct and indirect) are considered if not otherwise specified. Owing to accuracy population figures from 2013 are used.

Table 5. Summary of cost-of-illness studies presented in 2013 Euros

The relevance of mental health in specific population groups has been outlined. Dementias in the elderly population are a challenge to the health and social care systems, as life expectancy and prevalence have increased. The role of informal care is striking, raising the question how relatives can be supported faced with the burden of long term care and how care should be organised and financed respectively in times of limited resources.

With regard to the mental health of children and adolescents, the studies that have been discussed emphasize not only the burden on the patients, but also on the members of their families and carers.

A high share of the costs related to a child's mental disorder is borne by the parents. The health care and social care sector are affected in terms of costs, but in particular the educational services sector is stretched. Associated problems, such as poor education in adolescence, imply a worse socio-economic status and related adverse effects in adulthood [101].

Finally, the case of Austria illustrates that national cost data and epidemiology measures are scarce and scattered, impeding general statements on the current state of mental health of the population. On the one hand, cost data of several health insurance institutions indicate the burden of mental disorders in terms of the utilization of medical resources, health services as well as the impact on the number, duration and costs of taking sick-leave. Despite data insufficiencies, these cost estimates provide an initial overview of the importance of mental disorders at the societal level. On the other hand, the cost of illness information based solely on national primary data is currently not available, and thus prevents a more profound analysis of the role of specific mental disorders in the social and health care system.

12. Conclusion

Collectively, the studies mentioned in this review outline the critical role of mental health in European public health systems in terms of the provision of proper treatment as well as prevention programmes. Analyses of the single cost-of-illness studies have shown that estimates are often based on extrapolated data. Assumptions with regard to the epidemiology of a specific mental disorder affect study outcomes inevitably. The need for research and concerted action in mental health seems to be apparent. Appropriate data and health economic studies would lead to more informed decisions when it comes to the allocation of scarce resources in the health care system.

Author details

Denise Zak*

Address all correspondence to: denise.zak@tuwien.ac.at

Center of Public Finance and Infrastructure Policy, Department of Spatial Planning, Vienna University of Technology, Austria

References

[1] Frank, R.G. (2011). Economics and mental health: an international perspective. In: Glied S (Hrsg.). The Oxford handbook of health economics. Oxford Univ. Press, Oxford, 232-256.

[2] Büscher, G., Gerber, A. (2010). Gesundheitsökonomische Evaluationen als Ansatz zur Steurung der Ausgaben im Gesundheitswesen. In: Lauterbach, K. W., Lüngen, M., Schrappe, M. (Ed.). Gesundheitsökonomie, Management und Evidence based medicine: Handbuch für Praxis, Politik und Studium; mit 71 Tabellen. Schattauer Verlag, Stuttgart, 63-81.

[3] König, H. H., Friemel, S. (2006). Gesundheitsökonomie psychischer Krankheiten. Bundesgesundheitsblatt-Gesundheitsforschung-Gesundheitsschutz, 49(1), 46-56.

[4] Salize, H.J., Kilian, R. (2010). Gesundheitsökonomie in der Psychiatrie. Kohlhammer, Stuttgart

[5] Andlin-Sobocki, P., Jönsson, B., Wittchen, H. U., Olesen, J. (2005). Cost of disorders of the brain in Europe. European Journal of Neurology, 12(s1), 1-27.

[6] Wittchen, H. U., Jacobi, F. (2005). Size and burden of mental disorders in Europe-a critical review and appraisal of 27 studies. European neuropsychopharmacology, 15(4), 357-376.

[7] Wittchen, H. U., Jacobi, F., Rehm, J., Gustavsson, A., Svensson, M., Jönsson, B., Olesen, J., Allgulander, C., Maercker, A., van Os, J., Preisig, M., Salvador-Carulla, L., Simon, R., Steinhausen, H. C. (2011). The size and burden of mental disorders and other disorders of the brain in Europe 2010. European Neuropsychopharmacology, 21(9), 655-679.

[8] Gustavsson, A., Svensson, M., Jacobi, F., Allgulander, C., Alonso, J., Beghi, E., et al (2011). Cost of disorders of the brain in Europe 2010. European Neuropsychopharmacology, 21(10), 718-779.

[9] Olesen, J., Gustavsson, A., Svensson, M., Wittchen, H. U., Jönsson, B. (2012). The economic cost of brain disorders in Europe. European Journal of Neurology, 19(1), 155-162.

[10] Chevreul, K., Prigent, A., Bourmaud, A., Leboyer, M., Durand-Zaleski, I. (2012). The cost of mental disorders in France. European Neuropsychopharmacology, 28(8), 879-886.

[11] Tiainen, A., &Rehnberg, C. (2010). The economic burden of psychiatric disorders in Sweden. International journal of social psychiatry, 56(5), 515-526.

[12] Dilling, H., Mombour, W., Schmidt, M.H. (2011). International Klassifikation psychischer Störungen. ICD-10 Kapitel V (F) Klinisch-Diagnostische Leitlinien, 8.th ed., Verlag Hans Huber, Bern.

[13] Allgulander, C. (2006). Generalized anxiety disorder: What are we missing? European Neuropsychopharmacology, 16, Supplement 2, 101-108.

[14] Wittchen, H. U. (2002). Generalized anxiety disorder: prevalence, burden, and cost to society. Depression and anxiety, 16(4), 162-171.

[15] Revicki, D. A., Travers, K., Wyrwich, K. W., Svedsäter, H., Locklear, J., Mattera, M. S., Sheehan, D.V., Montgomery, S. (2012). Humanistic and economic burden of generalized anxiety disorder in North America and Europe. Journal of affective disorders, 140(2), 103-112.

[16] Hoffman, D. L., Dukes, E. M., Wittchen, H. U. (2008). Human and economic burden of generalized anxiety disorder. Depression and anxiety, 25(1), 72-90.

[17] Toghanian, S., DiBonaventura, M., Järbrink, K., Locklear, J. C. (2014). Economic and humanistic burden of illness in generalized anxiety disorder: an analysis of patient survey data in Europe. ClinicoEconomics and outcomes research: CEOR, 6, 151-163.

[18] Andlin-Sobocki, P., Wittchen, H. U. (2005). Cost of anxiety disorders in Europe. European Journal of Neurology, 12(s1), 39-44.

[19] Simon, G. E. (2003). Social and economic burden of mood disorders. Biological psychiatry, 54(3), 208-215.

[20] Paykel, E. S., Brugha, T., Fryers, T. (2005). Size and burden of depressive disorders in Europe. European neuropsychopharmacology, 15(4), 411-423.

[21] Sobocki, P., Lekander, I., Borgström, F., Ström, O., Runeson, B. (2007). The economic burden of depression in Sweden from 1997 to 2005. European Psychiatry, 22(3), 146-152.

[22] Thomas, C. M., Morris, S. (2003). Cost of depression among adults in England in 2000. The British Journal of Psychiatry, 183(6), 514-519.

[23] Friemel, S., Bernert, S., Angermeyer, M. C., König, H. H. (2005). Die direkten Kosten von depressiven Erkrankungen in Deutschland. Psychiatrische Praxis, 32(03), 113-121.

[24] Berto, P., D'Ilario, D., Ruffo, P., Virgilio, R. D., Rizzo, F. (2000). Depression: cost-of-illness studies in the international literature, a review. The Journal of Mental Health Policy and Economics, 3(1), 3-10.

[25] Wang, P. S., Simon, G., & Kessler, R. C. (2003). The economic burden of depression and the cost-effectiveness of treatment. International journal of methods in psychiatric research, 12(1), 22-33.

[26] Pini, S., de Queiroz, V., Pagnin, D., Pezawas, L., Angst, J., Cassano, G. B., Wittchen, H. U. (2005). Prevalence and burden of bipolar disorders in European countries. European Neuropsychopharmacology, 15(4), 425-434.

[27] Das Gupta, R., Guest, J. F. (2002). Annual cost of bipolar disorder to UK society. The British Journal of Psychiatry, 180(3), 227-233.

[28] Runge, C., & Grunze, H. (2004). Jährliche Krankheitskosten bipolarer Störungen in Deutschland. Der Nervenarzt, 75(9), 896-903.

[29] Kleine-Budde, K., Touil E, Moock, J., Bramesfeld, A., Kawohl, W., Rössler, W.(2013). Cost of illness for bipolar disorder: a systematic review of the economic burden. Bipolar Disorders 2013: Published by John Wiley & Sons Ltd.

[30] Fajutrao, L., Locklear, J., Priaulx, J., &Heyes, A. (2009). A systematic review of the evidence of the burden of bipolar disorder in Europe. Clinical Practice and Epidemiology in Mental Health, 5(3), doi:10.1186/1745-0179-5-3

[31] Lindström, E., Widerlöv, B., von Knorring, L. (1997). The ICD-10 and DSM-IV diagnostic criteria and the prevalence of schizophrenia. European psychiatry, 12(5), 217-223.

[32] Millier, A., Schmidt, U., Angermeyer, M. C., Chauhan, D., Murthy, V., Toumi, M., Cadi-Soussi, N. (2014). Humanistic burden in schizophrenia: A literature review. Journal of psychiatric research, 54, 85-93.

[33] Kitchen, H., Rofail, D., Heron, L., Sacco, P. (2012). Cognitive impairment associated with schizophrenia: a review of the humanistic burden. Advances in therapy, 29(2), 148-162.

[34] Awad, A. G., &Voruganti, L. N. (2008). The burden of schizophrenia on caregivers. Pharmacoeconomics, 26(2), 149-162.

[35] Beary, M., Hodgson, R., &Wildgust, H. J. (2012). A critical review of major mortality risk factors for all-cause mortality in first-episode schizophrenia: clinical and research implications. Journal of Psychopharmacology, 26(5 suppl), 52-61.

[36] Morden, N. E., Lai, Z., Goodrich, D. E., MacKenzie, T., McCarthy, J. F., Austin, K., Welsh, D.E., Bartels, S., Kilbourne, A. M. (2012). Eight-year trends of cardiometabolic morbidity and mortality in patients with schizophrenia. General hospital psychiatry, 34(4), 368-379.

[37] Laursen, T. M., Munk-Olsen, T., Vestergaard, M. (2012). Life expectancy and cardiovascular mortality in persons with schizophrenia. Current opinion in psychiatry, 25(2), 83-88.

[38] Kelly, D. L., McMahon, R. P., Liu, F., Love, R. C., Wehring, H., Shim, J. C., Warren, K.R., Conley, R. R. (2010). Cardiovascular Disease Mortality in Chronic Schizophrenia Patients Treated with Clozapine. The Journal of clinical psychiatry, 71(3), 304-3011.

[39] Hor, K., & Taylor, M. (2010). Review: Suicide and schizophrenia: a systematic review of rates and risk factors. Journal of Psychopharmacology, 24(4 suppl), 81-90.

[40] Bushe, C. J., Taylor, M., Haukka, J. (2010). Review: Mortality in schizophrenia: a measurable clinical endpoint. Journal of Psychopharmacology, 24(4 suppl), 17-25.

[41] Knapp, M., Mangalore, R., Simon, J. (2004). The global costs of schizophrenia. Schizophrenia bulletin, 30(2), 279-293.

[42] Oliva-Moreno, J., López-Bastida, J., Osuna-Guerrero, R., Montejo-González, A. L., & Duque-González, B. (2006). The costs of schizophrenia in Spain. The European Journal of Health Economics, 7(3), 179-184.

[43] Mangalore, R., & Knapp, M. (2007). Cost of schizophrenia in England. Journal of Mental Health Policy and Economics, 109(1), 23-41.

[44] WHO (2014). Global status report on alcohol and health. Luxembourg.

[45] Andlin-Sobocki, P., Rehm, J. (2005). Cost of addiction in Europe. European Journal of Neurology, 12(s1), 28-33.

[46] Baumberg, B. (2006). The global economic burden of alcohol: a review and some suggestions. Drug and alcohol review, 25(6), 537-551.

[47] Jane-Llopis, E. V. A., &Matytsina, I. (2006). Mental health and alcohol, drugs and tobacco: a review of the comorbidity between mental disorders and the use of alcohol, tobacco and illicit drugs. Drug and alcohol review, 25(6), 515-536.

[48] Rehm, J., Mathers, C., Popova, S., Thavorncharoensap, M., Teerawattananon, Y., Patra, J. (2009). Global burden of disease and injury and economic cost attributable to alcohol use and alcohol-use disorders. The Lancet, 373, 2223-2233.

[49] Room, R., Babor, T., &Rehm, J. (2005). Alcohol and public health. The lancet, 365, 519-530.

[50] Boden, J.M., Fergusson, D.M., Horwood, L. J. (2013). Alcohol misuse and criminal offending: Findings from a 30-year longitudinal study, Drug and Alcohol Dependence, 128(1–2), 30-36.

[51] Rehm, J., Room, R., van den Brink, W., & Jacobi, F. (2005). Alcohol use disorders in EU countries and Norway: an overview of the epidemiology. European Neuropsychopharmacology, 15(4), 377-388.

[52] Laramée, P., Kusel, J., Leonard, S., Aubin, H. J., François, C., Daeppen, J. B. (2013). The economic burden of alcohol dependence in Europe. Alcohol and alcoholism, 48(3), 259-269.

[53] Jarl, J., Johansson, P., Eriksson, A., Eriksson, M., Gerdtham, U. G., Hemström, Ö.,Selin, K.H., Lenke, L., Ramstedt, M., Room, R. (2008). The societal cost of alcohol consumption: an estimation of the economic and human cost including health effects in Sweden, 2002. The European Journal of Health Economics, 9(4), 351-360.

[54] Konnopka, A., & König, H. H. (2007). Direct and indirect costs attributable to alcohol consumption in Germany. Pharmacoeconomics, 25(7), 605-618.

[55] Laireiter, A. R., Messer, R., & Baumann, U. (2008). Alt und ohne Hilfe–Zur psychosozialen Versorgung alter Menschen. Zeitschrift für Gerontopsychologie &-psychiatrie, 21(1), 5-9.

[56] Wancata, J., Kaiser, G. (2008). Dimensionen der psychosozialen Versorgung alter Menschen. Zeitschrift für Gerontopsychologie &-psychiatrie, 21(1), 11-19.

[57] Berr, C., Wancata, J., Ritchie, K. (2005). Prevalence of dementia in the elderly in Europe. European neuropsychopharmacology, 15(4), 463-471.

[58] Jönnson, L., Wimo, A. (2009). The Cost of Dementia in Europe. A Review of the Evidence, and Methodological Considerations. Pharmacoeconomics, 27(5), 391-403.

[59] Connolly, S., Gillespie, P., O'Shea, E., Cahill, S., Pierce, M. (2014). Estimating the economic and social costs of dementia in Ireland. Dementia, 13(1), 5-22.

[60] Érsek, K., Kovács, T., Wimo, A., Kárpati, K., Brodszky, V., Péntek, M., Jönsson, L. Gustavvson, A. McDaid, D., Kenigsberg, P.E., Valtonen, H., Gulácsi, L. (2010). Costs of dementia in Hungary. The journal of nutrition, health & aging, 14(8), 633-639.

[61] Wimo, A., Jönsson, L., Gustavsson, A., McDaid, D., Ersek, K., Georges, J., Gulacsi, L., Karpati, K., Kenigsberg, P., Valtonen, H. (2011). The economic impact of dementia in Europe in 2008-cost estimates from the Eurocode project. International journal of geriatric psychiatry, 26(8), 825-832.

[62] Beecham, J. (2014). Annual Research Review: Child and adolescent mental health interventions: a review of progress in economic studies across different disorders. Journal of Child Psychology and Psychiatry, 55(6), 714-732.

[63] Rowland, A. S., Lesesne, C. A., & Abramowitz, A. J. (2002). The epidemiology of attention-deficit/hyperactivity disorder (ADHD): A public health view. Mental retardation and developmental disabilities research reviews, 8(3), 162-170.

[64] Schöffski, O., Sohn, S., Happich, M. (2008). Die gesamtgesellschaftliche Belastung durch die hyperkinetische Störung (HKS) bzw. Aufmerksamkeitsdefizit-/Hyperaktivitätsstörung (ADHS). Das Gesundheitswesen, 70(7), 398-403.

[65] De Ridder, A., De Graeve, D. (2006). Healthcare use, social burden and costs of children with and without ADHD in Flanders, Belgium. Clinical drug investigation, 26(2), 75-90.

[66] Le, H. H., Hodgkins, P., Postma, M. J., Kahle, J., Sikirica, V., Setyawan, J., Haim-Erder, M., Doshi, J. A. (2013). Economic impact of childhood/adolescent ADHD in a European setting: the Netherlands as a reference case. European child & adolescent psychiatry, 1-12.

[67] Tcheremissine, O. V., Lieving, L. M. (2006). Pharmacological aspects of the treatment of conduct disorder in children and adolescents. CNS Drugs, 20, 549-565.

[68] Ewest, F., Reinhold, T., Vloet, T. D., Wenning, V., Bachmann, C. J. (2013). Durch Jugendliche mit Störungen des Sozialverhaltens ausgelöste Krankenkassenausgaben. Kindheit und Entwicklung, 22(1), 41-47.

[69] Romeo, R., Knapp, M., & Scott, S. (2006). Economic cost of severe antisocial behaviour in children – and who pays it. The British Journal of Psychiatry, 188(6), 547-553.

[70] Knapp, M., Romeo, R., & Beecham, J. (2009). Economic cost of autism in the UK. Autism, 13(3), 317-336.

[71] Barrett, B., Byford, S., Sharac, J., Hudry, K., Leadbitter, K., Temple, K., Aldred, C., Slonims, V., Green, J. (2012). Service and wider societal costs of very young children with autism in the UK. Journal of autism and developmental disorders, 42(5), 797-804.

[72] Snell, T., Knapp, M., Healey, A., Guglani, S., Evans-Lacko, S., Fernandez, J. L., Meltzer, H., Ford, T. (2013). Economic impact of childhood psychiatric disorder on public

sector services in Britain: estimates from national survey data. Journal of child psychology and psychiatry, 54(9), 977-985.

[73] Heitzmann, K., Österle, A. (2008).Lange Traditionen und neue Herausforderungen: Das österreichische Wohlfahrtssyste In: Schubert, K., Hegelich, S., Bazant, U. (eds). Europäische Wohlfahrtssysteme. Ein Handbuch. VS Verlag, Wiesbaden, 47-70.

[74] Badelt C, Österle A. (2001). Grundzüge der Sozialpolitik. Spezieller Teil: Sozialpolitik in Österreich. 2nd ed., Manz, Wien

[75] Statistik Austria, Gesundheitsausgaben in Österreich. online (access 05.07.2014) http://www.statistik.at/web_de/statistiken/gesundheit/gesundheitsausgaben/ index.html

[76] GesundheitÖsterreich GmbH (2010). The Austrian health Care System. Key facts. Österreichisches Bundesministerium für Gesundheit,Wien

[77] Arbeitsmarktservice (2014). Rund um Arbeit und Behinderung. EineBroschürefürArbeitsuchende Menschen mitLernschwierigkeiten und/oder Behinderung. Wien

[78] Meise U, Wancata J, Hinterhuber H. Die Entwicklung der psychiatrischen Versorgung in Österreich. In: Rittmannsberger, H, Wancata, J. (eds.) Der österreichische Schizophreniebericht. Im Auftrag des Bundesministeriums für Gesundheit, Familie und Jugend, Linz, 2008, 134-145.

[79] Elgeti, H. (2013). Vorarlberger Psychiatriebericht. Im Auftrag des Amtes der Vorarlberger Landesregierung. Bregenz.

[80] Gesundheitsplattform Steiermark (2013). Psychiatriebericht 2012. Plattform Psyche zur psychosozialen Versorgung in der Steiermark. Online (access 10.07.2014) http://www.plattformpsyche.at/Documents/psychiatriebericht2012.pdf

[81] Katschnig, H., Denk, P., Scherer, M. (2004). Österreichischer Psychiatriebericht 2004.Analysen und Daten zur psychiatrischen und psychosozialen Versorgung der österreichischen Bevölkerung. Im Auftrag des Bundesministeriums für Gesundheit und Frauen, Wien.

[82] Gesundheit Österreich GmbH (2012). Österreichischer Strukturplan Gesundheit 2012 inklusive Großgeräteplan. Im Auftrag der Bundesgesundheitsagentur. Bundesministerium für Gesundheit. Wien.

[83] Hauptverband der österreichischen Sozialversicherungsträger (2012). Strategie psychische Gesundheit. Krankheit verhindern-Versorgung verbessern-Invalidität verringern. Salzburg.

[84] Kapusta, N. (2010). Aktuelle Daten und Fakten zur Zahl der Suizide in Österreich. Wien.

[85] Kapusta, N., Sonnecke, G. (2012). Suizide in Österreich: ein Update zur Entwicklung und aktueller Stand. neuropsychiatrie, 26(3), 103-105.

[86]   Watzka, C. (2012). Soziale Bedingungen von Selbsttötungen in Österreich. Eine Übersicht zu Risiko-und Schutzfaktoren. neuropsychiatrie, 26(3), 95-102.

[87]   Bundesministerium für Gesundheit (2011). SUPRA-Suizidprävention Austria. Wien, 2011.

[88]   Uhl, A., Bachmayer, S, Puhm, A., Strizek, J., Kobrna, U, Musalek, M. (2011). Handbuch Alkohol–Österreich. Statistiken und Berechnungsgrundlagen. Bundesministerium für Gesundheit, Wien.

[89]   Zechmeister I. (2005). Mental health care financing in the process of change: challenges and approaches for Austria. Lang, Frankfurt am Main ; Wien [u.a.] .

[90]   Österreichisches Institut für Gesundheitswesen (2010). Versorgung mit Psychotherapie. Eine Iststand-Erhebung mit einem Sonderkapitel zu Psychopharmaka. Eine Studie im Auftrag des Bundesministeriums für Gesundheit, Wien.

[91]   Thun-Hohenstein, L. (2008). Die Versorgungssituation psychisch auffälliger und kranker Kinder und Jugendlicher in Österreich. Kindermedizin-Werte versus Ökonomie. Springer, Wien, 163-173.

[92]   Thun-Hohenstein, L (2011). Kinder-und jugendpsychiatrische Versorgung in Österreich-ein Update. In: Kerbl, R., Thun-Hohenstein, L., Damm, L., & Waldhauser, F. (Eds.). Kinder und Jugendliche im besten Gesundheitssystem der Welt. 4. Jahrestagung Politische Kindermedizin 2010, Springer, Wien, 83-90.

[93]   Berger E, Aichhorn W, Friedrich MH, Fiala-Preinsperger, S., Leixnering, W., Mangold, G., Spiel, B., Tatzer, E., Thun-Hohenstein, L. (2006). Kinder-und Jugendpsychiatrische Versorgung in Österreich. Neuropsychiatrie 20(2), 86–90.

[94]   Hauptverband der österreichischen Sozialversicherungsträger, Salzburger Gebietskrankenkasse (2011). Analyse der Versorgung psychisch Erkrankter. Projekt „Psychische Gesundheit. Abschlussbericht. Wien/ Salzburg.

[95]   Wancata, J., Sobocki, P., Katschnig, H. (2007). Die Kosten von "Gehirnerkrankungen" in Österreich im Jahr 2004. Wiener klinische Wochenschrift, 119(3-4), 91-98.

[96]   Haberfellner, E.M. (2008): Kosten der Schizophrenie. In: Rittmannsberger, H., Wancata, J. (Hrsg.): Österreichischer Schizophreniebericht 2008, Bundesministerium für Gesundheit, Wien, 191-198.

[97]   Czypionka, T., Pock, M., Röhrling, G., Sigl, C. (2013). Volkswirtschaftliche Effekte der Alkoholkrankheit. Eine ökonomische Analyse für Österreich. Research Report, Institute for Advanced Studies, Vienna.

[98]   Yang, B., Lester, D. (2007) Recalculating the Economic Cost of Suicide. Death Studies, 31(4), 351-361.

[99]   EUROSTAT (2014). Ausgaben der Leistungserbringer der Gesundheitsversorgung nach Kostenträgern der Gesundheitsversorgung-EUR, Einheiten Landeswährung,

KKS [hlth_sha3m] . http://appsso.eurostat.ec.europa.eu/nui/submitViewTableAction.do [access 04.09.2014]

[100] EUROSTAT (2014). Bevölkerung am 1. Januar nach Alter und Geschlecht [demo_pjan] http://appsso.eurostat.ec.europa.eu/nui/show.do?dataset=demo_pjan&lang=de [access 04.09.2014]

[101] Knapp, M., King, D., Healey, A., & Thomas, C. (2011). Economic outcomes in adulthood and their associations with antisocial conduct, attention deficit and anxiety problems in childhood. Journal of Mental Health Policy and Economics, 14(3), 137-147.

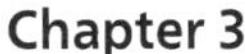

Chapter 3

Alcohol Consumption Among Adolescents — Implications for Public Health

Francisca Carvajal and Jose Manuel Lerma-Cabrera

Additional information is available at the end of the chapter

http://dx.doi.org/10.5772/58930

1. Introduction

Alcohol is the most commonly used and abused drug worldwide [1]. The highest level of alcohol consumption occurs in the developed world. This fact is not surprising since the history of alcoholic beverages is linked to the history of mankind. For centuries, alcohol consumption has been part of our culture and society. Drinking alcohol is a social activity, embedded today in traditional and sociocultural contexts. Probably, the main reason for alcohol consumption is its ability to produce positive moods and stress-relieving effects. In the last twenty years, worldwide per capita consumption of alcohol has remained stable. Currently, every person in the world aged 15 years or older drinks on average approximately 6 liters of pure alcohol per year. However, not all people in the world drink alcohol. Specifically, 61.7% of world population aged 15 years or older has not drunk alcohol in the past 12 months. This mean that those who drink alcohol consume on average 14.63 liters of pure alcohol annually. However, according to data from the Global Information System on Alcohol and Health [2], there are significant geographical variations in total per capita alcohol consumption. Thus, Chad (African WHO region) has the highest level of worldwide consumption at more than 33 liters per year. In comparison, alcohol consumption per capita in Pakistan (Eastern Mediterranean WHO region) averaged 1.2 liters per year (see Table 1).

Every year, a large amount of money is spent on alcohol worldwide. In fact, Europeans spend about 100 billion euros per year on alcoholic beverages. This is reflected in the region's high rate of alcohol consumption per capita: 15 liters of pure ethanol per year. Consuming and abusing these huge amounts of alcohol is clearly a problem, with enormous health and socioeconomic effects worldwide. Thus, harmful use of alcohol is a major public health problem. Drinking alcohol is socially acceptable and associated with relaxation and pleasure,

---

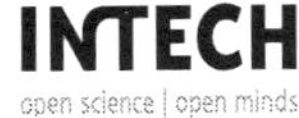

WHO region	Males (15+)	Females (15+)	Both sexes (15+)
Africa	20.12	10.44	16.91
America	16.66	8.86	13.47
Eastern Mediterranean	18.57	6.52	15.31
Europe	19.93	9.41	15.44
South-East Asia	19.41	4.13	15.73
Western Pacific	14.84	4.43	10.95
Total	**18.25**	**7.29**	**14.63**

Table 1. Total alcohol per capita consumption, drinkers only, 2010 (in liters of pure alcohol; aged 15+). Data from Global Status Report on Alcohol and Health (WHO, 2014)

and some people drink alcohol without experiencing harmful effects. However, alcohol does cause a growing number of people to experience physical, social and psychological harmful effects. Alcohol has important effects on our body, even when consumed in small amounts. The effects of alcohol intoxication are greatly influenced by gender, drinking speed, type and amount of food consumed, etc. Physiological changes appear as a function of Blood Alcohol Concentration (BAC) (see Table 2). BAC refers to the milligrams of alcohol per 100 milliliters of blood, and is usually expressed as a percentage. For instance, having a BAC of 0.10 means that a person has 1 part alcohol per 1000 parts blood. As the amount of alcohol consumed in a single sitting increases, the BAC increases proportionately.

BAC level (%)	Physiological effects
0.02 – 0.09	Mood changes (euphoria, increased sociability, talkativeness and more expansive personality), loss of inhibition, impaired coordination
0.1 – 0.19	Lack of coordination, impaired judgment, difficulty in walking and standing steadily
0.2 – 0.29	Marked ataxia (staggering; slurred speech), major motor impairment, nausea
0.30 – 0.39	Increased sedation/hypnosis, marked decreases in responsiveness to environmental stimuli, partial amnesia ("blackout") likely
0.4 or more	Alcohol poisoning, coma, risk of death (lethal dose for 50% of people)

Table 2. BAC levels and their effects for a typical person

As indicated in Table 2, excessive alcohol use has immediate physiological and psychological effects that increase the risk of many harmful health conditions. These effects vary from mood changes to alcohol poisoning and coma. Over time, excessive alcohol use can lead to chronic diseases (cardiovascular problems, liver diseases…), neurological impairment and social problems, including unemployment and family problems. Also, people who drink too much or too often, or are unable to control alcohol consumption, can develop an alcohol use disorder.

Alcohol dependence and harmful alcohol use are recognized as mental health disorders in the *Diagnostic and Statistical Manual of Mental Disorders* (DSM-5) [3] and the *International Statistical Classification of Diseases and Related Health Problems* (ICD-10) [4]. The Diagnostic and Statistical Manual of Mental Disorders (DSM-5) defines Alcohol Use Disorder (AUD) as the presence of at least 2 of 11 criteria within a 12-month period, defined by a cluster of behavioral and physical symptoms organized in four groups:

1. *Impaired control:* (1) alcohol is often taken in large amounts or over longer period than was intended, (2) unsuccessful efforts to stop or cut down alcohol use, (3) spending a great deal of time obtaining, using, or recovering from alcohol use, (4) craving for the substance.

2. *Social impairment:* (5) failure to fulfill major obligations due to use, (6) continued use despite problems caused or exacerbated by use, (7) important social, occupational or recreational activities given up or reduced because of alcohol use.

3. *Risky use:* (8) recurrent alcohol use in hazardous situations, (9) continued use despite physical or psychological problems caused or exacerbated by alcohol use.

4. *Pharmacological dependence:* (10) tolerance to substance effects, (11) withdrawal symptoms when not using or using less.

According to the DSM-5, the severity of the alcohol use disorder (mild, moderate and severe) is based on the number of criteria met. Anyone meeting 2 or 3 criteria would receive the mild AUD diagnosis. Anyone meeting 4 or 5 criteria would receive the moderate AUD diagnosis. Finally, anyone meeting 6 or more criteria would receive the severe AUD diagnosis.

Although a large proportion of the population consumes alcohol, not all of them become alcohol dependent. Research shows that people who drink moderately may be less likely to experience AUD. Thus, only 3.6% of alcohol users worldwide are alcohol dependent, a condition implying a degree of addiction that makes it difficult for them to abstain or reduce their drinking in spite of increasingly serious harm [2] (see Figure 1). When comparing different WHO regions, the following conclusion can be made. The highest lifetime prevalence of alcohol use disorder occurs in Europe (6.1%) and the Americas (5.4%). The lowest prevalence rates of alcohol use disorders occurs in South-East Asia (2.1%) and Eastern Mediterranean countries (0.4%)

Specifically, alcohol use is ranked as the third leading risk factor for disease and disability in the world. It is the leading risk factor in the Western Pacific and the Americas, and the second largest in Europe. According to 2012 data from the Global Information System on Alcohol and Health [2], harmful use of alcohol kills 3.3 million people annually and represents 4.5% of the global disease burden. Also, alcohol has been shown to be causally related to more than 60 different types of diseases and injuries [5]. For example, 33.4% of all deaths caused by cardiovascular disease (i.e. hypertension, atrial fibrillation and hemorrhagic stroke [6] and diabetes mellitus [7] are causally related to ethanol consumption; also, alcohol has been related to gastrointestinal diseases such as liver cirrhosis and pancreatitis in 16.2% of cases [8]. Generally, the risk of suffering these disease is related to the volume of alcohol consumed: the higher the

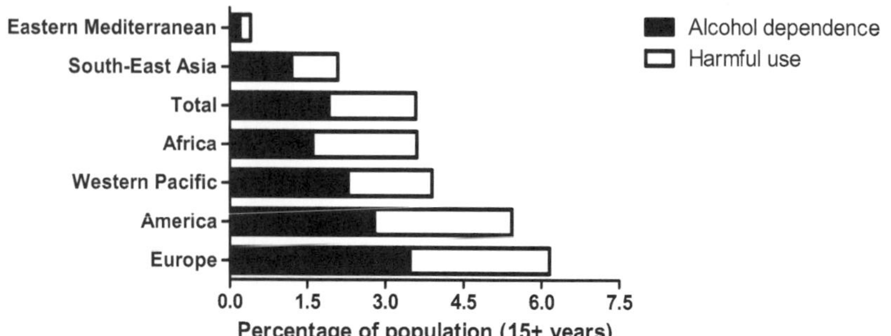

Figure 1. Prevalence of alcohol use disorders (AUDs) by WHO region, 2010. Data from Global Status Report on Alcohol and Health (WHO, 2014)

volume, the larger the risk of these diseases. Recently, drinking alcohol has been related to the incidence of infectious diseases such as tuberculosis and HIV/AIDS [9].

The impact of harmful use of alcohol is not just personal, it may also impose significant social and economic costs on society. The economic cost of ethanol abuse is estimated at more than $235 billion every year [10]. More than 70 percent of the estimated cost of alcohol abuse is attributed to lost productivity. Other costs are largely the result of alcohol-related health care, motor vehicle accidents, and law enforcement and other criminal justice expenses.

Adolescents are a particularly vulnerable to the harmful effects of alcohol. In fact, ten years ago, the National Institute on Alcohol Abuse and Alcoholism (NIAAA) formed an interdisciplinary working group on underage drinking in order to intensify research, evaluation and outreach efforts on the underage drinking problem. Alcohol is the most common drug of abuse in adolescence, more than tobacco and other illicit drugs. Misuse of alcohol among adolescent is an international problem. In fact, 320.000 young people aged 15 to 29 die each year from alcohol-related causes—9% of all deaths in that age group [11].

Bearing in mind all these data, in 2010 the World Health Assembly approved a resolution to urge countries to strengthen national responses to public health problems caused by the harmful use of alcohol.

2. Present situation

In general, adolescence can be defined as the transitional period between childhood and adult maturity characterized by behavioral, hormonal and neurochemical changes designed to prepare the body for independent survival. It is derived from the Latin *adolescere-*. The present participle *adolescens* means growing up; the past participle *adultus* means grown up. The World Health Organization (WHO) defines adolescents as people between 10 and 19 years of age. However, different definitions of adolescence have been used in scientific literature. Thus, whereas some clinical researchers define human adolescence as the age span from approximately 9 to 18 years of age [12], others consider the entire second decade of life as "adolescence" [13]. In spite of conceptual term differences, all studies agree with the idea that adolescence is a time of marked change, a time of transition into adulthood. Therefore, at this age, people experiment with adult aspects of life: they establish their own identities, make close relationship outside the family, and want to try out new things, some of which may be risky or even dangerous. Many teenagers experiment with alcohol and illegal drugs.

Epidemiological studies have detected the development of a new pattern of alcohol consumption in adolescents. This pattern is characterized by drinking large amounts of alcohol over a short period of time, especially in leisure time and weekends, with periods of abstinence between drinking episodes. In spite of the fact that young people drink less often than adults, on average they consume more drinks per drinking occasion than adult drinkers. Specifically, compared to adults, adolescents drink more than twice as much per drinking episode [14].We can say that they show a pattern of binge drinking.

In 2004, the NIAAA defined binge drinking as a pattern of drinking that brings Blood Alcohol Concentration (BAC) to 0.08 grams percent or above. For adults, this pattern corresponds to drinking five or more drinks (male), or four or more drinks (female), in about two hours. For adolescents, an important debate has developed over the definition of binge and whether that definition must be different for adults and adolescents due to alcohol absorption differences. Thus, according to recent research estimates, reaching a given BAC level takes fewer drinks for young people.

Although it has declined in the last decade, underage drinking (ages 12-20) is still an important public health problem. Despite the fact that these teens are under the legal age for purchasing alcohol, many adolescents engage in underage drinking in general and binge drinking in particular. However, the levels and patterns of alcohol consumption vary widely between countries. According to the Global Status Report on Alcohol and Health [2] the prevalence of heavy episodic drinking in 15-19 year-olds ranged from 50.6% in Germany to zero in some Eastern Mediterranean countries, such as Afghanistan, Morocco or Tunisia. Particularly, in the African, Eastern Mediterranean and South-East Asia regions, young people (15 to 19) are less likely to engage in heavy episodic drinking (see Table 3). By contrast, adolescent alcohol use is common in many European and American countries. Thus, in a US study, 10% of 8th graders, 22% of 10th graders and 26% of 12th graders reported that they had consumed five or more drinks in a row within the previous 2 weeks [15]. Clearly, underage alcohol use increases with age. Specifically, the percentage of the population who drinks at least one whole drink rises steeply during adolescence. In Europe, the binge-drinking rates are even twice or three times higher than in United States [16]. Thus, 50–70% of 16-year olds have consumed alcohol once in their lives, and >35–70% of European adolescents who have ever drunk report at least one heavy drinking episode in the previous month [17].

Table 3 shows clear differences in alcohol use between genders. Underage males report more alcohol use than underage females, independently of WHO region. Similarly, previous studies in adults have shown that women drink less than men and also, that they have more alcohol-related problems than men [18]. Studies have shown that adolescent girls suffer more adverse cognitive effect related to alcohol than adolescent boys, especially in working memory and visual-spatial functions. Multiple factors can contribute to gender differences in risk factors for alcohol use. For example, hormonal fluctuation, differences in alcohol metabolism, or gender-specific drinking patterns. In agreement with these data showing gender differences in alcohol use profile, alcohol prevention should take these sub-group differences into account.

WHO region	Males	Females	Both sexes
Africa	6.43	1.84	4.16
America	23.89	5.58	14.88
Eastern Mediterranean	0.24	0.07	0.15
Europe	35.00	18.19	26.80
South-East Asia	0.5	0.06	0.29
Western Pacific	18.00	6.65	12.47
Total	14.01	5.39	9.79

Table 3. Heavy episodic drinking prevalence* (%, 15-19 year-olds), 2010. *Consumed at least 60 grams or more of pure alcohol on at least one occasion in the past

2.1. Binge drinking and short-and long-term outcomes

Binge drinking has many negative short-and long-term outcomes. In a 2004 global mortality patterns report, 3.2 million deaths were attributed to alcohol use among people aged 15 to 29. That is 19% of all deaths—the highest mortality risk factor in the age group. Binge drinking is associated with increased risk of:

- *unsafe sexual activity* [19,20]. Underage alcohol use has been associated to risky sexual behavior (unwanted, unintended and unprotected sexual activity) and multiple sex partners. For example, 32% of adolescent who started drinking at 13 reported having unplanned sex because of drinking, and 10% reported having unprotected sex because of drinking [21]. Such behavior increases the risk of unplanned pregnancy and sexually transmitted disease infection [19]. Also, young people who drink are more likely to carry out or be the victim of physical or sexual assault [21].

- *criminal and aggressive behavior* [22]. Hazardous alcohol use can reduced physical control and ability to recognize warning signs in potentially dangerous situation, therefore increasing the risk of becoming a victim of violence [22,23]. Similarly, reduced self-control and ability to process incoming information and assess risks can make some drinkers perpetrate acts of violence [24]. Recently, it has been proposed that a common risk factor (i.e. anti-social personality disorder) could explain the relationship between violence and heavy alcohol drinking [25, 26].

- *suicide ideation and suicide attempts* [27]. Thus, individuals with suicide ideation and attempts are more likely to engage in heavy episodic drinking and have greater alcohol problem [28].

Also, binge drinking has been associated with successful suicide [29]. Every year in the United Stated, about 300 young people under 21 commit suicide as result of underage drinking.

- *drunk driving or riding in a vehicle driven by a drunk driver* [30]. 24 percent of drivers aged 15 to 20 involved in fatal motor vehicle accidents had been drinking. Alcohol has a range of effects on reaction time, cognitive processing, coordination, alertness, vision, and hearing, all of which increase accident risk.

- *alcohol intoxication and accidental death.* Consuming alcohol can cause a range of physical consequences, from hangovers to death from alcohol poisoning. Alcohol intoxication is manifested by such signs as slurred speech, loss of coordination, unsteady gait, euphoria, confusion, impaired judgment or stupefaction. Also, it can lead to complications such as trauma, dehydration, delirium, heart attack or convulsions. In the most severe cases, alcohol poisoning can lead to coma and even death.

Finally, we know that the adolescent brain undergoes neurodevelopmental changes. These changes can be influenced by genetic, environmental and sexual hormone factors. Thus, drinking alcohol early in the adolescence has adverse effects on the brain [31].

2.2. The adolescent brain and substances of abuse

The transition to adolescence is characterized by a rapid biological transformation, including the hormonal and physiological changes of puberty. During this period, the body grows (height and weight), secondary sex characteristics emerge, and sex hormones reach adult levels. Adolescence is a time of substantial neuromaturation involving important changes in numerous brain regions, including the hippocampus, the prefrontal cortex, and limbic system structures. Although the human brain does reach approximately 90% if its adult weight by age 6 [32], structural changes continue throughout adolescence. Specifically, the prefrontal cortex, which plays an important role in executive control functions (i.e. planning, emotional regulation, decision making…) starts to develop early in life and continues after adolescence and into the early 20s. In contrast, the limbic system—the site that governs reward processing, appetite and pleasure seeking— develops earlier than the prefrontal cortex. This maturation disparity between limbic system and prefrontal cortex might explain the preponderance of behaviors driven by emotion and reward over more rational decision making in adolescents.

Changes observed in the adolescent brain are characterized not only by continued neural system maturation, but also by changes in the synaptic connection in these neural regions. During adolescence, the brain is highly plastic and shaped by experience. It has been shown that gray matter volume and density decrease during adolescence. Developmental declines in gray matter occur first in the sensory and motor regions of the cortex and then in the prefrontal cortex (PFC) and other cortical association areas [33, 34]. Such reduction in gray matter is largely due to the loss of weak or unused synapses via synaptic pruning. As the person matures into adulthood, this process makes these areas more efficient and promotes speed, overall efficiency, and enhanced information processing capacity. Conversely, white matter increases during the transition from childhood to young adulthood, first in the occipital regions and then in the frontal, temporal and parietal association areas. Myelination has been related to increased cognitive efficiency. In general, this neural pruning may serve to refine the abundance of brain connections and increase brain efficiency during adolescence.

Similarly, throughout adolescence there are rapid changes in neurotransmission and plasticity. These changes have a particularly strong effect on dopamine (DA) and serotonin. Both neurotransmitters are dynamically changing in the adolescent brain. The dopaminergic system undergoes marked transitional changes during development. During adolescence, the brain shows elevated basal levels of extracellular DA in comparison with adulthood [35]. Also, dopamine D1 and D2 [36], but not dopamine D3 [37] receptor levels increase in the striatum during early adolescence. The activity levels of these dopaminergic receptors are 30-40% greater than in adults, measured as an increase in D1 and D2 receptor binding [38]. Moreover, the density of DA transporter (DAT), which removes DA from the synapses, is greater in adolescence than in adulthood [39, 40]. Bearing in mind the role of dopamine in reward and euphoria, these changes in the dopaminergic system could be related to the euphoric behaviors showed by adolescents.

Several studies have shown that the serotonergic system undergoes reorganization during postnatal development (from childhood through adolescence). Specifically, brain serotonin (5-hydroxytryptamine or 5-HT) concentration peaks early in life and then decreases to adult levels levels [41, 42]. 5-HT$_{2A}$ subtype receptor levels behave similarly [43]. Moreover, the 5-HT turnover has been reported to be approximately 4 times lower in adolescents than in adults [44]. In addition, serotonin transporters—involved in neurotransmitter inactivation—steadily increase until adulthood [40, 45] and decrease synaptic 5-HT concentration. The low level of 5-HT has been associated with impaired impulse control, anxiety, and aggressive behavior. In summary, evidence indicates that during adolescence, there is relatively greater activity in the dopamine system than in the inhibitory serotonin (5-HT) system, potentially resulting in an imbalance in the reward (DA-mediated) and suppression (5-HT-mediated) mechanisms [38, 46].

Others neurotransmitters (acetylcholine, glutamate, GABA…) also undergo brain changes during development. Relative to adults, adolescents exhibit developmentally enhanced activity of the glutamatergic system in certain brain regions [47], while at the same time displaying developmentally immaturity of the gamma-aminobutyric acid (GABA) system [48,49]. On the other hand, the maturation of the central cholinergic system, which plays an important role in both memory/learning and anxiety, occurs in this critical period [50].

The neurochemical, cellular and structural organization of the adolescent brain makes it more vulnerable than the adult brain to disruption from activities such as binge drinking. The brains of adolescents that consume alcohol show a reduction on myelin fiber tracts with frontal connections as well as altered white matter integrity, events that might underlie dysfunctions in learning, memory and executive functions [51]. In addition, since alcohol interacts with some neurotransmitter systems that are essential for brain development, drug exposure during adolescence may be particularly harmful to the still developing brain. For example, binge drinking results in altered serotoninergic innervation and increased transporter density in several brain regions, including the forebrain [52]. Thus, underage drinking could contribute to altered sleep patterns, impulsivity, satiation and other behaviors associated with serotoninergic function. In the same way, given that acetylcholine is an important neurotrophic agent implicated in cholinergic target cell proliferation and differentiation [53, 54], ethanol consumption during adolescence could evoke neurodevelopmental abnormalities by disrupting the timing or intensity of neurotrophic actions. In addition, the alteration of cholinergic system could be mediating the learning and memory deficits shown by adolescent who consume alcohol.

Binge-drinking adolescents suffer volume reduction in several brain areas, such as the prefrontal cortex, the hippocampus and the left middle and inferior temporal gyrus [55-57]; this reduction is positively correlated with the duration of alcohol use. Several studies have shown cognitive impairments in adolescents with alcohol use disorder [58]. As such, neuropsychological studies have revealed that binge-drinking adolescents exhibit poor performance in tasks assessing verbal and nonverbal memory, problem solving, attention, working memory, and visual-spatial skills [58-61]. Furthermore, adolescent binge drinkers were faster in speed test response, confirming the hypothesis of increased impulsivity in this population [62]. Interestingly, a recent study has demonstrated that old people and young people who consume excessive alcohol show similar deterioration in executive function [63]. These data suggest that, as a consequence of alcohol consumption, the area of the brain undergoing deterioration is similar in both adolescents and old people. However, additional research could help clarify if alcoholism produces cognitive aging.

Finally, the changes in the adolescent brain have consequences not only at the time but also later in life. Recent studies have demonstrated that exposure to alcohol during adolescence has long-term effects on the brain that persist into adulthood. There is evidence that ethanol exposure during adolescence might also alter neuropeptide systems critically involved in voluntary ethanol intake. Thus, following binge-like ethanol exposure during adolescence, adult animals show increased mRNA expression of basal corticotrophin releasing factor (CRF) in the paraventricular nucleus of hypothalamus [64], decreased overall hippocampal neuropeptide Y (NPY) immunoreactivity in Wistar rats [65], and reduced α-MSH expression in the hypothalamus and the amygdala of adult rats [66]. Given the role of these neuropeptides in ethanol consumption and the fact binge-like ethanol exposure during adolescence increases the probability of ethanol consumption during adulthood, the changes observed in these studies might contribute to increased vulnerability to ethanol consumption during adulthood. However, additional studies are necessary to check this hypothesis.

3. Risk factors for alcohol consumption among adolescents

Alcohol consumption among adolescents has a multifaceted etiology. In this section, we will address the reasons why adolescents drink large amounts of alcohol, focusing on age-dependent alcohol sensitivity. Research literature has shown that, in general, adolescents are more sensitive than adults to the stimulating effects of alcohol, and less sensitive to some of the aversive effects of acute alcohol intoxication. Finally, and given that both environmental and genetic factors are found to affect levels of alcohol use from adolescence to adulthood [67], we will dedicate a subsection to this topic.

3.1. Adolescents and adults respond differently to the effects of alcohol

Ethanol use increases throughout adolescence and is often associated with relatively high consumption levels. Although the exact cause of the increase in ethanol consumption during adolescence is not known, age-dependent sensitivity differences to some ethanol effects may play a contributory role. Mainly, two complementary explanations are given as to why adolescents drink more alcohol than adults. First, they are more sensitive to the positive effects of alcohol, i.e. the social loss of inhibition effect of alcohol when compared with adults [68], which may serve to reinforce or promote excessive intake. In fact, on average and per occasion, adolescents consume more alcohol than adults. In agreement with these behavioral data, it has been demonstrated that in adolescence a single ethanol exposure causes a robust and pronounced increase in dopamine release in comparison with adults [69]. This enhancement in dopamine release is consistent with the greater rewarding effects of alcohol in adolescents [70]. Thus, the increased sensitivity to alcohol's rewarding effects could contribute to increased susceptibility to alcoholism in the adolescent population.

Secondly, numerous studies have demonstrated that adolescents are less sensitive to the negative effects of alcohol than adults, such as sedation, loss of coordination and hangover effect. This decreased sensitivity may allow adolescents to continue drinking longer than their adult counterparts, thereby increasing the risk of acute cognitive impairment and brain damage.

Because it is unethical and illegal to provide alcohol to minors for the purpose of research, the majority of research on this topic have been performed on laboratory animals, primarily rodents. Findings from several studies using animal adolescence models support the hypothesis that adolescents are less sensitive to the negative effects of alcohol than adults, including hypnotic [71], hypothermic [72,73], motor impairing [74,75] and anxiolytic effects [76].

For instance, adolescent rats are markedly less sensitive than adult rats to alcohol-induced sedation. Sedation refers to the calming or tranquilizing effect of a drug. In rats, sedation is measured by the loss of the righting reflex. After a large acute dose of ethanol, adolescent rats regained their righting reflex and woke up more quickly at higher blood alcohol levels (BAC) than adult animals [71]. These authors suggest that the same differences should exist in humans. Consequently, adolescents may experience minimal hypnotic effect from ethanol consumption, thus receiving less negative feedback as a result of drinking. In addition, adolescents appeared more sensitive to high doses of ethanol when examining ethanol's hypothermic effects [72]. In general, adolescent showed a greater magnitude of ethanol-induced hypothermia than adults; even though adults showed more rapid and sustained ethanol-induced hypothermia than adolescents [73].

It is well known that alcohol disrupts motor coordination. Numerous studies suggest that adolescent rats display age-related differences in the development of motor impairment [74, 75], suggesting that the disruption is less pronounced in adolescents than in adults. Similarly, human adolescents might drink more because of their relative insensitivity to motor cues signaling intoxication.

One important motivation for alcohol use is the fact that alcohol has anxiety-reducing properties. The evidence for the anxiolytic effect of ethanol in human [77] and animal models [78] has been demonstrated. Studies carried on adolescent rats have shown that they are less sensitive than adults to the anxiolytic effect of alcohol. Specifically, some investigators have found that, due to tolerance development, adolescent rats require greater quantities of alcohol than adults to reach anxiolytic effects [76].

Likewise, adolescent rats are less sensitive than adults to consequences associated with ethanol withdrawal. The signs of ethanol withdrawal include physiological (headache, fatigue, tremor, …) and psychological (anxiety, guilt, depression,…) symptoms. Adolescent rats show less anxiogenic signs of acute withdrawal as measured in the elevated plus maze [79], in the open field test [80] or in a social interaction test [81]. The results of these studies suggest that even when using different behavioral test to examine anxiety, adolescents fail to exhibit the withdrawal-induced anxiety seen in adults. Human studies have shown that, compared to adults, adolescents who commonly abuse alcohol, rarely report withdrawal symptoms upon drinking cessation [82].

In summary, findings derived from basic research indicate that adolescents and adults experience alcohol differently. In general, adolescents are less sensitive to the negative aspects of alcohol consumption (sedation, motor impairment, anxiety), but more sensitive to its positive and rewarding effects. Thus, adolescents are "resistant" to the negative effects of ethanol that limit consumption progression. In general, during adolescence, more drinks are necessary to elicit a signal that it is time to stop. Conversely, adolescents are more sensitive to the effects that facilitate the maintenance, progression and escalation of alcohol consumption. This pattern of response to alcohol would be a vulnerability factor for adolescents to engage in problematic drinking trajectories. However, there are environmental and genetic factors that may also contribute to alcohol consumption among adolescents.

3.2. Environment and heritability factors

The environment and heritability factors play a dramatic role in controlling individual predisposition to developing alcohol abuse [83, 84]. Knowing the characteristics that increase the risk of adolescent alcohol use disorder can be helpful in preventing or attenuating such risk.

The relationship between early use of alcohol during adolescence and the increased risk of excessive alcohol drinking and alcohol disorder in adulthood has been well documented. Several studies have reported that alcohol consumption before 14 years of age is associated with a fourfold increase in the risk of alcohol dependence in adulthood [85, 86]. Similarly, 10 years after alcohol initiation, 14% of adolescent who started to drink at early ages, versus 2% of those who delayed the drinking onset, met alcohol dependence criteria [87]. Also, early alcohol use is associated with more mental health and social negative effects [88] or even with increased later use and abuse of other substances (tobacco, marijuana or other illicit drugs) [89].

Another important risk factor associated with using alcohol for the first time at an earlier age is a family history of alcoholism [90-92]. Having a family history of alcohol drinking problems is associated with greater underage drinking [90, 91] and greater frequency of alcohol-use problems [92]. Several studies have reported that only the father's drinking had a direct effect on adolescent drinking [93, 94] while the mother's didn't. Further research is needed to clarify the real impact of parental drinking on adolescent drinking. It is known that alcohol use disorder tends to be repeated within families. For example, 60% of people with alcohol dependence and a family history of alcohol (i.e., an alcoholic parent) initiated drinking at age 13. By contrast, when they did not have a family history of alcohol, only 28% initiated drinking at age 13 [95]. However, it is difficult to draw clear conclusions about this factor because this predisposition may be due to children inheriting certain genes that determine an underlying predisposition or because they learn certain behavioral patterns that lead to the development of alcoholism. Moreover, we should consider that other studies have shown no family history [96] and no offspring and/or parent gender dependence [94] on young adult problematic drinking. Given the non-conclusive data, additional research is needed to understand the relationship between family history of alcoholism and early use of alcohol during adolescence.

Other environmental factors recognized as important risk factors in excessive alcohol use among adolescents are: the influence of a stressful life event [97] and peer substance use on initiation and intensity of alcohol use. The exposure to stress is strongly associated with the initiation and prolongation of alcohol drinking which most often evolves into alcohol dependence. In other words, and given that adolescents are highly vulnerable to social influence and they tend to copy what their friends do to feel accepted, peer effects on risk-taking are strong in this age group. For example, having friends who drink increases the likelihood that an adolescent will drink too. According to the National Survey on Drug Abuse and Health (2012), the probability of ethanol consumption if a few friends have consumed alcohol within the past 30 days is 7.3%, 25% if most of them consumed alcohol and 41.4% if all of them consumed alcohol. Similarly, adolescents are also influenced by how much their friends drink [98].

It has been shown that intrapersonal risk factors predict alcohol-related problems among adolescents and young adults. Some of them are poor behavioral regulation and Attention Deficit Hyperactivity Disorder (ADHD) [99-101], delinquency and personality traits, like sensation seeking, impulsivity [102] and neuroticism [103]. All of them have been shown to be positively related to drug use among youth.

In addition, recent data have highlight the existence of protective factors, such as parental control and a supportive environment [104, 105]. Studies have consistently found that the parenting style significantly protects against adolescent drinking behavior. Specifically, both indulgent and authoritative parenting styles have been hypothesized to be a major source of influence on protection against adolescent substance use [106]. It seems that fostering an environment of acceptance, dialogue and affection is a good strategy to prevent adolescent alcohol consumption. For example, adolescents from authoritative households (i.e. harmonious, warm and responsive parents that exert concurrently firm control and maturity demands) use less illegal drugs [107]. As well as parental control, involvement in social activities is another protective factor in adolescent alcohol use [108]. Adolescents who demonstrate a high involvement in social activities (sports, extracurricular and/or academic activities…), are less likely to consume alcohol or other drugs.

Studies have shown that alcohol use among adolescents could also be influenced by genetic factors. Behavioral genetic studies carried on twins have shown a significant genetic component in alcohol dependence (58%), regular alcohol use (43%) and alcohol-related problems (38.5%) [109, 110]. By analyzing the genetic makeup of adolescents who consume alcohol, researchers have found specific chromosome regions that correlate with this consumption pattern. One recent study found that a serotonin transporter polymorphism (5-HTTLPR) predicted adolescent increase in alcohol use over time [111]. In spite of having a similar initial level of alcohol consumption, adolescents with the 5-HTTLPR showed larger increases in alcohol consumption. Other genes associated with the risk of developing alcohol use disorder (AUD) during youth is μ-opioid receptor (OPRM1) polymorphism [112, 113]. Thus, adolescents who met criteria for an AUD diagnosis had a higher prevalence of this polymorphism. Finally, genes involved in gamma-aminobutyric (GABA) receptors have also been widely studied because of their role in alcohol use disorders in adolescence and young adulthood. The most frequently studied polymorphism included the GABA receptor subunits GABRA2 [114] and GABRG3 [115]. Further research is needed to identify the actual genes involved in the early alcohol consumption and their contribution to alcohol problems in adolescents.

In summary, studies have clearly shown that both genetic and environmental factors contribute to the risk of alcohol dependence in adolescence and later in adulthood, and it is likely that the interplay between these factors is critical in determining the risk of alcohol abuse and dependence. For example, twin studies have found that initiation on alcohol use is largely influenced by the environmental risk factor [116]. Once initiation has occurred, genetic factors explain a large amount of alcohol use frequency variations (34–72%) especially as adolescents get older [116]. Thus, studies that tested interactions between environmental factors and genes implicated in alcohol drinking in adolescence are necessary. We cannot forget that, in spite of the fact that certain genetic polymorphism may increase the probability to develop alcohol dependence, the manifestation of the disorder might depend on environmental factors.

4. Prevention programs

Alcohol dependence is a chronic disorder that causes high direct and indirect costs to public health and has important social and family implications. Moreover, it ranks among the first on the list of disorders that cause higher rates of death in the world. However, it has remained a relatively low priority in public policy, including in public health policy. Considering all these data, in 2010 the World Health Assembly approved a resolution to urge countries to strengthen national responses to public health problems caused by the harmful use of alcohol.

At 1.8 billion, adolescents and young adults represent more than a quarter of the world's population. According to data from the WHO's Global Burden of Disease study, 7.4% of all disability and premature deaths in people aged 10-24 are alcohol-attributable, followed by unsafe sex (4%) or illicit drug use (2%) [117]. Also, it should be noted that most of the mental disorders begin before age 25. This finding suggest that public health strategies should focus on child and adolescent health, paying special attention to adolescent drinking. Given that early initiation of alcohol use has been frequently associated with later alcohol-related problems [87], delaying the initiation of drinking from early adolescence to late adolescence or adulthood is an important prevention goal [118]. Understanding the precursors and etiology of drinking behavior is necessary to limit premature and excessive drinking among adolescents.

However, before we start to set up alcohol consumption prevention plans for adolescents, we must identify alcohol consumption determinants, i.e. why do young people drink? Numerous studies have demonstrated that both alcohol expectations and drinking motives are related to alcohol use [119, 120]. However, it seems that drinking motives are the most proximate factor preceding alcohol use. Adolescents appear to drink because of social motives being either positive (social camaraderie) or negative (peer pressure, not to feel left out). Thus, most adolescents drink alcohol to relax, to have fun or to belong to the group. In general, alcohol is used to gain social recognition [119]. Another factor that influences alcohol consumption among adolescents is alcohol expectations. Several studies have shown that high positive alcohol expectations predict alcohol consumption and alcohol problems among adolescents [121, 122]. In agreement with these data, alcohol use prevention programs may benefit from addressing adolescent perceptions about the positive consequences of alcohol use. In essence, knowing drinking motivations and alcohol expectations may lead to designing more effective preventive strategies.

Governments and other stakeholders can support and empower communities to use their local knowledge and cultural expertise to adopt effective approaches to prevent and reduce harmful use of alcohol [123]. Generally, government support for community action takes the form of training programs and policies for subgroups at particular risk, such as adolescents. There is a great variety of governmental initiatives to prevent alcohol use and abuse during adolescence from school-to parents-based programs. Because early adolescence is a time when alcohol use experimentation often begins to occur, middle high school age student are most often targeted in this prevention programs. As well as school-based program, there are programs to teach parents effective ways to monitor and communicate with their children about the use of alcohol. Mainly, the majority of these programs focus on giving information about the negative health, social and behavioral outcomes of drinking alcohol during adolescence. These approaches considered that people make decisions about alcohol use and abuse based on their knowledge of the adverse consequences involved. However, it has been demonstrated that prevention programs based solely on providing information about the negative consequences of alcohol have little influence on alcohol consumption [124, 125]. Thus, the World Health Organization (WHO) suggested promoting prevention campaigns focused on affective and conative components of attitudes and not just cognitive components. In addition to the educational component, a section to induce changes in attitudes towards excessive alcohol consumption should be included in prevention programs. As is generally acknowledged, adolescent drinking behavior is strongly influenced by peers. For that, workshops where adolescents learn effective strategies of self-control based on the ability to say "no" in social pressure situations are very effective to prevent alcohol consumption. Amongst the generic prevention programs, those based on psychosocial approaches demonstrated significantly greater reductions in alcohol use. Among the effective psychosocial and developmental alcohol misuse prevention programs currently used in schools, we would like to highlight the Like Skills Training Program, the Unplugged Program and the Good Behaviour Game. For example, the Unplugged Program is based on a social influence approach and addresses social and personal skills, knowledge, and normative beliefs about alcohol. Reviews of the literature dealing with school-based programs support the idea that this kind of programs based on a social influence model may prevent juvenile alcohol use through attitude modification, refusal skills and normative perceptions [126].

Community-based alcohol abuse prevention programs include some combination of school, family and public policy. Among public policies aimed at reducing alcohol consumption among adolescents, one of the measures proposed is the prohibition of selling alcohol to individuals under a certain age or the consumption of alcohol under this age. In 2012, most countries (69.27%) determined that the minimum legal drinking age (MLDA) is 18 years. However, some countries have no age limit or a 16-year age limit. Studies evaluating the minimum legal drinking ages showed a statistically significant inverse relationship with alcohol consumption. Thus, it seems that greater MLDA's were associated with slight reductions in the prevalence of alcohol consumption [127]. Another policy to reduce adolescent alcohol consumption is increasing the price of alcohol. Several studies have shown that, as the price of alcohol increases, alcohol consumption and alcohol-related problems decline among the general population [128]. Specific studies to evaluate the real impact of the price of alcohol on adolescent populations is needed. Besides price, other controls on alcohol availability, such as restriction of the hours and days of alcohol purchasing or numbers and types of alcohol outlets, have been shown to affect levels of drinking.

Recent research has demonstrated that presenting a coordinated, comprehensive message across multiple delivery component is most effective in terms of changing behavior. We have mentioned some effective prevention programs in schools, families and communities. By implementing evidence-based strategies, governments can reduce excessive alcohol consumption and the many health and social costs related to it. Moreover, prevention programs for adolescent alcohol use could have a positive impact in preventing other common risks often associated to alcohol drinks, such as violent behavior or unprotected sex. At the same time, adolescent personal and social well-being will be promoted.

5. Conclusion

At 1.8 billion, adolescents and young adults represent more than a quarter of the world's population. Many health-related behaviors usually starting in adolescence (i.e. alcohol use) contribute to disease in adulthood. Several studies have indicated that a considerable amount of adolescents drink alcohol, and this number is continually growing. Nevertheless, the increase in alcohol use and abuse among adolescents has been coupled with increasing social, health and economic consequences. Adolescents who drink alcohol may experience a range of adverse short-and long-term consequences, including physical and mental health problems, violent and aggressive behavior, and adjustment problems in school and at home. Clearly, underage drinking and its consequences present a significant public health problem that must command our attention.

Acknowledgements

The writing of this chapter was supported by CONICYT, Fondecyt Regular, Grant 1140284. We thank Ruy Burgos for reviewing the English version of the manuscripts. Correspondence concerning this chapter should be addressed to Maria Francisca Carvajal, Department of Psychology, Universidad Autonoma de Chile, Carlos Antúnez, 1920, Santiago de Chile (Chile) CP 7500566; e-mail: maria.carvajal@uautonoma.cl

Author details

Francisca Carvajal* and Jose Manuel Lerma-Cabrera

*Address all correspondence to: mcr246@ual.es

Department of Psychology/Universidad Autonoma de Chile, Santiago de Chile, Chile

References

[1]   Koob GF, Le Moal M. Plasticity of reward neurocircuitry and the "dark side" of drug addiction. Nature Neuroscience 2005; 8(11): 1442-1444.

[2]   World Health Organization. Global Status Report on Alcohol and Health. Geneva: WHO; 2014.

[3]   American Psychiatric Association (APA). Diagnostic and Statistical Manual of Mental Disorders, Fifth Edition. Washington DC: APA; 2013.

[4]   World Health Organization (WHO). Inter-national Statistical Classification of Diseases and Related Health Problems. Tenth Revision. Geneva: WHO; 1993.

[5]   Rehm J, Room R, Graham K, Monteiro M, Gmel G, Sempos CT. The relationship of average volume of alcohol consumption and patterns of drinking to burden of disease—an overview. Addiction 2003; 98(9): 1209–1228.

[6]   Roerecke M, Rehm J. Alcohol intake revisited risks and benefits. Current Atherosclerosis Reports 2012; 14(6): 556–562.

[7] Baliunas DO, Taylor BJ, Irving H, Roerecke M, Patra J, Mohapatra S, Rehm J. Alcohol as a risk factor for type 2 diabetes: A systematic review and meta analysis. Diabetes Care 2009; 32(11): 2123–2132.

[8] Rehm J, Taylor B, Mohapatra S, Irving H, Baliunas D, Patra J et al. Alcohol as a risk factor for liver cirrhosis: a systematic review and meta-analysis. Drug and Alcohol Review 2010; 29(4): 437–445.

[9] Parry C, Rehm J, Poznyak V, Room R. Alcohol and infectious diseases: an overlooked causal linkage? Addiction 2009; 104 (3): 331-332.

[10] Rehm J, Mathers C, Popova S, Thavorncharoensap M, Teerawattananon Y, Patra J. Global burden of disease and injury and economic cost attributable to alcohol use and alcohol-use disorders. The Lancet 2009; 373(9684): 2223–2233.

[11] World Health Organization. Global Information System on Alcohol and Health. Geneva: WHO; 2011.

[12] Buchanan CM, Eccles JS, Becker JB. Are adolescents the victims of raging hormones? Evidence for activational effects of hormones on moods and behavior. Psychology Bulletin 1992; 111(1): 62 –107.

[13] Petersen AC, Silbereisen RK, Sörensen S. Adolescent development: A global perspective. In: Hurrelmann K, Hamilton SF. (eds.) Social Problems and Social Contexts in Adolescence. New York: Aldine de Gruyter, 1996. pp. 3–37.

[14] Substance Abuse and Mental Health Services Administration. National Survey on Drug Use and Health: National Findings. Rockville: SAMHSA; 2007.

[15] Johnston LD, O'Malley PM, Bachman JG, Schulenberg JE. Monitoring the future: National results on adolescent drug use. Overview of key findings, 2007. Bethesda: National Institutes of Health; 2008.

[16] Ahlström SK, Österberg EL. International perspectives on adolescent and young adult drinking. Alcohol Research and Health 2004; 28(4): 258–268.

[17] Danielsson AK, Wennberg P, Hibell, Romelsjö A. Alcohol use, heavy episodic drinking and subsequent problems among adolescents in 23 European countries: Does the prevention paradox apply? Addiction 2012; 107(1): 71–80.

[18] Khan MR, Cleland CM, Scheidell JD, Berger T. Gender and racial/ethnic differences in patterns of adolescent alcohol use and associations with adolescent and adult illicit drug use. American Journal of Drug and Alcohol Abuse 2014; 40(3): 213-224.

[19] Cooper ML. Alcohol use and risky sexual behavior among college students and youth: Evaluating the evidence. Journal of Studies on Alcohol and Drugs 2002; 14: 101-117.

[20] Lomba L, Apóstolo J, Mendes, F. Consumo de drogas, alcohol y conductas sexuales en los ambientes recreativos nocturnos de Portugal. Adicciones 2009; 21(4): 309-326.

[21] Hingson R, Heeren T, Winter M, Wechsler H. Magnitude of alcohol related mortality and morbidity among U.S. college students age 18-24: Changes from 1998 to 2001. Annual Review of Public Health 2005; 26: 259– 279.

[22] Siciliano V, Mezzasalma L, Lorenzoni V, Pieroni S, Molinaro S. Evaluation of drinking patterns and their impact on alcohol-related aggression: a national survey of adolescent behaviours. BMC Public Health 2013; 13(1): 950.

[23] Room R, Babor T, Rehm J. Alcohol and public health. The Lancet 2005; 365(9458): 519-530.

[24] Abbey A, Zawacki T, Buck PO, Clinton M, McAuslan P. et al. Alcohol and sexual assault. Alcohol Research and Health 2001; 25(1): 43-51.

[25] Moeller FG, Dougherty DM. Antisocial personality disorder, alcohol and aggression. Alcohol Research and Health 2001, 25(1): 5-11.

[26] White HR, Brick J, Hansell S. A longitudinal investigation of alcohol use and aggression in adolescence. Journal of Studies on Alcohol and Drugs 1993; 11:62-77.

[27] Randall JR, Doku D, Wilson ML, Peltzer K. Suicidal behavior and related risk factor among school aged yout in the Republic of Benin. Plos One. 2014; 9(2): 88233.

[28] Stephenson H, Pena-Shaff J, Quirk P. Predictors of college student suicidal ideation: gender differences. College Student Journal 2006; 40(1):109-117.

[29] Cherpitel CJ, Borges GLG, Wilcox HC. Acute alcohol use and suicidal behavior: A review of the literature. Alcoholism: Clinical and Experimental Research 2004; 28(Suppl 1):18S–28S.

[30] Center for Disease Control and Prevention. Health, United States, 2008, with special feature on the health of young adults. United States: National Center for Health Statistics Health; 2008

[31] Nixon K, McClain JA. Adolescence as a critical window for developing an alcohol use disorder: current findings in neuroscience. Currents Opinion in Psychiatry 2010; 23(3): 227–232.

[32] Casey BJ, Galvan A, Hare TA. Changes in cerebral functional organization during cognitive development. Current Opinion in Neurobiology 2005; 15(2): 239-244.

[33] De Bellis MD, Clark DB, Beers SR, Soloff PH, Boring AM, Hall J et al. Hippocampal volume in adolescent-onset alcohol use disorders. American Journal of Psychiatry 2002; 157(5):737– 744.

[34] Huttenlocher PR. Morphometric study of human cerebral cortex development. Neuropsychologia 1990; 28(6):517–527.

[35] Badanich KA, Adler KJ, Kirstein CL. Adolescents differ from adults in cocaine conditioned place preference and cocaine induced dopamine in the nucleus accumbens septi. European Journal of Pharmacology 2006; 550(1): 95–106.

[36] Andersen SL, Thompson AT, Rutstein M, Hostetter JC, Teicher MH (2000). Dopamine receptor pruning in prefrontal cortex during the periadolescent period in rats. Synapse 2000; 37(2): 167–169

[37] Stanwood GD, McElligot S, Lu L, McGonigle P. Ontogeny of dopamine D3 receptors in the nucleus accumbens of the rat. Neurosciente Letters 1997; 223(1):13-16.

[38] Spear LP. The adolescent brain and age-related behavioral manifestations. Neuroscience and Biobehavioral Reviews 2000; 24(4): 417-463.

[39] Meng SZ, Ozawa Y, Itoh M, Takashima S. Developmental and age-related changes of dopamine transporter, and dopamine D1 and D2 receptors in human basal ganglia. Brain Research 1999; 843(1): 136–144.

[40] Tarazi FI, Tomasini EC, Baldessarini RJ. Postnatal development of dopamine and serotonin transporters in rat caudate-putamen and nucleus accumbens septi. Neuroscience Letters 1998; 254(1): 21–24.

[41] Kalsbeek A, Voorn P, Buijs RM, Pool CW, Uylings HB. Development of the dopaminergic innervation in the prefrontal cortex of the rat. The Journal of Comparative Neurology 1988; 269(1):58 –72.

[42] Rosenberg DR, Lewis DA. Changes in the dopaminergic innervation of monkey prefrontal cortex during late postnatal development: a tyrosine hydroxylase immunohistochemical study. Biological Psychiatry 1994; 36(4): 272–277.

[43] Morilak DA, Ciaranello RD. Ontogeny of 5-hydroxytryptamine2 receptor immunoreactivity in the developing rat brain. Neuroscience 1993; 55(3): 869–880.

[44] Teicher MH, Andersen SL. Limbic serotonin turnover plunges during puberty. Poster presented at the meeting of the Society for Neuroscience, Miami Beach, Forida; 1999.

[45] Monti PM, Miranda R, Nixon K, Sher KJ, Swartzwelder S, Tapert SF, White A, Crews FT. Adolescence: Booze, brains, and behavior. Alcoholism: Clinical and Experimental Research 2005; 29(2): 207-220.

[46] Ernst M, Pine DS, Hardin M. Triadic model of the neurobiology of motivated behavior in adolescence. Psychological Medicine 2006; 36(3):299–312.

[47] Kasanetz F, Manzoni OJ. Maturation of excitatory synaptic transmission of the rat nucleus accumbens from juvenile to adult. Journal of Neurophysiology 2009; 101(5): 2516–2527.

[48] Brooks-Kayal AR, Shumate MD, Jin H, Rikhter TY, Kelly ME, Coulter DA. gamma-Aminobutyric acid (A) receptor subunit expression predicts functional changes in

hippocampal dentate granule cells during postnatal development. Journal of Neurochemistry 2001; 77(5): 1266–1278.

[49] Yu ZY, Wang W, Fritschy JM, Witte OW, Redecker C. Changes in neocortical and hippocampal GABAA receptor subunit distribution during brain maturation and aging. Brain Research 2006; 1099(1): 73–81.

[50] Zahalka E, Seidler FJ, Lappi SE, Yanai J, Slotkin TA. Differential development of cholinergic nerve terminal markers in rat brain regions: implications for nerve terminal density, impulse activity and specific gene expression. Brain Research 1993; 601(1): 221–229.

[51] Bava S, Jacobus J, Thayer RE, Tapert S. Longitudinal changes in white matter integrity among adolescent substance users. Alcoholism: Clinical and Experimental Research 2013; 37(Suppl 1):E181–189.

[52] Coleman LG, Liu W, Oquz I, Styner M, Crews FT. Adolescent binge ethanol treatment alters adult brain region volumes, cortical extracellular matrix protein and behavioral flexibility. Pharmacology, Biochemistry and Behavior 2014; 116: 142-151.

[53] Hohmann CF, Berger-Sweeney J. Cholinergic regulation of cortical development and plasticity: new twists to an old story, Perspectives on Developmental Neurobiology 1998; 5(4): 401–425.

[54] Lauder JM, Schambra UB, Morphogenetic roles of acetylcholine, Environmental Health Perspective 1999; 107 (Suppl.1): 65–69.

[55] De Bellis MD, Narasimhan A, Thatcher DL, Keshavan MS, Soloff P, Clark DB. Prefrontal cortex, thalamus, and cerebellar volumes in adolescents and young adults with adolescent-onset alcohol use disorders and comorbid mental disorders. Alcoholism: Clinical and Experimental Research 2005; 29(9):1590–1600.

[56] Nagel BJ, Schweinsburg AD, Phan V, Tapert SF. Reduced hippocampal volume among adolescents with alcohol use disorders without psychiatric comorbidity. Psychiatry Research: Neuroimaging 2005; 139(3):181–190.

[57] Squeglia LM, Rinker DA, Bartsch H, Castro N, Chung Y, Dale AM, Jernigan TL, Tapert SF. Brain volume reductions in adolescent heavy drinkers. Developmental Cognitive Neuroscience 2014; 9:117-25.

[58] Brown SA, Tapert SF, Granholm E, Delis DC. Neuroconitive functioning of adolescents: effects of protracted alcohol use. Alcoholism, Clinical and Experimental Research 2000; 24(2): 164-171.

[59] Ferrett HL, Carey PD, Thomas KG, Tapert SF, Fein G. Neuropsychological performance of south African treatment-naïve adolescents with alcohol dependence. Drug and Alcohol Dependence 2010; 110(1-2): 8-14.

[60] Tapert SF, Baratta MV, Abrantes AM, Brown SA. Attention dysfunction predicts substance involvement in community youths. Journal of the American Academy of Child & Adolescent Psychiatry 2002; 41(6):680-686

[61] García-Moreno LM, Expósito J, Sanhueza C, Angulo MT. Actividad prefrontal y alcoholismo de fin de semana en jóvenes. Adicciones 2008; 20(3): 271-280.

[62] Scaife JC, Duka T. Behavioural measures of frontal lobe function in a population of young social drinkers with binge drinking pattern. Pharmacology, Biochemistry, and Behavior 2009; 93(3): 354-362.

[63] Sanhueza C, García-Moreno LM, Expósito J. Weekend alcoholism in youth and neurocognitive aging. Psicothema 2011; 23(2): 209-214.

[64] Przybycien-Szymanska MM, Mott NN, Paul CR, Gillespie RA, Pak TR. Binge-pattern alcohol exposure during puberty induces long-term changes in HPA axis reactivity. PLoS One 2011; 6(4):e18350.

[65] Gilpin NW, Roberto M. Neuropeptide modulation of central amygdala neuroplasticity is a key mediator of alcohol dependence. Neuroscience & Biobehavioral Reviews 2012; 36(2):873–888.

[66] Lerma-Cabrera JM, Carvajal F, Alcaraz-Iborra M, de la Fuente L, Navarro M, Thiele TE, Cubero I. Adolescent binge-like ethanol exposure reduces basal α-MSH expression in the hypothalamus and the amygdala of adult rats. Pharmacology, Biochemistry and Behavior 2013; 110: 66-74.

[67] Meyers JL, Dick DM. Genetic and environmental risk factors for adolescent-onset substance use disorders. Child and Adolescent Psychiatric Clinics of North America 2010; 19(3): 465-477.

[68] Spear LP. Alcohol's effects on adolescents. Alcohol Reseach and Health 2002; 26(4): 287-291.

[69] Pascual M, Boix J, Felipo V, Guerri C. Repeated alcohol administration during adolescence causes changes in the mesolimbic dopaminergic and glutamatergic systems and promotes alcohol intake in the adult rat. Journal of Neurochemistry 2009; 108(4): 920-931.

[70] Doremus-Fitzwater TL, Varlinskaya EI, Spear LP. Motivational systems in adolescence: Possible implications for age differences in substance abuse and other risk-taking behaviors. Brain and Cognition 2010; 72(1):114–123.

[71] Silveri MM, Spear LP. Decreased sensitivity to the hypnotic effects of ethanol early in ontogeny. Alcoholism: Clinical and Experimental Research 1998; 22(3):670– 676.

[72] Silveri MM, Spear LP. Ontogeny of ethanol elimination and ethanol-induced hypothermia. Alcohol 2000; 20(1): 45-53.

[73] Ristuccia RC, Spear LP. Autonomic responses to ethanol in adolescent and adult rats: a dose-response analysis. Alcohol 2008; 42(8): 623–629.

[74] Silveri MM, Spear LP. Acute, rapid, and chronic tolerance during ontogeny: observations when equating ethanol perturbation across age. Alcoholism. Clinical and Experimental Research 2001; 25(9): 1301-1308.

[75] White AM, Bae JG, Truesdale MC, Ahmad S, Wilson WA, Swartzwelder HS. Chronic-intermittent ethanol exposure during adolescence prevents normal developmental changes in sensitivity to ethanol-induced motor impairments. Alcoholism: Clinical and Experimental Research 2002; 26(7): 960-968.

[76] Varlinskaya EI, Spear LP. Differences in the social consequences of ethanol emerge during the course of adolescence in rats: social facilitation, social inhibition, and anxiolysis. Developmental Psychobiology 2006; 48(2): 146-161.

[77] Zimmermann P, Wittchen HU, Höfler M, Pfister H, Kessler RC, Lieb R. Primary anxiety disorders and the development of subsequent alcohol use disorders: a 4-year community study of adolescents and young adults. Psychological Medicine 2003; 33(07): 1211–1222.

[78] Pohorecky LA. Interaction of ethanol and stress: research with experimental animals —an update. Alcohol and alcoholism 1990; 25(2-3):263-276.

[79] Doremus TL, Brunell SC, Varlinskaya EI, Spear LP. Anxiogenic effects during withdrawal from acute ethanol in adolescent and adult rats. Pharmacology, Biochemistry and Behavior 2003; 75(2): 411-418.

[80] Slawecki CJ, Roth J. Comparison of the onset of hypoactivity and anxiety-like behavior during alcohol withdrawal in adolescent and adult rats. Alcoholism: Clinical and Experimental Research 2004; 28(4): 598-607.

[81] Varlinskaya EI, Spear LP. Changes in sensititivy to ethanol-induced social facilitation and social inhibition from early to late adolescence. Annals of the New York Academy of Science 2004; 1021:459-461.

[82] Martin CS, Winters KC. Diagnosis and assessment of alcohol use disorders among adolescents. Alcohol Health and Research World 1998; 22(2): 95–105.

[83] Clark DB, Winters KC. Measuring risks and outcomes in substance use disorders prevention research. Journal of Consulting and Clinical Psychology 2002; 70(6): 1207–1223.

[84] Lovinger DM, Crabbe JC. Laboratory models of alcoholism: treatment target identification and insight into mechanisms. Nature Neuroscience 2005; 8(11): 1471-1480.

[85] Dawson DA, Goldstein RB, Chou SP, Ruan WJ, Grant BF. Age at first drink and the first incidence of adult-onset DSM-IV alcohol use disorders. Alcoholism: Clinical and Experimental Research 2008; 32(12):2149-2160.

[86] Hingson RW, Zha W. Age of drinking onset, alcohol use disorders, frequent heavy drinking, and unintentionally injuring oneself and others after drinking. Pediatrics 2009; 123(6): 1477-1484.

[87] DeWit D, Adlaf EM, Offord DR, Ogborne AC. Age at first alcohol use: risk factors for the development of alcohol disorders. American Journal of Psychiatry 2000; 157(5): 745–750.

[88] McCambridge J, McAlaney J, Rowe R. Adult consequences of late adolescent alcohol consumption: a systematic review of cohort studies. PLoS Medicine 2011; 8(2): e1000413.

[89] Kirby T, Barry AE. Alcohol as a gateway drug: a study of US 12th graders. Journal of School Health 2012; 82(8): 371-379.

[90] LaBrie JW, Kenney SR, Lac A, Migliuri S. Differential drinking patterns of family history positive and family history negative first semester college females. Addictive Behaviors 2009; 34(2):190–196.

[91] Labrie JW, Migliuri S, Kenney SR, Lac A. Family history of alcohol abuse associated with problematic drinking among college students. Addictive Behaviors 2010; 35(7): 721–725.

[92] Leeman RF, Fenton M, Volpicelli JR. Impaired control and undergraduate problem drinking. Alcohol and Alcoholism 2007; 42(1): 42–48.

[93] Barnes GM, Reifman AS, Farrell MP, Dintcheff BA. The effects of parenting on the development of adolescent alcohol misuse: a six-wave latent growth model. Journal of Marriage and the Family 2000; 62(1): 175–186.

[94] Zhang L, Welte JW, Wieczorek WF. The influence of parental drinking and closeness on adolescent drinking. Journal of Studies on Alcohol and Drugs 1999; 60(2): 245–251.

[95] Grant BF, Dawson DA. Age at onset of alcohol use and its association with DSM-IV alcohol abuse and dependence: Results from the National Longitudinal Alcohol Epidemiologic Survey. Journal of Substance Abuse 1997; 9:103–110.

[96] Bennett ME, McCrady BS, Johnson V, Pandina RJ. Problem drinking from young adulthood to adulthood: patterns, predictors and outcomes. Journal of studies on alcohol 1999; 60(5): 605-614.

[97] Enoch MA. The role of early life stress as a predictor for alcohol and drug dependence. Psychopharmacology (Berlin) 2011; 214(1):17-31.

[98] Bremner P, Burnett J, Nunney F, Ravat M, Mistral W. Young People, Alcohol and Influences. New York: Joseph Rowntree Foundation; 2011.

[99] Knop J, Penick EC, Nickel EJ, Mortensen EL, Sullivan M, Murtaza S, Jensen P, Manzardo AM, Gabrielli WF. Childhood ADHD and conduct disorder as independent

predictors of male alcohol dependence at age 40. Journal of studies on alcohol and drugs 2009; 70(2): 169-177.

[100] Lopez B, Schwartz SJ, Prado G, Huang S, Rothe EM, Wang W, Pantin H. Correlates of early alcohol and drug use in Hispanic adolescents: examining the role of ADHD with comorbid conduct disorder, family, school, and peers. Journal of Clinical Child and Adolesc Psychology 2008; 37(4): 820–832.

[101] Tucker JS, Orlando M, Ellickson PL. Patterns and correlates of binge drinking trajectories from early adolescence to young adulthood. Health Psychology 2003; 22(1): 79–87.

[102] Bates ME, Labouvie EW. Adolescent risk factors and the prediction of persistent alcohol and drug use into adulthood. Alcoholism: Clinical and Experimental Research 1997; 21(5): 944–950.

[103] Grabe HJ, Mahler J, Witt SH, Schulz A, Appel K, Spitzer C, Stender J, Barnow S, Freyberger HJ, Teumer A, Volzke H, Rietschel M. A risk marker for alcohol dependence on chromosome 2q35 is related to neuroticism in the general population. Molecular Psychiatry 2011; 16(2): 126–128.

[104] Moore GF, Rothwell H, Segrott J. An exploratory study of the relationship between parental attitudes and behaviour and young people's consumption of alcohol. Substance Abuse Treatment, Prevention and Policy 2010; 5: 6.

[105] Velleman R, Templeton L. Substance misuse by children and young people: the role of the family and implications for intervention and prevention. Current Paediatrics 2007; 17(1): 25-30.

[106] Calafat A, García F, Juan M, Becoña E, Fernandez-Hermida JR. Which parenting style is more protective against adolescent substance use? Evidence within the European context. Drug and Alcohol Dependence 2014; 138: 185-192.

[107] Bahr SJ, Hoffmann JP. Parenting style, religiosity, peers, and adolescent heavy drinking. Journal of Studies on Alcohol and Drugs 2010; 71(4): 539–543.

[108] Kristjansson AL, James JE, Allegrante JP, Sigfusdottir ID, Helgason AR. Adolescent substance use, parental monitoring, and leisure-time activities: 12-year outcomes of primary prevention in Iceland. Preventive Medicine 2010; 51(2): 168–171.

[109] Goldman D, Oroszi G, Ducci F. The genetics of addictions: uncovering the genes. Nature Reviews Genetics 2005; 6(7): 521–532.

[110] Prescott C, Hewitt JK, Truett KR, Heath AC, Neale MC, Eaves LJ. Genetic and environmental influences on lifetime alcohol-related problems in a volunteer sample of older twins. Journal of Studies on Alcohol and Drugs 1994; 55(2): 184–202.

[111] van der Zwaluw CS, Engels RC, Vermulst AA, Rose RJ, Verkes RJ, Buitelaar J, Franke B, Scholte RH. A serotonin transporter polymorphism (5-HTTLPR) predicts the de-

velopment of adolescent alcohol use. Drug and Alcohol Dependence 2010; 112(1): 134–139

[112] Dick DM, Pagan JL, Viken R, Purcell S, Kaprio J, Pulkinnen L et al. Changing environmental influences on substance use across development. Twin Research and Human Genetics 2007; 10(02): 315–326.

[113] Miranda R, Ray L, Justus A, Meyerson L, Knopik V, McGeary J et al. Initial evidence of an association between OPRM1 and adolescent alcohol misuse. Alcoholism: Clinical and Experimental Research 2010; 34(1):112–122.

[114] Dick DM, Aliev F, Latendresse S, Porjesz B, Schuckit M, Rangaswamy M et al. How phenotype and developmental stage affect the genes we find: GABRA2 and impulsivity. Twin Research and Human Genetics 2013; 16(03): 661–669.

[115] Dick DM, Edenberg HJ, Xuei X, Goate A, Kuperman S, Schuckit M et al. Association of GABRG3 with alcohol dependence. Alcoholism: Clinical and Experimental Research 2004; 28(1): 4–9.

[116] Rose RJ, Dick DM, Viken RJ, Pulkkinen L, Kaprio J. Drinking or abstaining at age 14? A genetic epidemiological study. Alcoholism: Clinical and Experimental Research 2001b; 25(11):1594-1604.

[117] Gore FM, Bloem PJN, Patton GC, Ferguson J, Joseph V, Coffey C et al. Global burden of disease in young people aged 10–24 years: a systematic analysis. The Lancet 2011; 377(9783): 2093-2102.

[118] Pitkänen T, Lyyra AL, Pulkkinen, L. Age of onset of drinking and the use of alcohol in adulthood: a follow-up study from age 8-42 for females and males. Addiction 2005; 100(5): 652-661.

[119] Kuntsche E, Knibbe R, Engels R. Why do young people drink? A review of drinking motives. Clinical psychology reviews 2005; 25(7): 841-861.

[120] Kuntsche E, Knibbe R, Engels R, Gmel G. Drinking motives as mediators of the link between alcohol expectancies and alcohol use among adolescents. Journal of Studies on Alcohol and Drugs 2007; 68(1): 76-85.

[121] Randolph KA, Gerend MA, Miller BA. Measuring alcohol expectancies in youth. Journal of Youth and Adolescence 2006; 35(6): 939-948.

[122] Zamboaga BL. Alcohol expectancies and drinking behaviors in Mexican American college students. Addictive Behaviors 2005; 30(4): 673-684.

[123] Ramstedt M, Leifman H, Müller D, Sundin E, Norström T. Reducing youth violence related to student parties: Findings from a community intervention project in Stockholm. Drug and Alcohol Review 2013; 32(6): 561–565.

[124] Canning U, Millward L, Raj T. Drug use prevention: A review of reviews. Londres: Health Development Agency; 2003.

[125] Tobler NS, Roona MR, Ochshorn P, Marshall DG, Streke AV, Stackpole KM. School-based adolescent drug prevention programs: 1998 meta-analysis Journal of Primary Prevention 2000; 20(4): 275-336.

[126] Giannotta F, Vigna-Taglianti F, Rosaria Galanti M, Scatigna M, Faggiano F. Short-term mediating factors of a school-based intervention to prevent youth substance use in Europe. Journal of Adolescent Health 2014; 54(5): 565-573.

[127] Wagenaar AC, Toomey TL. Effects of minimum drinking age laws: review and analyses of the literature from 1960 to 2000. Journal of Studies on Alcohol and drugs 2002; (Suppl. 14): 206-225.

[128] Elder RW, Lawrence B, Ferguson A, Naimi TS, Brewer RD, Chattopadhyay SK, Toomey TL, Fielding JE. Task Force on Community Preventive Services. The effectiveness of tax policy interventions for reducing excessive alcohol consumption and related harms American Journal of Preventive Medicine 2010; 38(2): 217–229.

Chapter 4

Variables that May Affect the Transmission of Dengue – A Case Study for Health Management in Asia

Muhiuddin Haider and Jamie Turner

Additional information is available at the end of the chapter

http://dx.doi.org/10.5772/59983

1. Introduction

Dengue, an emergent viral infection, has increased exponentially since the 1960s [1]. In spite of the alarming escalation of cases reported, the WHO still believes the disease is significantly underreported [2]. The effects of climate change are expected to dramatically increase the global incidence and geographic locations of dengue. According to the WHO, the number of countries reporting dengue cases has increased from nine countries before 1960 to more than 64 countries in 2007 [2]. Dengue cases continue to climb despite numerous interventions globally to halt the progression. Climate change allows the primary dengue vectors to thrive in more geographical locations; increased population, urbanization and deforestation have also provided favorable conditions for vectors. In areas with poor or nonexistent infrastructure, sanitation, and unreliable water supplies, water storage systems provide ideal breeding grounds for mosquitos. These issues are compounded by intercontinental commerce, specifically the transport of tires, which harbor rainwater and mosquito larvae, allowing introduction of non-native mosquitos to other countries.

No cure currently exists for dengue and vaccine development has been fraught with difficulties. Dengue should be categorized as one of the most imperative global health issues in need of effective solutions. Drastic changes need to occur in public health approaches and health management policies for dengue. Without serious and immediate attention to the escalation of dengue the global burden of disease will significantly intensify.

2. Background

Dengue is believed to be an ancient disease, one with unclear origins. Early Chinese medical records first describe a dengue-like outbreak as early as 400 AD, and later historical docu-

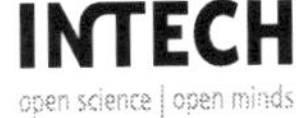

mentation in Asia, Africa, and North America made record of a dengue-like epidemic in the seventeenth century. Dengue has often been referred to as "break bone fever"; it was given this name due to the onset of high fever accompanied by agonizing bone and joint pain. The word "Dengue" was first recorded in the nineteenth century derived from the Spanish word meaning "fastidious" possibly to describe the way infected individuals carefully walked while experiencing horrendous bone pain [3].

Dengue is an infection passed from person to person by vector transmission. The predominant vectors for dengue are *Aedes aegypti* and *Aedes albopictus*. The vectors become infected after the female mosquito takes a blood meal from an infected human. Once the mosquito has been infected the virus incubates inside the mosquito host for approximately 8-10 days [4]. Upon completion of the incubation period the infected mosquito is capable of transmitting dengue to any human that it feeds on, for the remainder of its life. Four primary serotypes of dengue exist, DEN-1, DEN-2, DEN-3, DEN-4. Recently the Center for Infectious Disease and Research Policy reported a fifth serotype [5].

The most severe manifestations of the disease are dengue shock syndrome, and dengue hemorrhagic fever. Infection with one serotype does not impart complete or lasting immunity to other serotypes of dengue. Following recuperation from dengue infection, of a specific serotype, an individual has immunity from that serotype however immunity to other serotypes transitory and incomplete leaving individuals at a significantly increased risk of infection with a more severe serotype of dengue [2]. Unlike other vector-transmitted diseases, concurrent dengue infections increase an individual's susceptibility to a more life threatening serotype of dengue. Some cases of dengue are asymptomatic, however the classic symptoms include malaise, severe muscle and joint pain all accompanied with a high fever. The only treatment option currently administered for dengue infection is fluid replacement and rest. More severe cases of dengue cause capillaries in the body to leak blood plasma. This can progress to internal hemorrhaging, organ failure, and death [2].

According to estimates from the Centers for Disease Control and Prevention (CDC) three billion people globally are at risk of contracting dengue [4]. Although accurate assessments of dengue are difficult to ascertain, one undeniable observation is that Asia bears an unequal burden of dengue cases, with an approximate seventy percent of cases arising in Asian countries [6]. Findings from a recent study reveal that dengue is universal throughout tropical regions. Researchers estimate that there are 390 million dengue infections annually, all around the globe [6]. This is more than triple the WHO's most recent estimates of 100 million infections each year [2]. Another 16 million infections are attributed to Africa's burden of disease, which rivals that of the Americas and is significantly larger than previously predicted [6]. It is assumed that these numbers still underestimate the true incidence of dengue. Several factors likely add to the underreporting of dengue. Many tropical regions have various other diseases with symptomatically similar illnesses, which people may not seek treatment for or, if treatment is sought, misdiagnosis can occur. There are also potential economic impacts of reporting dengue for both individuals and countries as a whole.

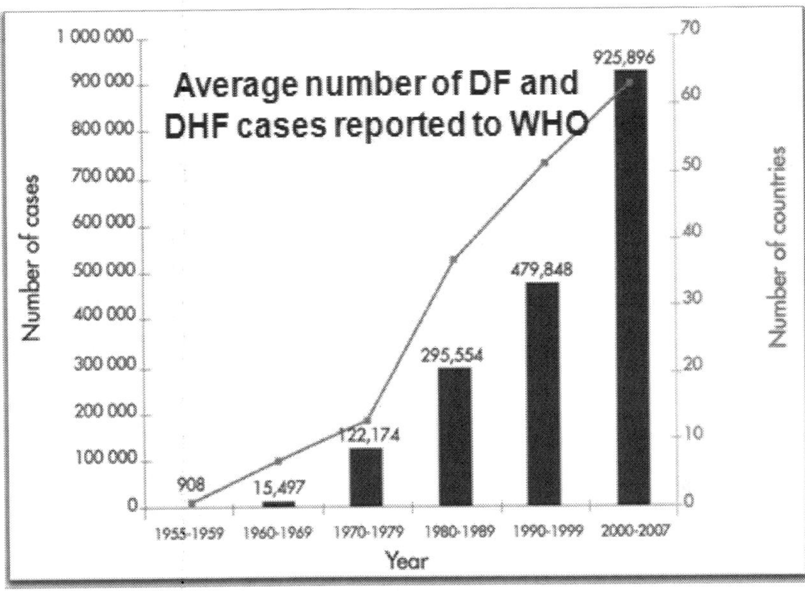

http://www.who.int/entity/csr/disease/dengue/dengue2008.jpg

Figure 1. World Health Organization

Climate and population growth are important factors for predicting the current risk of dengue around the world. With population explosion, globalization, and constant urbanization, dramatic shifts in the distribution of the disease are anticipated. The virus may be introduced to areas that previously were not at risk, and those, that are currently affected, may experience enormous increases in the number of cases. Endemic transmission in Africa and the Americas, recent outbreaks in Portugal, and the ever-increasing incidence in Asia are proof of the challenges that plague an effective dengue control and the issues surrounding vector control [6]. This is a pivotal moment in the fields of global health and health management systems. Efforts to combat dengue appear stuck. However, recent vaccine developments appear to be more effective at delivering a more feasible vaccine Strategies for tackling dengue need to be rethought in order to maximize the value and cost-effectiveness of health management systems, by indicating where resources can be targeted to achieve maximum and sustainable impact.

Humans have known for a long time that climatic conditions affect epidemic diseases. Today there is a worldwide increase in many infectious diseases and this reflects the combined impacts of rapid demographic changes, as well as social and environmental changes in human living conditions. Important determinants of vector-transmitted disease include: vector survival, reproduction, and the vector's biting habits. Vectors can survive and reproduce within a range of optimal climatic conditions, which include factors such as temperature, rainfall, proximity to large bodies of water, amount of daylight and elevation. There is a large body of evidence demonstrating associations between climatic conditions and infectious diseases. Dengue is of great public health concern and may be very sensitive to long term climate change. Dengue varies seasonally in highly endemic areas. Excessive rainfall and high humidity are major contributing factors to enhancing mosquito breeding sites and thus overall mosquito populations. Mathematical modeling methods have been used to demonstrate the relationship between climatic variables and biological parameters such as breeding, survival, and biting rates. Landscape modeling is also used because climate also influences habitats. Combining climate bases models with spatial analytical methods to study the effects of both climatic and environmental factors are beginning to be used to predict how climate induce changes would affect mosquito populations.

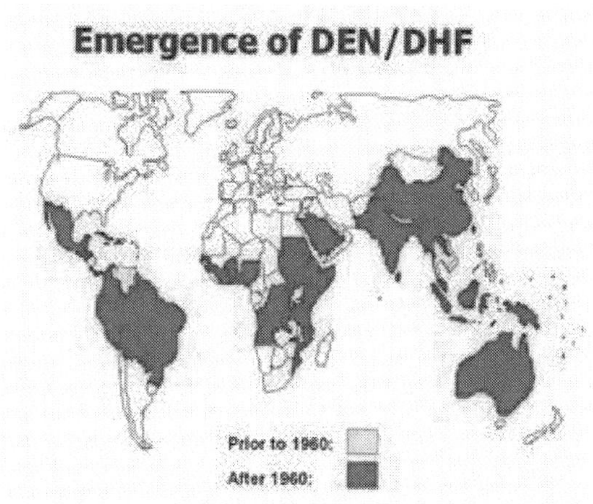

http://www.who.int/entity/csr/disease/dengue/dehngueemergence.jpg

Figure 2. World Health Organization

3. Burden of Disease

The burden of disease due to dengue started in Asia after the commencement of World War II [7]. Major factors contributing to the post war dengue proliferation include: worldwide rapid population expansion, urbanization, and globalization of markets. These factors coupled with new modes of human transportation could have facilitated the dissemination of both people and disease [7].

In order to initiate successful health management policies and programs it is important to understand the economic impact of dengue on Southeast Asia. Several articles have been published about this topic as well as assessments from the WHO. The overwhelming consensus

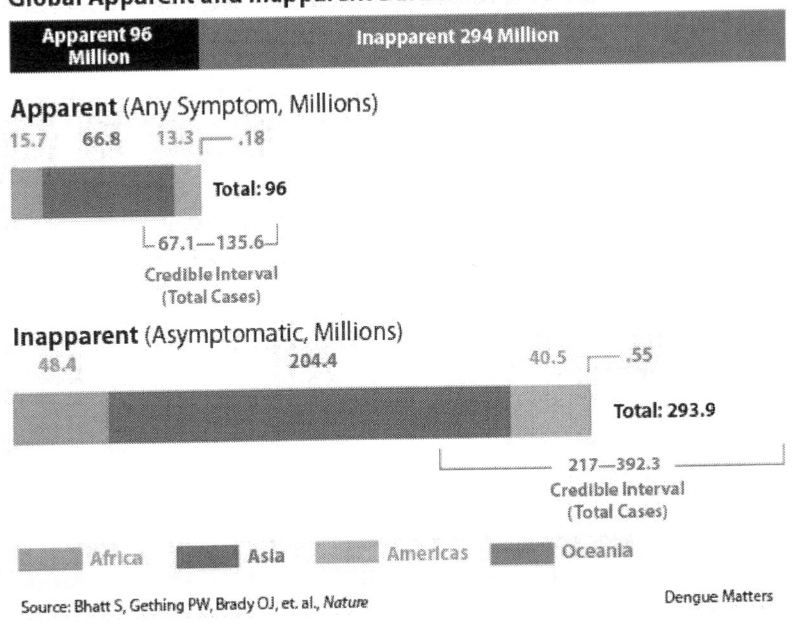

http://www.denguematters.info/content/issue-14-dengue-updates-december-2013

Figure 3. Dengue matters

reports that dengue is one of the most critical infectious diseases in tropical and subtropical regions. Dengue represents a monumental burden in Southeast Asia where it is endemic. Studies conducted from 2001 – 2005 have reported dengue specific cases in Cambodia to be three million dollars annually, Malaysia at forty-two million dollars annually, and Thailand fifty-three million dollars annually [8]. Another study estimated annual costs for Cambodia to be eight million dollars [9]. In 2009 the officially reported dengue cases were estimated to cost Malaysia one hundred million dollars [10]. The estimates of SEA burden of disease due to dengue are available only for a fraction of countries in the region. Estimates vary depending on methodology of studies and variance in officially reported cases. Although dengue is a reportable disease there is a considerable amount of underreporting [11, 12]. The total number of dengue related cases is difficult to ascertain due to inconsistency in surveillance methods and unreliability of surveillance reporting. Unreliability is due to a variety of factors including method and certainty of diagnosis as well as when and where the data were collected. To better illustrate the current estimates for the burden of disease the following graphs from Dengue Matters are provided: figure 3 and figure 4.

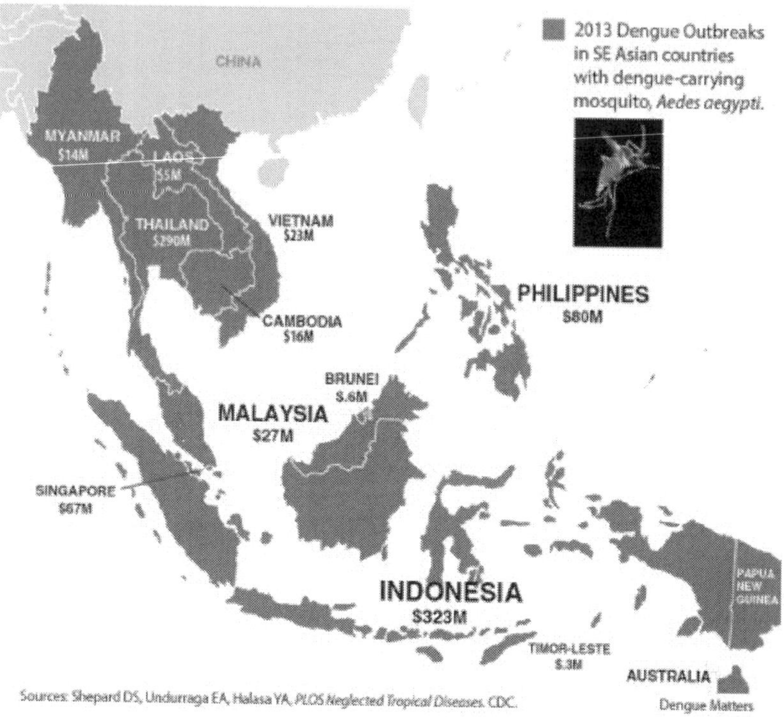

http://denguematters.info/content/issue-15-spotlight-dengue-southeast-asia

Figure 4. 'Dengue Matters'

The rapid urbanization and development of Asian cities has a drastic effect on the transmission of infectious disease. Currently, millions of people inhabit several cities in Asia. This coupled with a lack of wastewater infrastructure, insufficient housing, and unhygienic societal conditions promote the propagation of dengue infection. These factors are some of the major contributors to the proliferation of dengue in Asia [87].

Various global issues impact the delicate balance between environment and development. This balance has serious ramifications for controlling vector-transmitted diseases. The most profound impact on the encroachment of the environment is the explosion in human population. According to the United States Census Bureau, the world population is currently seven billion individuals. A human population that continues to grow will have a number of impacts on the surrounding environment and mosquito ecology including depletion of natural resources, opportunistic breeding sites, decreased biodiversity.

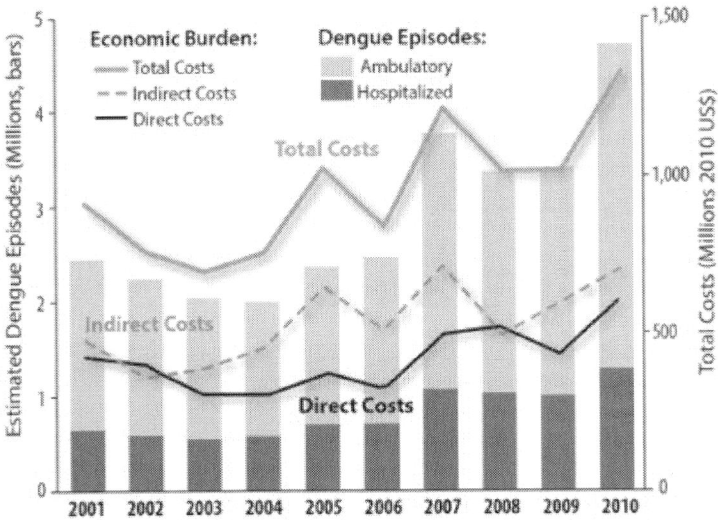

http://denguematters.info/content/issue-15-spotlight-dengue-southeast-asia

Figure 5. 'Dengue Matters'

The perpetual demand for commercial goods, food, and energy compels nations to develop vast quantities of land and water resources for agricultural and energy harvesting purposes. In the process of land development, deforestation and soil degradation decimate the natural habitats of mosquito populations. These processes are then compounded by man-made water reservoirs and irrigation systems designed to facilitate land development. Such large stagnant bodies of water may be providing generous breeding grounds for vector populations. Mitigation of such ecological impacts may be addressed by allowing cooperative consultation during construction planning phases. Construction plans can be coupled with adequate health risk assessment plans to facilitate improved environmental safeguards to prevent future vector ecological problems and health concerns. Areas developed for their natural resources undergo significant alterations in human population living conditions and density, which correlate to the incidence of infectious diseases [13]. Land development tends to create population migration due to potential economic opportunities and the need for seasonal labor. Settlement of individuals in a new area without competent infrastructure of water systems can introduce new unexposed individuals into a high-risk situation that has the potential to spread vector-transmitted illnesses rapidly. Living conditions may also degrade the overall health of the population and promote the spread of viral variations [13].

Expeditious urbanization entices rural individuals to relocate to urban environments based on potential economic opportunities. As this occurs urban settings tend to be ill prepared for the increased demand of basic water services. Sewage, sanitation and drinking water supplies rarely match the populations' needs and consequently result in increased incidence of infectious diseases. Historical patterns of rapid urbanization coupled with observable correlations of increased infectious disease, specifically vector-transmitted diseases, highlight the dramatic need for resources in urban settings.

Vector transmitted diseases such as dengue increase as biodiversity decreases. When natural habitats are destroyed by land development projects, habitats become simplified. The breakdown of habitats facilitates the growth of mosquito populations over their natural predators. Exacerbating the situation is the excessive use of pesticides, which can select for mutations, and lead to insecticide resistant mosquitos. Of particular concern are the agricultural applications of indiscriminate pesticide application that can release chemical residue into the environment affecting a wide variety of other insects. Natural predators of mosquitos, like dragonflies, tend be unintended victims of pesticide overuse and in turn lead to the acceleration of insecticide resistance.

The effects of climate change on global disease patterns and geographical expansion are still speculative. By reflecting on the observable patterns in the last few decades, some trends become apparent. A few of the global climate change issues have the potential for impacting vector ecology and thus vector transmitted diseases. Increased temperatures may expand the geographical endemic areas for infectious diseases. Warmer temperatures may also allow vector migration to occur at higher altitudes. Shifts in global wind patterns may impact the passive migration of vectors. Increased rainfall introduces stagnant water issues to new areas and plays an important role in the life cycle of a mosquito. Most dengue transmitting vectors breed in small pools of water. The existence of potential vector breeding grounds depends not only upon rainfall but also on evaporation. The patterns, frequency, and amounts of rainfall globally are expected to change and will impact temperature, evaporation and humidity thereby making clear predictions regarding vector migrations complex. Increased temperatures are anticipated to increase sea levels, natural disasters, and rainfall all of which could lead to greater vector breading site opportunities Climate change is predicted to increase the quantity and intensity of natural disasters. Natural disaster areas are ideal sites for the dissemination of infectious disease and give ample opportunities for vectors to propagate.

Various time series studies explore the relationship between average temperatures in conjunction with rainfall rates. It has been hypothesized that increasing temperatures could be part of the reason why dengue can now survive in a greater range of areas. Many other confounding factors, however, could be causing the increase in dengue in these areas. Further investigations into whether climate change could drive the geographical spread of the disease and produce an increase in incidence would be beneficial. Other studies consider the impact temperature and deforestation have on vector transmitted diseases. Assessing the biological significance of the warming trend on mosquito populations some scientists suggest that the observed temperature changes will be significantly amplify the mosquito population. The effects of climate change on the health of human societies are already evident however these effects are expected to increase. Direct assessment of climate related effects are difficult to definitively ascertain due to the complexity of interrelated variables. Challenges arise when attempting to distinguish which variables most directly affect climate change but a few influences are clear. Human population explosion, the use and development of land, and naturally occurring variability are some of the most influential factors in climate change. Current data can be used to influence future policy and public information. Many agree that climate change exacerbates weather related issues, droughts from a dearth of rainfall or once manageable seasonable rainfall causing widespread flooding conditions [88]. Affects suffered as a result of climate change would include weather-related disasters. Condition can be temporary or permanent, ranging from short-term displacement from a natural disaster to living with severe water scarcity. Currently the best estimates of the level of impact of climate on health trends are just predictions based on possibilities. Gradual environmental degradation due to climate change also affects long-term water quality and quantity in various parts of the world. Water related issues could trigger increases in vector-transmitted diseases such as dengue. Environmental degradation is a contributing factor to poverty, and can expel people from their homes. Individuals affected by water scarcity, poverty, disease, or displacement also tends to have worse health outcomes. Climate change can be expected to disproportionally affect developing countries. Effects brought on by climate change could further reduce health outcomes and increase food and water insecurity leading to more displacement and greater proportions of populations subjected to poverty and disease. Increases in poverty would result in competition for scarce resources and greater burdens on economically limited governments. Deteriorating conditions could ultimately lead to increases in conflicts. Therefore, health outcomes are employed as a foundation for climate change associated influences [88]. Employing this tactic, WHO assesses the global burden of disease related to climate change factors to have longitudinal effects on millions of individuals currently [1]. Climate change is anticipated to significantly increase food and water quality and insecurity [1]. Climate change is expected to produce an increase in chronic diseases, respiratory diseases, and vector-transmitted diseases, all of which could overburden the current public health system. A warmer and more variable climate leads to increased levels of air pollutants and increased transmission of diseases through unclean water. It compromises agricultural production and it increases the hazards of weather-related disasters. Climate change together with the changes vector habitats as well as water supplies can increase the incidence of many diseases particularly dengue.

Dengue incidence, particularly dengue epidemics, has been currently associated with rainy season. Despite the number of studies, convincing data or models supporting this hypothesis is limited in small countries [14]. A study in Thailand found that climatic factors play a role in transmission cycle of DHF, but relative importance of these factors varied with geographical areas [15]. Ecological studies related to *Aedes aegypti* have shown that *Aedes aegypti* is a humidity loving species and is governed by the conditions to which it has adapted. It avails all available opportunities in the peridomestic domain during this rainy season when temperature falls down and humidity increases. The association between flooding caused by precipitation and an increase in vector breeding sites is multifaceted. It is generally believed that increased rainfall will increase the number of breeding sites particularly for mosquitos

[16]. Flooding is typically followed by an immediate dip in vector populations, due to excess water clearing out existing breeding sites, however as waters recede mosquito populations tend to bounce back in areas where the water pools [17]. The relationship between dengue and increased precipitation is not always proportional because transmission of dengue requires the disease be prevalent in the population for vectors to be able to transmit the disease [16]. Although increased precipitation can cause more areas of pooled water, which can increase mosquito population density or increase exposure to mosquito populations through housing damage. Increased rainfall or flooding situations do not always affect the incidence of dengue infections in populations [18]. It is postulated that with an increase of mosquitos the incidence of potential dengue transmission is increased [18]. Typically after a natural disaster occurs an increase in infectious disease follows, this can occur for several reasons: lack of access to clean water, crowding living conditions, disruptions in vector elimination programs, and increase in time spent outdoors which increases the exposure to vectors [18]. Addressing some of the known risk factors and bolstering public health infrastructure can mitigate potentially preventable vector transmitted disease. Particular attention should be paid to post natural disaster situations. When individuals travel to avoid the effects of natural disasters it can lead to congregations in areas without proper water supply or sewage infrastructure both of which can rapidly increase the incidence of infectious disease [19]. Another consideration of a shift in human settlements is the potential upsurge in stress and mental illness, and human struggle, which can aggravate infectious diseases like dengue [20].

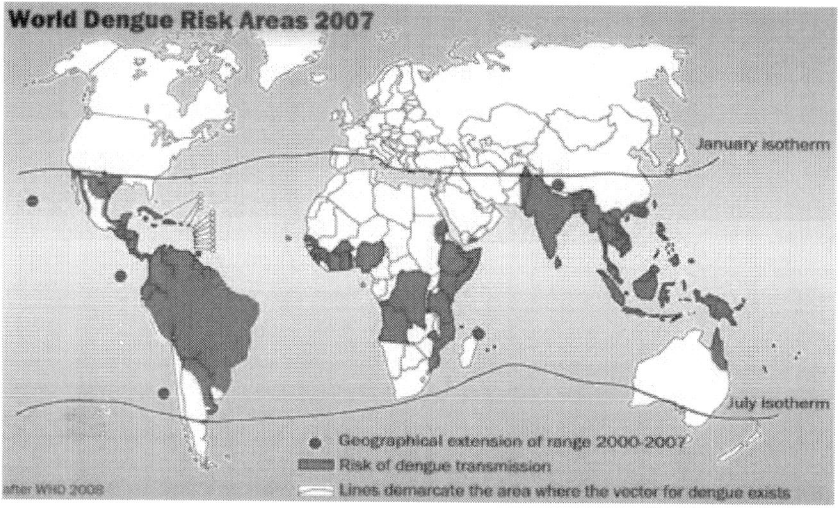

http://www.who.int/entity/csr/disease/dengue/dengue2006.jpg

Figure 6. World Health Organization

Although dengue is currently a global concern, approximately seventy-five percent of individuals living in Asia have been exposed to dengue [21, 22]. More than one billion high-risk individuals, like children, live in a dengue endemic country in Southeast. In SEA the leading cause of child hospitalizations and child mortality are attributed to dengue [22, 23]. The WHO has a clear documentation of the development of dengue in the last few decades. Eight SEA countries reported dengue related illnesses in 2003; within six years all SEA countries reported endemic dengue [21, 22]. The number of dengue cases in SEA continues to climb in quantity and severity. Currently eight SEA countries are categorized as hyper-endemic, meaning all four stains of dengue exist simultaneously [22].

Dengue infections in children aged 5 years or younger, mostly in developing countries could see a sharp increase in incidence. Other severely affected population groups could include women, the elderly and people living in small islands, and other coastal regions. These groups are the most affected due to social factors such as immune susceptibility and geographic areas of high risk. Immune susceptibility affects the very young and the very old while geographical high-risk areas are those prone to natural disasters and areas lacking water and sewage infrastructure. Southeast Asia disproportionally experiences a great burden of disease due to these factors [88]. Overall, the per capita mortality rate from vector borne diseases is exponentially greater in developing nations than in developed regions.

There is increasing incidence of dengue incidence in older age groups, and this age shift has been reported in Singapore, Indonesia, Bangladesh and Thailand [24, 25]. Thailand, cases of dengue in small infants as young as 1-2 months and in adults have been reported with increasing frequency [26]. During the first known outbreak in Nepal the majority of the cases occurred between the age of 16 and 45 years [27]. The first recorded outbreak in Bangladesh affected the age group of 18-33 years were the most affected [28]. Sri Lanka with chronological overview shows that modal age group affected by dengue has shifted from less than 15 years of age to 15-34 years of age. It has been hypothesized that the time interval between two sequential infections could be the reason to explain this phenomenon [29, 30]. There are many studies from South-East Asia region that suggest higher ratio of males than females in dengue hospitalized and only few studies suggest no difference in sexes [24, 26, 28]. However, almost all of these studies were hospital-based suggesting they represent those who had access healthcare rather than the infected population [29]. Gender bias is still abundant in many countries and health-seeking behavior is linked to this issue. Further research into determining the sex differences both in infection and severity of the disease is needed to understand the biological and cultural factors that drive disease pattern in communities.

4. Objective

Explore the potential for cooperative health management policy to effectively combat the eminent threat of dengue epidemics due to climate change. In order to measure and evaluate past interventions and current health management system responses, a review of dengue literature was performed. Along with reporting successful and non-successful interventions, insight into response and treatment options available for dengue outbreaks in Asia was also assessed. All evaluations were performed with the intention of highlighting areas of health management in critical need of change to attain progress in the battle against vector-transmitted disease in Asia.

5. Methodology

A systematic review of dengue history, transmission, prevention, diagnosis, treatment, control, surveillance, response, intervention outcomes and vaccine development was performed. The purpose was to explore the potential complex causal links of effective health management strategies to combat the occurrence of dengue pandemics due to global climate change. Through the use of evidence-based literature the following paper will discuss current challenges of dengue prevention, transmission, control and vaccine development; successful and unsuccessful interventions in endemic areas, future predictions of dengue endemic areas due to climate change, and future role of health management policies globally. The research issues we address in this paper include prior intervention methods and their effectiveness, treatments, and implications on health management policies. This paper is divided into subsections with the purpose of addressing each of the research questions. A variety of intervention methods including some unconventional approaches are explained. The treatment subsection brings to light the lack of treatments available. Implications of health management and policy examine the methods of surveillance, existing infrastructure, potential sustainable approaches, and technological developments. Through the conclusion section we provide a summation and identify gaps in current public health management approaches. Although data from other sources has been used the majority of the articles focus on responses in Southeast Asia. This paper is limited to a public health management approach rather than a site management or medical management approach

6. Interventions

When assessing the dengue vector control methods in Asia the predominant types included chemical, environmental, and biological. Most interventions focused on evaluating their effectiveness based on reduction of adult vector population rather than decreased incidence of disease. Although adult vector control reduces the mosquito populations, it often does not appear to reduce the rate of dengue infections. Vector control must also be continually maintained which can cause imposition to the human population and additional costs to governments. Chemical means of vector control seem to have a better effect, when compared to other methods, for control of outbreak situations. Insecticide treated netting (ITN), or curtains, seem to be less sustainable predominantly due to non-use or improper use of ITN by indigenous populations. Bed nets used while sleeping, provide some protection but are not as effective against dengue vectors like they are in malaria; this is because the mosquitoes that transmit the dengue virus often bite during the day rather than at night. Insecticide resistance to chemical means of vector control is a problematic issue that has arisen and must be factored into any future chemical campaigns to control vector populations. Dengue is believed to be a primarily urban disease as the vectors are well adapted to human habitation. The urbanization of South East Asia that started after World War II for economic purpose has led to population growth that contributes to the increase of susceptible hosts. However, dengue has spread into rural areas from where it had not been reported before. During the first half of the 21st century, piped water supply was restricted to urban towns, and now that supply system has been introduced into rural areas, water storage practices have changed. Modern transport system has also connected the rural areas better, and, finally, solid waste disposal also became a consequence from all this development. These are most cited reasons for rural dengue spread [30, 31]. In Singapore, successful vector control programs have brought down dengue incidence between 1974 and 1985. However, there was a major resurgence of dengue with more adult cases being reported. Serological studies indicated changes in the transmission sites and that the transmission was occurring in work sites rather than in residential houses [32].

Resistance to insecticides, specifically dichlorodiphenyltrichlorethane (DDT), presents a significant challenge to the control of dengue vectors. DDT was first introduced during World War II to protect troops and control vector- borne disease, such as malaria. After World War II, the indiscriminant agricultural use of DDT greatly increased vector resistance. The World Health Organization launched a program to eradicate malaria in 1955. This program, based partially on the use of DDT was initially successful; however, the success was not sustained in lower socioeconomic areas. Today indoor residual spraying (IRS) is used to control vector populations [33]. IRS is the application of DDT to the internal walls of domiciles to repel or eliminate mosquitos. This method is effective, long lasting, and reduces both DDT resistances in vector populations as well as diminishes environmental destruction due to DDT contamination [34].

Health education to control dengue ensures that community members understand the process of dengue infection and the critical behaviors that need to be altered to prevent transmission and decrease the incidence of morbidity and mortality.

Interventions with a primary focus on behavior modification, through educational means, seem to have better, long lasting effects on the incidence of dengue. Educational campaigns involving the community are well received and sustainable. The cost is comparatively low compared to vector control measures. These programs allow for community involvement and ownership, which are the proven foundation to any successful intervention. Appointment of a community leader, with involvement from inception through the intervention, compared with communities without involvement prior to commencement of the intervention had better reduction of dengue vectors and dengue infection rates [35]. The most highly involved communities reported the most intervention success [36, 37]. Requiring the involved communities to take and maintain ownership of the interventions seems to play a significant role in intervention effectiveness [38, 39]. Additional benefits to high levels of community involvement included increased community efficacy, community pride, and an overall increase in well being [36].

Educational programs delivered through schools seemed to have the greatest impact on behavioral changes to reduce vector populations [35, 39, 40, 41, 42]. These interventions suggest educational programs delivered through schools are more effective than other methods of distributing educational information. In Colima, Mexico a study highlighted the effectiveness of a combined approach with a focus on uninterrupted health education to reduce the breeding sites of vectors [43]. The aforementioned study demonstrated community targeted health education combined with larvicide treatment had a greater impact on decreasing mosquito habitats than larvicide treatment alone. [43] This combined approach is not universally accepted. (Some argue that too much variation occurs between the acquisition of knowledge and implantation [44, 45]. Individuals with sound comprehension of preventive measures were most often successful in incorporating new behaviors to prevent dengue disease and transmission [50]. It is important to understand that in cultures where the indigenous people lacked sufficient understanding of disease transmission, changes to their personal and household behaviors were met with resistance. Their resistance stemmed from a belief that vector control should be a governmental responsibility rather than a personal responsibility [52, 52]. Education programs based in schools enhance community education programs because of the transference of information and utility from classrooms to domicile. A main factor for the success of school based education programs stems from the fact that dengue predominantly affects children; therefore, education directed at the young population can help maintain changes in attitudes and behaviors [53]. In Thailand, [54, 55], school based education programs have demonstrated children's increase in understanding and prevention of dengue. Although knowledge of mosquitos and habitat reduction methods are beneficial, they must be incorporated into a health belief and behavioral change model to ensure success. The incorporation of behavioral change models to introduce educational information is pivotal to community acceptance and participation [56]. Current gaps in research insufficiently explain the best mode of delivery and most effective length of continuous education program. Educational programs' variance is dependent upon adequate funding, convenient health care centers, human capacity, political involvement, and availability of additional resources.

In Cambodia, the National Dengue Control Program provides dengue education in the school system and at local health centers [52]. Although these programs can be effective they are not given financial priority nor are they routinely evaluated for effectiveness. Materials provided for educational purposes can be complicated and therefore misunderstood. The individuals tasked to oversee the distribution of educational material are teachers and health care workers [52]. These workers are often inadequately trained and lack guidelines that recommend practical and effective methods of preventing vector bites. Insufficient funding for new and updated educational materials leads to a culture of familiarity and lapse into old behaviors and habits that propagate dengue infections. Community involvement in the control and prevention of dengue is essential, but will not be substantially effective until proper resources are consistently allocated [52].

Some of the environmental interventions discussed in this article include the use of natural predators as vector control. Dragonfly larvae used in an experiment to reduce the abundance of *A. aegypti* mosquitos, in Myanmar, showed positive results [57]. Virtually all A. *aegypti larvae* disappeared immediately after two dragonflies were placed in each container, and the density of adult mosquitos declined within six weeks [57]. The use of Copepods, natural mosquito larvae predators, in an intervention in Viet Nam proved to be inexpensive and community- accepted [58]. Environmental interventions are best suited for large communal water storage containers. The use of predators may be useful in reducing vector populations, particularly where communities lack water and sewage infrastructure. Global warming is said to affect the disease pattern, and it is essential for epidemiologists to understand such patterns in relation to biodiversity. Such an approach can have a dramatic impact on the public health strategies for disease prevention and control. Climate change may have variable effects on different diseases; some diseases may be sensitive to climatic changes, while others may be less responsive [59]. Climate change may actually expand the range of vector borne diseases from the tropical zone, where the species diversity of hosts is comparatively high in contrast to the temperate climatic zone, where species diversity is very low [60, 61]. It is too early to predict the impact of biodiversity and global warming on the propagation of vector borne disease as the vector behavior and transmission mechanisms of the host differ [62]. It is also necessary to initiate innovative research and systematic monitoring programs to obtain first hand information about the patterns of disease occurrence and relate it with biodiversity.

Biodiversity plays an important role in the transmission of diseases. However, the mechanism by which the biodiversity disease relationship is controlled is still ambiguous, as biodiversity and disease pattern show varied degrees of complexities, which need to be, addressed in future studies. Extensive studies on biodiversity–disease relationships in different ecological zones would be helpful in order to demystify the associations with this relationship. The task is not easy for ecologists as the dynamic nature of ecosystems poses difficulties in understanding various eco-based relationships. The need for increased precision in estimates presents an opportunity for investment in research on the social implications of climate change.

7. Immunizations

Currently no vaccine exists to protect against dengue. Specific challenges in vaccine development are due to three major factors. The first difficulty arises from the fact that dengue has four distinct serotypes each with the ability to cause disease. The second and more challenging obstacle is each infection increases an individual's risk of contracting a more severe strain of dengue. Therefore an effective vaccine must protect against all serotypes simultaneously. Lastly, there are no known animal hosts for dengue. Without an animal host, the only viable candidates for vaccine trials are human beings themselves. Testing the effectiveness of a trial vaccine poses serious ethical issues.

8. Implications on health management policy

Increased burning of fossil fuels by the world's developed nations and the continued course of industrialization and development are attributed with great impacts to the world's climate.

Developing nations will face an unequal burden of disease caused by climate change. Individuals in impoverished areas have enormous morbidity and mortality rates in relation to infectious diseases when compared with developed nations [88]. More concretely, both climate change and disease affect human vulnerability. In addition to the known factors of dengue, such as variation in seasonal weather, vector control programs, and socioeconomic status, climate change is extremely likely to influence current vector-borne disease epidemiology. While the effects could manifest in several ways ranging from, an increase in short term epidemics to a gradual change in long term disease tendencies. Currently there are limited amounts of published articles that provide information containing predictions. There is currently a dearth of substantiated information regarding the exact percentage of climate change influenced infectious disease. This can prove challenging to making new public health policies [18]. Clear indications of climate change on dengue, will be easier to detect than overall climate change, due to the slow rate of transformation. Climate change variability will depend on the level of health infrastructure in the affected areas. The cost and efficacy of prevention and potential cures or vaccines will be essential to disease management.

Making headway in the fight against vector-transmitted diseases ideally will incorporate a multidisciplinary approach. Working together with mosquito experts to understand mosquito attraction and control vector populations, future development that considers ecological balance and mitigates human impact on the environment, unified and structured rapid disease identification surveillance reporting and treatment of diseases, well-funded and continually evolving community education programs are all vital parts of a holistic approach.

High-risk populations for contraction of the more serious forms of dengue, dengue hemorrhagic fever and dengue shock syndrome, are individuals who have recently been infected with a less severe stain of dengue. Children in impoverished areas are at particularly elevated risk. They often become infected early with less severe stains of dengue, which puts them at a much higher risk of contracting a more severe type of dengue and thus more likely to die. Little to no research has been completed to assess the ability to transmit the dengue through breast milk. This could potentially shed new light on transmission risk factors.

Surveillance of disease is one of the most critical factors for assessing and responding to disease outbreaks. Once surveillance indicates an emerging infectious disease, treatment, containment, and prevention of new cases becomes the focus of effective health management. The existing surveillance systems in Asia are woefully inadequate to address the urgency of dengue. Lack of emerging disease surveillance, in Asia, must be given greater priority. The use of surveillance to forecast the risk of vector borne disease more accurately could greatly alter the impact of emerging disease. Traditional health management resources are insufficiently funded; focused efforts to develop more effective, and more accurate tools could greatly aid early detection of increased infection rates.

Strong health systems are also important to maintain. Dengue outbreaks can be worsened when health systems are not strong enough to adequately respond to the increased demands of epidemics. Viruses are continually evolving to outwit control measures. Public health and health systems must be ever vigilant in maintaining set priorities to tackle infectious diseases, such as dengue. Training of community- based individuals in assessing; treating, reporting, and containing outbreaks of dengue are of great importance. There is an imperative need for point of care testing. Many areas of Asia with endemic dengue lack access to proper laboratory testing. Even in the presence of laboratory facilities testing for dengue can be time consuming. Point of care (POC) testing would allow health care workers in the communities to rapidly assess and accurately diagnose dengue infections. One of the major challenges to preventing the spread of dengue infections is the amount of time needed to confirm the presence of antibodies in the host system; however, with POC testing this could be significantly mitigated.

The need for sustainable development in sanitation and water availability is pivotal to alleviating the burden of disease in Asia. The establishment of a consistent water supply to homes would decrease the need for water storage and thus decrease available breeding sites for vectors, bacteria, and other pathogens. The WHO conducted a cost benefit analysis of establishing such systems in developing countries. The outcome of the analysis discussed the financial gain that could be achieved. The report suggests a minimal return of 3 to 1 for each dollar invested, and up to thirty-four times the return on investment [63]. This would also directly reduce the burden of various diseases and drastically reduce the need for economic funding to combat preventable diseases. Although exact funding estimates are variable depending on regions, the application of new ideas or innovations to tackling the engineering obstacles could prove financially profitable [63]. In addition to potential profitability, establishing or improving sanitation and water supply could reduce the average days lost due to illness. There would also be a decrease in money spent by patients seeking treatment. The benefits to improving and establishing these systems would behoove nations globally. The increase in production of developing countries coupled with more consistent attendance in schools would also allow these countries to establish and maintain ownership of high health management improvements at a cost significantly less than the current burden of disease [63].

Public health principals are rooted in the idea of community involvement. This involvement has been proven effective for sustainable interventions. Communities that do not understand, support, or have a clear understanding of the importance of the intervention undermine intervention success. Community health and well-being are multifactorial and equally affect individuals quality of life. Community based changes should be made to the current system with the intention of improving the health of the entire community and should be evidence based. Approaching these changes from a community level and paying acute attention all aspects of the social, political, and economic factors of each community in an effort to reduce health disparities [89].This is important to eliminate or reduce factors that contribute to health problems or introduce new elements that promote better health.

Mosquitos can fly distances equivalent to about thirty miles; this includes open ocean distances, like those found between islands and mainland. They can smell humans from a distance of fifty yards. Mosquito eradication would significantly decrease the global burden of disease;, however the magnitude and complexity of such a project would not only be impractical but potentially have unintended consequences on global ecology. Scientists are however, employing innovative techniques to battle vector transmitted diseases, and some of the most groundbreaking processes can be found in the fight against malaria. Malaria research is developing new ways to combat vector populations: genetically altered mosquitos, mosquito attraction and repulsion factors, the use of animals to detect mosquito breeding sites, and human pharmaceutical interventions for exterminating adult mosquitos.

There are hundreds of scientists whose entire lives and careers have been devoted to working on the problems caused by mosquitoes. They follow their breeding habits, study them to understanding their sense of smell, and decipherer their DNA. Bart Knols, a malariologist, is a leader in the fight against mosquito-transmitted disease. Although insecticides are making a comeback, new modern and radical versions are in the forefront of this battle. Genetically altered mosquitos offer a potential middle ground to complete mosquito eradication. The normal process inside mosquitos involves the release of a repressor chemical to prevent protein (tTA) from binding to the complementary site [64]. Genetic modification alters this process by removing the repressor and allowing the tTA to bind to the tetO-binding site. This binding process triggers more tTA proteins to be released and bond to tetO creating a continuous cycle [64]. The tTA protein damages the normal mosquito cells and causes larvae to die [64]. The following image illustrates the aforementioned process. This genetic alteration does not allow the larvae to survive to adulthood. Male and female mosquito genes are necessary for successful breeding of genetically altered offspring, but only male mosquitoes are released after the modification process is complete. Release of only the male mosquitos is done to prevent any genetically altered mosquitoes from biting humans, thereby eliminating the potential of genetically altered genes being transferred to humans. Careful consideration has been given to ethical and safety concerns where genetic modification techniques are applied. Advocates for genetically modified mosquitos argue that mosquito transmitted disease could be drastically lowered with very little disruption in the ecology. Others have suggested that the so-called Asian tiger mosquito, which also carries dengue, could fill the vacuum left by the Aedes aegypti.

Mosquito traps are another potential low cost high impact innovation that may impact the number of dengue related illnesses. Traps specifically designed for this purpose have been developed with a variety of users in mind: researcher, private consumers, and commercial consumers. Through a combination of light and dark contrasting color combinations these traps visual simulate objects that naturally attract mosquitos. The traps also are made with chemical compounds meant give off an odor similar to human skin. Some traps additionally have CO2, which is another attractant for mosquitos. These traps reduce adult mosquito populations without the need for insecticides or pesticides [65].

Smartphones may help increase the ability to halt outbreaks of dengue fever. Mobile phones are increasingly being used across the developing world to collect data and improve health outcomes. Mobile phones have penetrated the majority of markets worldwide and South East Asia is one of the mobile phones fastest growing markets.

The potential of integrated mobile services could better serve rural communities by providing the ability to communicate health related information. Rural communities tend to face unnecessary health related hardships that could be greatly mitigated with mobile access to health experts and necessary information services. Mobile connectedness would also allow for more accurate assessments of the prevalence of diseases [87]. A range of educational services could be provided via mobile phones for health education in remote villages and communities.

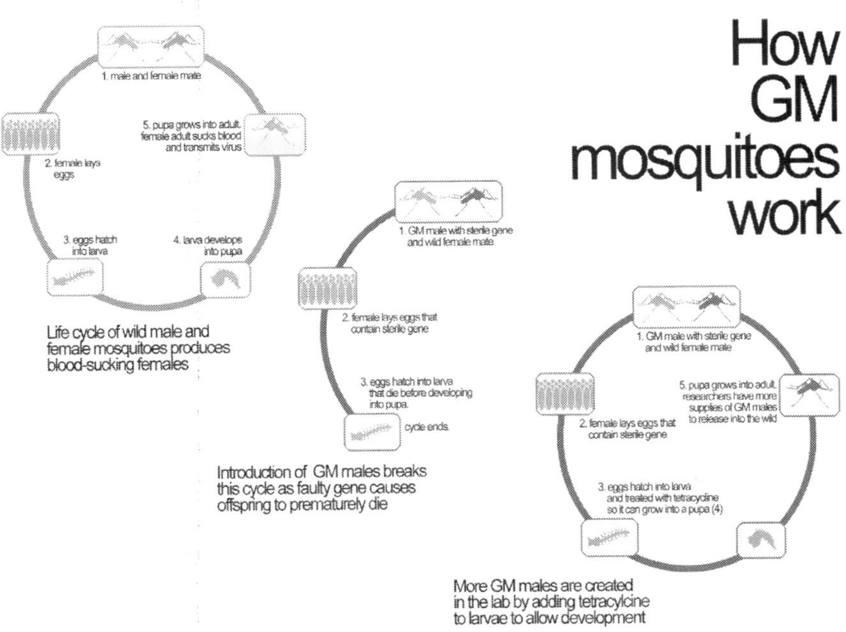

https://oneinsevenpeople.wordpress.com/tag/dengue/

Figure 7. How GM mosquitos work

Mobile phone can be used to collect and analyze data regarding disease outbreaks faster, which would allow for faster response time and containment. This is particularly important for communities that have been displaced due to a natural disasters or conflict.

In Sri Lanka in a brief experiment morning and evening newspapers were printed using ink infused with citronella, a natural insect repellent. The experiment began by handing out newspapers on World Health Day and although no long lasting effects were expected. This type of approach may be more cost effective than other approaches and may serve as a bridge while waiting for an effective vaccine to be developed. Another possible use of such a low-tech approach may allow for dissemination of health related educational pamphlets or newspapers treated with natural insect repellant [66].

9. Conclusion

The first step in effective dengue prevention and control should be recognizing it as a priority and understanding its characteristics.[67] Factors that may have contributed to rapid changing epidemiology of dengue in South East Asia region are the challenges that need to be addressed

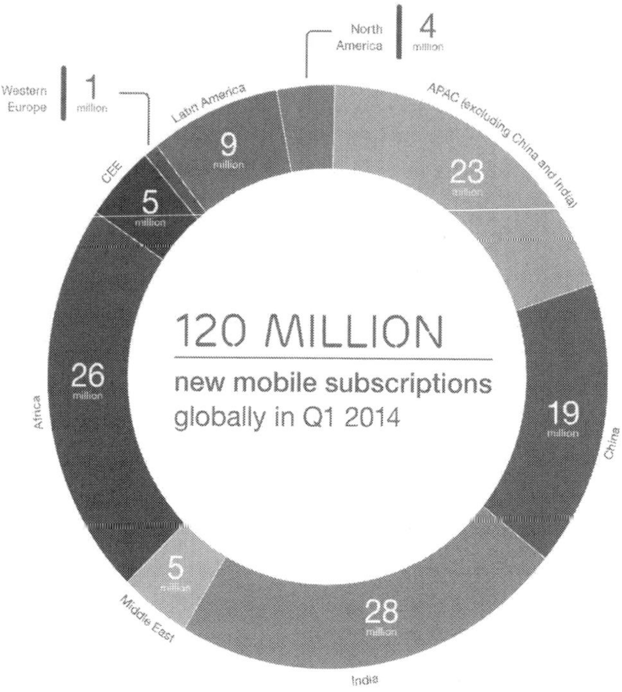

http://www.ericsson.com/news/1790097

Figure 8. Ericsson Mobile

in designing operational research and implementation strategies. Operational research is needed to answer research questions on how the efficacy, cost-effectiveness, sustainability and scaling-up of existing and promising new control methods can be enhanced. Complementary to basic research, operational and implementation research are important in achieving progress. Dengue is a rising threat globally and requires actions of prevention and control in an urgent manner. Some of the major factors influencing changes in dengue epidemiology include: viral subtypes with increased virulence, lack of information on vector ecology in microclimatic conditions, time interval in sequential infection. Greater resources and efforts will be essential to containing the expected changes in disease epidemiology. Climate variability has the potential to produce multiple disease epidemics simultaneously. Climate change has extensive consequences that reach well beyond health concerns. Human health and survival is contingent upon the effects of climate change. Future health policies are related to climate change and therefore policy changes for both should be interwoven. The complex relationship of socioeconomic status, climate changes and the proliferation of infectious disease like dengue should be addressed as a global issue. Climate change is expected to affect vector breeding sites and global dissemination in addition to human immunology, migration, and behavior. Impoverished areas have heightened environmental risk and decreased resources to prevent or manage dengue infection [88]. Community based interventions employing education and natural predators may be of particular use in rural and urban areas. However for long lasting declines in infectious disease major infrastructure must be undertaken. Changes in water security and wastewater are integral for public health programs to wholly address the propagation of dengue [88]. Most of the structural improvements could reduce the incidence of other infectious diseases.

Resources and knowledge must be harnessed at a community level through integrated programs. Having aid workers trained in effective responses and prevention for dengue infections is paramount and will make a substantial contribution toward reducing dengue related illness. Much needed behavior changes can only come about by empowering communities with critical knowledge concerning hygiene, sanitation, and the environment. Funding and continual training needs to be given priority this will allow community health workers to identify and treat suspected dengue cases. Integration of community needs and aspirations with overall health outcomes will improve the overall community-based surveillance.

Economic growth opportunities, of Asian countries, can be bolstered if endemic dengue infections can be tackled, treated, and effectively managed. Opportunities exist for stakeholders and financial investors to better utilize their contributions by investing in holistic sustainable and innovative health management policies and public health practices. Equilibrium needs to be reached between communities, sustainability, infrastructure, technological advances, ecofriendly approaches, and effective solutions. Educational and community based programs should be a central focus on all future dengue control and prevention measures. The most effective methods of educational programs were those based out of the primary schools within communities. A means of rapid on site testing should be utilized for detection and diagnosis of dengue. Once dengue is diagnosed in a community, better reporting and surveillance must occur to prevent epidemics. Addressing the lack of accurate surveillance systems in Asia could significantly impact response time and limit the occurrence of epidemic episodes of dengue. Future innovations focused on natural deterrents to target mosquitos may have useable implications for other vector transmitted diseases. These issues are important to the field of public health and health management systems further research, analysis, and monitoring is warranted to fully understand the effects of interconnected, sustainable, innovative ways to reduce the global burden of dengue infections.

Pharmaceuticals designed to treat dengue have made progress and could potentially develop more rapidly due to the enormity of dengue's impact on a global scale. The continued increase of vector-transmitted diseases might make the drug markets for a dengue cure economically viable. Morbidity issues as they relate to economies can be drastically affected by sudden epidemics; here is where antivirals could potentially have a complementary role to vaccines for dengue. The challenges that remain with dengue pharmaceuticals are due to the need for human clinical trials.

Author details

Muhiuddin Haider* and Jamie Turner

*Address all correspondence to: mhaider@umd.edu

School of Public Health, University of Maryland, USA

References

[1] Impact of Dengue. *WHO*. Retrieved May 17, 2014, from http://www.who.int/csr/disease/dengue/impact/en/

[2] World Health Organization, Retrieved May 16, 2014 from http://www.who.int/topics/dengue/en/

[3] Halstead, S. B. "Dengue: Overview and History." In Dengue: Tropical Medicine: Science and Practice, vol. 5, eds. G. Pasvol & S. L. Hoffman (London: Imperial College Press, 2008): 1–28.

[4] Dengue Clinical Lab. (2014, May 16). *Centers for Disease Control and Prevention*. Retrieved May 20, 2014, from http://www.cdc.gov/dengue/, http://www.cdc.gov/dengue/clinicalLab/clinical.html, http://www.cdc.gov/dengue/clinicalLab/caseDef.html

[5] Researchers identify fifth dengue subtype. *CIDRAP*. Retrieved May 15, 2014, from http://www.cidrap.umn.edu/news-perspective/2013/10/researchers-identify-fifth-dengue-subtype

[6] Dash, A., Bhatia, R., Sunyoto, T., & Mourya, D. (2013). Emerging and Reemerging arboviral diseases in Southeast Asia. *Journal of vector borne disease, 50*(June 2013), 77-84.

[7] Ooi, E., & Gubler, D. J. (2009). Dengue in Southeast Asia: epidemiological characteristics and strategic challenges in disease prevention. *Cadernos de Saude Publica, 25*, S115-S124.

[8] Suaya JA, Shepard DS, Siqueira JB, Martelli CT, Lum LCS, et al. (2009) Cost of dengue cases in eight countries in the Americas and Asia: A prospective study. Am J Trop Med Hyg 80: 846–855

[9] Beaute J, Vong S (2010) Cost and disease burden of dengue in Cambodia. BMC Public Health 10: 1–6

[10] Lim LH, Vasan SS, Birgelen L, Murtola TM, Gong H-F, et al. (2010) Immediate cost of dengue to Malaysia and Thailand: An estimate. Dengue Bulletin 34: 65–76

[11] Undurraga EA, Halasa YA, Shepard DS (2012) Use of expansion factors to estimate the burden of dengue in Southeast Asia: a systematic analysis. PloS Negl Trop Dis 7: e2056

[12] Undurraga EA, Halasa YA, Shepard DS (2011) Expansion factors: a key step in estimating dengue burden and costs in Southeast Asia. Am J Trop Med Hyg 85: 318.

[13] Therawiwat M, Fungladda W, Kaewkungwal J, Imamee N, Steckler A. Community-based approach for prevention and control of dengue hemorrhagic fever in Kanchanaburi Province, Thailand. *The Southeast Asian Journal Of Tropical Medicine And Public Health.* 2005;36(6):1439-1449.

[14] Hales (2002); J. A. Patz, D. Campbell-Lendrum, T Holloway, et al., "Impact of regional climate change on human health, " *Nature* (2005), pp. 310-317.

[15] Colón-González (2013); M. Hagenlocher, E. Delmelle, I. Casas et al., "Assessing socio-economic vulnerability to dengue fever in Cali, Colombia: Statistical vs expert-based modeling, " *International Journal of Health Geographics* 12/1 (2013), p. 36; M. Johansson, D. Cummings, and G. Glass, "PLOS medicine: Multiyear climate variability and Dengue—El Niño Southern Oscillation, weather, and dengue incidence in Puerto Rico, Mexico, and Thailand: A longitudinal data analysis, " *PLoS Medicine* 6/11 (2009), pp. 1-9.; M. A. Johansson, F. Dominici, and G. E. Glass. "Local and global effects of climate on dengue transmission in Puerto Rico, " *PLoS Neglected Tropical Diseases* (2009), pp. 1-5.

[16] McMichael (2006); C. P. Diman, and W. Tahir, "Potential of stagnant water due to dam flooding, " *Innovation Management and Technology Research, 2012 International Conference* (2012), pp. 609-612.; J. T. Watson, M. Gayer, and M. A. Connolly, "Epidemics after natural disasters, " *Emerging Infectious Diseases* (2007), pp. 1-5.

[17] Centers for Disease Control and Prevention, "Emergency mosquito control associated with Hurricane Andrew–Florida and Louisiana, 1992, " *Morbidity Mortality Weekly Report.* (1993), pp. 240-242.

[18] R. S. Nasci, and C. G. Moore, "Vector-borne disease surveillance and natural disasters, " *Emerging Infectious Disease* (1998), pp. 333-334.

[19] Millennium Ecosystem Assessment Report on Ecosystems and human well-being. Vol 5 (2005).

[20] McMichael., pp. 401-413.

[21] Rodhain F, Rosen L. Mosquito vectors and dengue virus-vector relationships. In: Gubler DJ, Kuno G, editors. Dengue and Dengue Hemorrhagic Fever. New York: CAB International; 1997. p. 45-60.

[22] Gubler DJ. The changing epidemiology of yellow fever and dengue, 1900 to 2003: Full circle? Comp Immunol Microbiol Infect Dis 2004;27:319-30.

[23] Nimmanutya S. Dengue haemorrhagic fever: Current issues and future research. Asia-Oceanian. J Pediatr Child Health 2002;1:1-22.

[24] Kalayanarooj S, Nimmannitya S. Guidelines for dengue hemorrhagic fever case management. Bangkok: Bangkok Medical Publisher; 2004.

[25] Chareonsook O, Foy HM, Teeraratkul A, Silarug N. Changing epidemiology of dengue haemorrhagic fever in Thailand. Epidemiol Infect 1999;122:161-6.

[26] SedhainA, Adhikari S, Bhattarai GR, Regmi S, Subedee LR, Chaudhary SK, et al. A clinicoradiological and laboratory analysis of dengue cases during an outbreak in central Nepal in 2010. Dengue Bull 2012;36:134-48.

[27] Rahman M, Rahman K, Siddque AK, Shoma S, Kamal AH, Ali KS, et al. First outbreak of dengue hemorrhagic fever in Bangladesh. Emerg Infect Dis 2002;8:738-40.

[28] Gupta E, Dar L, Kapoor G, Broor S. The changing epidemiology of dengue in Delhi, India. Virol J 2006;3:92.

[29] Guha-Sapir D, Schimmer B. Dengue fever: New paradigms for a changing epidemiology. Emerg Themes Epidemiol 2005;2:1.

[30] Ooi EE. Changing pattern of dengue transmission in Singapore. Dengue Bull 2001;25:40-4.

[31] Zargar, U.R., 2011. Proceed with caution on disease eradication. Science and Development Network. http://www.scidev.net/en/ health/health-policy/editor-letters/ proceed-with-caution-on-dis- easeeradication-1.html (accessed 10/12/2014).

[32] Dobson, A., Carper, R., 1992. Global Warming and Potential Changes in Host–Parasite and Disease–Vector Relationship. Yale University Press, Connecticut, pp. 201–217.

[33] Harvell, C.D., Mitchell, C.E., Ward, J.R., Altizer, S., Dobson, A.P., et al, 2002. Ecology – climate warming and disease risks for terrestrial and marine biota. Science 296, 2158–2162.

[34] Miller, E., Huppert, A., 2013. The effects of host diversity on vector- borne disease: the conditions under which diversity will amplify or dilute the disease risk. PLoS ONE 8, e80279.

[35] Ooi EE, Gubler DJ. Dengue in South East Asia: Epidemiological

[36] World Health Organization (WHO) Global Strategy for Dengue Prevention and Control, 2012–2020. Geneva: WHO Press; 2012.

[37] WHO Regional Office for South-East Asia Comprehensive Guidelines for Prevention and Control of Dengue and Dengue Haemorrhagic Fever, Revised and Expanded Edition. New Delhi: World Health Organisation South East Asia Regional Office; 2011.

[38] Gubler DJ. Epidemic dengue/dengue hemorrhagic fever as a public health, social and economic problem in the 21st century. Trend Microbiol. 2002;10(2):100–103. [PubMed]

[39] Report of the Third Expert Group Meeting on DDT, UNEP/POPS/DDT-EG.3/3, Stockholm Convention on Persistent Organic Pollutants, November 12, 2010. http://chm.pops.int/Programmes/DDT/Meetings/DDTEG32010/tabid/1108/mctl/ViewDetails/EventModID/1421/EventID/116/xmid/4037/language/en-US/Default.aspx

[40] "Is DDT still effective and needed in malaria control?". Malaria Foundation International. Archived from the original on November 18, 2010. Retrieved March 15, 2006. http://www.webcitation.org/5uKxTzvxt

[41] Nam VS, Yen NT, Kay B, Marten GG, Reid JW. Eradication of Aedes aegypti from a village in Vietnam using copepods and community participation. *The American Journal of Tropical Medicine and Hygiene.* 1998;59:657-660.

[42] Crabtree SA, Wong CM, Mas'ud F. Community participatory approaches to Dengue prevention in Sarawak, Malaysia. *Human Organization.* 2001;60(3):281-287.

[43] Suwanbamrung C, Dumpan A, Thammapalo S, Sumrongtong R, Phedkeang P. A model of community capacity building for sustainable dengue problem solution in Southern Thailand. *Health.* 2011;3(9):584-601.

[44] Nam VS, Nguyen TY, Tran VP, Truong UN, Le QM, Le VL, et al. Elimination of dengue by community programs using Mesocyclops(Copepoda) against Aedes aegypti in central Vietnam. *The American Journal Of Tropical Medicine And Hygiene.* 2005;72(1): 67-73.

[45] Kay B, Nam VS. New strategy against Aedes aegypti in Vietnam. *Lancet.* 2005; 365(9459):613- 617.

[46] Phatumachinda B, Phanurai P, Samutrapongse W, Chareonsook OA. Studies on community participation in Aedes aegypti control at Phanus Nikhom district, Chonburi Province, Thailand. *Mosquito-Borne Diseases Bulletin.* 1985;2:1-8.

[47] Suroso H, Suroso T. Aedes aegypti, control through source reduction by community efforts in Pekalongan, Indonesia. *Mosquito-Borne Diseases Bulletin.* 1990;7:59-62.

[48] Swaddiwudhipong W, Chaovakiratipong C, Nguntra P, Koonchote S, Khumklam P, Lerdlukanavonge P. Effect of health education on community participation in control of dengue hemorrhagic fever in an urban area of Thailand. *The Southeast Asian Journal Of Tropical Medicine And Public Health.* 1992;23(2):200-206.

[49] Espinoza-Gomez F, Hernandez-Suarez CM, Coll-Cardenas R (2002) Educational campaign versus malathion spraying for the control of Aedes aegypti in Colima, Mexico. Journal of Epidemiology and Community Health 56(2): 148–152.

[50] Lloyd L, Winch P, Ortega-Canto J, Kendall C (1992) Results of a community based Aedes aegypti control program in Merida, Yucatan, Mexico. American Journal of Tropical Medicine and Hygiene 46: 635–642.

[51] Swaddiwudhipong W, Lerdlukanavonge P, Klumklam P, Koonchote S, Nguntra P, et al. (1992) A survey of knowledge, attitudes and practice of the prevention and control of dengue hemorrhagic fever in an urban community in Thailand. Southeast Asian Journal of Tropical Medicine and Public Health 23(2): 207–211.

[52] Rosenbaum J, Nathan M, Ragoonanansingh R, Rawlins S, Gayle C (1995) Community participation in dengue prevention and control: A survey of Health Education for Dengue Control in Cambodia PLoS Neglected Tropical Diseases | www.plosntds.org 9 2007 | Volume 1 | Issue 3 | e143 knowledge, attitudes and practices in Trinidad and Tobago. The American Society of Tropical Medicine and Hygiene 53(2): 111–117.

[53] Whiteford LM (2000) Local identify, globalization and health in Cuba and the Dominican Republic. In: Whiteford LM, Manderson L, eds. Global Health Policy, Local Realities: The fallacy of a level-playing field. Boulder, CO: Lynne Rienner Publishers. pp 57–78.

[54] Perez-Guerra CL, Seda H, Garcia-Rivera EJ, Clark GG (2005) Knowledge and attitudes in Puerto Rico concerning dengue prevention. Pan-American Journal of Public Health 17(4): 243–253.

[55] Win KT, Nang SZ, Min A (2004) Community-based assessment of dengue related knowledge among caregivers. Dengue Bulletin 28: 189–195.

[56] Serufo JC, Souza AM, Avares VA (1993) Dengue in the South-Eastern Region of Brazil – Historical analysis and epidemiology. Revista de Saude Publica 27(3): 157–167.

[57] Wangroongsarb Y (1997) Dengue control in Thailand. Public Health 14: 32–38.

[58] Chau T, Fortin J, Khun S, Nguyen H (2000) Practise what is preached? Dengue health education in Muan District, Khon Kaen Province, Thailand: Primary school children's knowledge and reported practice, in Australian Centre for International & Tropical Health and Nutrition. Brisbane: The University of Queensland.

[59] Lennon J (2005) The use of health belief model in dengue health education. Dengue Bulletin 29: 217–219.

[60] Samways, M. J. (1996, May 22). Insects in the Urban Environment: Pest Pressures versus Conservation Concerns. *International Conference on Urban Pests*, pp. 129-133.

[61] Kay BH, Nam VS, Tien TV, Yen NT, Phong TV, Diep VTB, et al. Control of aedes vectors of dengue in three provinces of Vietnam by use of Mesocyclops (Copepoda) and community-based methods validated by entomologic, clinical, and serological surveillance. *The American Journal Of Tropical Medicine And Hygiene*. 2002;66(1):40-48.

[62] Costs and benefits of water and sanitation improvements at the global level (Evaluation of the). *WHO*. Retrieved May 20, 2014, from http://www.who.int/water_sanitation_health/wsh0404summary/en/

[63] Fu, G., A. A. James, D. Aw, D. Nimmo, R. S. Lees, L. Alphey, N. Jasinskiene, O. Marinotti, H. Kim Phuc, S. Scaife, H. White-Cooper, T. U. Berendonk, P. Gray, and L. Jin. "Female-specific flightless phenotype for mosquito control." *Proceedings of the National Academy of Sciences* 107.10 (2010): 4550-4554.

[64] "Mosquito Trap Product Range Helps Prevent Malaria, Dengue or Yellow Fever." *The256Com RSS*. Web. 22 July 2014. http://the256.com/mosquito-trap-product-range-helps-prevent-malaria-dengue-or-yellow-fever.html

[65] "This Sri Lankan Newspaper Repels Mosquitos While You Enjoy Reading." *Wonderful Engineering*. N.p., n.d. Web. 24 July 2014. http://wonderfulengineering.com/this-sri-lankan-newspaper-repels-mosquitos-while-you-enjoy-reading/

[66] Ang LW, Foong B, Ye T, Chow A, Chew S. Impact of 'carpet-combing' vector control operations in terminating the 2005 dengue outbreak in Singapore. *Epidemiological News Bulletin*. 2007;33(3):31-36.

[67] Beckett CG, Kosasih H, Tan R, Widjaja S, Listianingsih E, Ma'roef C, et al. Enhancing knowledge and awareness of dengue during a prospective study of dengue fever. *The Southeast Asian Journal Of Tropical Medicine And Public Health*. 2004;35(3):614-617.

[68] Butraporn P, Saelim W, Sitapura P, Tantawiwat S. Establishment of an environmental master team to control dengue haemorrhagic fever by local wisdom in Thailand. *Dengue bulletin*. 1999;23: 99-104.

[69] Eamchan P, Nisalak A, Foy HM, Chareonsook OA. Epidemiology and control of dengue virus infections in Thai villages in 1987. *The American Journal Of Tropical Medicine And Hygiene*. 1989;41(1):95-101.

[70] Hien Tran V. Application of mosquito—proof water containers in the reduction of dengue mosquito population in a dengue endemic province of Vietnam. *Asian Pacific Journal of Tropical Disease*. 2011;1(4):270-274.

[71] Igarashi A. Impact of dengue virus infection and its control. *FEMS Immunology And Medical Microbiology*. 1997;18(4):291-300.

[72] Kay BH, Tuyet Hanh TT, Le NH, Quy TM, Nam VS, Hang PVD, et al. Sustainability and cost of a community-based strategy against Aedes aegypti in northern and central Vietnam. *The American Journal Of Tropical Medicine And Hygiene*. 2010;82(5): 822-830.

[73] Kittayapong P, Yoksan S, Chansang U, Chansang C, Bhumiratana A. Suppression of dengue transmission by application of integrated vector control strategies at seropositive GIS-based foci. *The American Journal Of Tropical Medicine And Hygiene*. 2008;78(1):70-76.

[74] Madarieta SK, Salarda A, Benabaye MRS, Bacus MB, Tagle R. Use of permethrin-treated curtains for control of Aedes aegypti in the Philippines. *Dengue Bulletin*. 1999;23:51-54.

[75] Osaka K, Ha DQ, Sakakihara Y, Khiem HB, Umenai T. Control of dengue fever with active surveillance and the use of insecticidal aerosol cans. *The Southeast Asian Journal Of Tropical Medicine And Public Health*. 1999;30(3):484-488.

[76] Pengvanich V. Family leader empowerment program using participatory learning process for dengue vector control. *Journal Of The Medical Association Of Thailand = Chotmaihet Thangphaet*. 2011;94(2):235-241.

[77] Phan-Urai P, Kong-ngamsuk W, Malainual N. Field trial of Bacillus thuringiensis H-14 (Larvitab) against Aedes aegypti larvae in Amphoe Khlung, Chanthaburi Province, Thailand. *Journal of Tropical Medicine and Parasitology*. 1995;16:35-41.

[78] Suaya JA, Shepard DS, Caram M, Hoyer S, Nathan MB. Cost-effectiveness of annual targeted larviciding campaigns in Cambodia against the dengue vector Aedes aegypti. *Tropical Medicine and International Health*. 2007;12(9):1026-1036.

[79] Tan C-C. SARS in Singapore--key lessons from an epidemic. *Annals Of The Academy Of Medicine, Singapore*. 2006;35(5):345-349.

[80] Tun-Lin W, Lenhart A, Nam VS, Rebollar-Téllez E, Morrison AC, Barbazan P, et al. Reducing costs and operational constraints of dengue vector control by targeting productive breeding places: a multi-country non-inferiority cluster randomized trial. *Tropical Medicine & International Health: TM & IH*. 2009;14(9):1143-1153.

[81] Umniyati SR, Umayah SS. Evaluation of community-based Aedes control programme by source reduction in Perumnas Condong Catur, Yogyakarta, Indonesia. *Dengue Bulletin*. 2000;24:1-3.

[82] Van Kerkhove MD, Ly S, Guitian J, Holl D, San S, Mangtani P, et al. Changes in poultry handling behavior and poultry mortality reporting among rural Cambodians in areas affected by HPAI/H5N1. *Plos One*. 2009;4(7):e6466.

[83] Vanlerberghe V, Villegas E, Jirarojwatana S, Santana N, Trongtorkit Y, Jirarojwatana R, et al. Determinants of uptake, short-term and continued use of insecticide-treated curtains and jar covers for dengue control. *Tropical Medicine & International Health: TM & IH*. 2011;16(2):162-173

[84] Wolbachia. *FAQs*. Retrieved May 19, 2014, from http://www.eliminatedengue.com/faqs/index/type/wolbachia

[85] Oxitec Limited. *Dengue Fever Information Centre*. Retrieved July 26, 2014, from Oxitec: http://www.oxitec.com/our-targets/dengue-fever-and-chikungunya/

[86] United States Census Bureau. Retrieved July 20, 2014 from http://www.census.gov/popclock/

[87] Best Practices for supporting internet and development initiatives. http://www.fao.org/docrep/W6840E/w6840e06.htm

[88] United Nations. Housing the poor in Asian cities, Urbanization: The role the poor play in urban development. http://www.citiesalliance.org/sites/citiesalliance.org/files/QG1-Urbanization%5B2%5D.pdf

[89] CDC http://www.cdc.gov/phppo/pce/part1.htm

Developments in Potable Water Testing

Microbial Health Risks of Regulated Drinking Waters in the United States — A Comparative Microbial Safety Assessment of Public Water Supplies and Bottled Water

Stephen C. Edberg

Additional information is available at the end of the chapter

http://dx.doi.org/10.5772/58879

1. Introduction

The quality of drinking water in the United States (U.S.) is extensively monitored and regulated by federal, state and local agencies, yet there is increasing public concern and confusion about the safety and quality of drinking water — both from public water systems and from bottled water products. In the U.S., tap water and bottled water are regulated by two different agencies: the Environmental Protection Agency (EPA) regulates public water system water (tap water) and the Food and Drug Administration (FDA) regulates bottled water. Federal law requires that the FDA's regulations for bottled water must be at least as protective of public health as EPA standards for tap water [1].

The *quantity* of publically supplied water which is directly consumed as drinking water is estimated by the American Water Works Association to be less than four tenths of one percent (<0.4%) of the total produced [2]. As a food product, however, 100% of bottled water is intended for human consumption.

With respect to public water supplies, researchers estimate that more than 500 boil alerts occurred in the United States in 2010 [3]. In addition, the Centers for Disease Control and Prevention (CDC) reports that waterborne diseases, such as *Cryptosporidiosis* and *Giardiasis*, cost the U.S. healthcare system as much as $539 million a year in hospital expenses [4]. In 2006, EPA researchers reported an estimated 16.4 million cases of acute gastrointestinal illness per year are caused by tap water [5]. Subsequent research has estimated that the number of illnesses to be closer to 19.5 million cases per year [6].

In contrast, a survey of state bottled water regulatory authorities, dated June, 2009 and conducted by the Government Accountability Office (GAO), found there were zero outbreaks

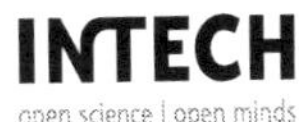

of foodborne illness from bottled water over a 5-year period. Moreover, in testimony before a July 9, 2009 Congressional hearing, a FDA official stated that the agency was aware of no major outbreaks of illness or serious safety concerns associated with bottled water in the past decade [7]. In addition, a review of the FDA's recall database reveals that only two Class I recalls of bottled water products have occurred since 1990. The first, occurring in Puerto Rico in June, 1990, was a recall of isopropyl alcohol that was labeled as "distilled water." The second recall, in 2007, involved five Armenian mineral water products imported into the U.S. with excessive arsenic levels, as discovered by testing completed by the FDA.

Drinking water experts have begun turning their attention to the distribution systems that carry the EPA-regulated public system drinking water from treatment plants to consumers. Emerging research has found that microbial issues in distribution systems are causing significant waterborne illness outbreaks, and that the outbreak incidence has been steadily increasing since the late 1980s [8].

The purpose of this review and position paper is to help educate the public about the importance of access to safe drinking water and inform policy makers and the general public about issues such as water distribution systems, infrastructure repair, safe water availability, and the EPA's regulation of public water systems for microbial contaminants and how this compares with the FDA's regulation of bottled water. All of these topics combined are potentially major contributing factors to impending health concerns and risks related to drinking water in the United States.

2. Comparison of regulations, standards, monitoring and advisories

2.1. Regulations

Public drinking water and bottled water are both regulated extensively. These regulations include an array of international, federal, state, and local agencies, and in some cases, trade associations. There are health-based standards for both tap and bottled waters, and these standards are, with few exceptions, the same [9].

Unlike tap water compliance failures, which generally result in monetary fines and requirements for corrective action, under the Park Doctrine, the failure of a bottled water product to meet the FDA Standards of Quality can result in criminal liability for the responsible person(s) in the manufacture and distribution of a food product that causes adverse health consequences to the public [10].

2.2. Standards

There are notable differences in standards for microbiological contaminants between bottled water and tap water. With the promulgation of the FDA's "Bottled Water Microbial Rule," effective December 1, 2009, bottled water now has standards specifically regulating total coliform (TC) and Escherichia coli (E. coli) in both non-Public Water System (PWS) source water and all finished product water. There are specific requirements for follow-up monitoring in the event of a positive test result for total coliform, i.e., each positive TC result must be evaluated for presence of E. coli. The FDA Rule also makes clear that:

1. If E. coli is detected and confirmed in non-PWS source water, that source water is not of a safe and sanitary quality for bottling, and must not be used as a source for bottled water. If that water is used for bottling, the finished product is considered by the FDA to be adulterated.

2. If E. coli is detected and confirmed in finished product water at any level, that product is also deemed adulterated under provisions of the Federal Food, Drug, and Cosmetic Act (FFDCA).

The EPA currently has no enforceable standard for either total coliform or E. coli in source waters. Under the EPA Groundwater Rule (GWR), groundwater-sourced PWSs must engage in additional source water testing and implement a sanitary survey, specified levels of treatment, and other corrective actions, but the source is not removed from service. However, the U.S. EPA published the revised Total Coliform Rule (rTCR) as a final rule on February 13, 2013. Although not yet promulgated, the Rule will affirm a new standard for E. coli in public drinking water, and will also require an investigation and corrective action at groundwater sources that test positive for E. coli. The revised TCR removes the standard for total coliform, while the FDA continues to regulate bottled water for both total coliform and E. coli.

With regard to response when a microbial standard is exceeded, bottled water compliance is determined from each individual test result in both the source and the finished product. When one sample exceeds the standard of quality for E. coli, and the bottler continues to use the source for bottling, the finished product is considered by the FDA to be adulterated and subject to recall. The FDA also clearly stated its policy on adulterated finished product in the 2009 Bottled Water Microbial Rule.

"If E. coli is present in bottled water, then the bottled water is deemed to be adulterated under section 402(a)(3) of the act (§ 165.110(b)(2)(i)(B); § 165.110(d))." 74 Fed. Reg. 25651 (May 29, 2009)

Public water systems are currently required to collect a specified number of samples per month, as is discussed in the monitoring section. The current EPA TCR maximum contaminant level (MCL) for total coliform is "no more than 5% of monthly samples are valid for total coliform." For example, if a small groundwater-sourced community water system collects only the required minimum of 25 samples per month, one of those samples may test positive for total coliform, but the system would be in compliance with the TCR. The TCR requires positive test results for total coliform to be confirmed for presence of E. coli. If any of the coliform samples are positive for E. coli, a public notification, usually with a boil water order, is issued to consumers. The new USEPA revised Total Coliform Rule will require public notification only for E. coli when it becomes effective (date to be determined).

The comparison of microbiological standards for bottled water and tap water is presented in the table.

Microbiological Contaminants	FDA SOQ	EPA MCL
Total coliform	If positive for total coliform, follow-up testing required to determine presence of E. coli in source water.	No MCL in source water.
	Finished product: MPN: <2.2 organisms per 100 ml. (8) MF: <4 CFU per 100 ml; arithmetic mean shall not exceed 1 coliform organism per 100 ml. (8)	No MCL in finished water.
Escherichia coli (E. coli)	None detected in source water. If detected, source water not of a safe, sanitary quality.	No MCL in source water. [11]
	None detected in finished product. If detected, product is deemed adulterated.	None detected in finished water. None detected in any of the follow-up samples if initial sample is positive.

Table 1. Comparison of microbiological standards

In addition, the EPA has established a guideline for heterotrophic plate count (HPC) bacteria of 500 CFU/ml as a means of demonstrating adequate levels of disinfection in the distribution system. This is not a health-based standard, and it is only used to indicate adequate disinfection in the distribution system. There are no standards or guidelines for HPC in bottled water. However, in 2002, the World Health Organization published a report on HPC bacteria in drinking water, concluding that "The available body of evidence supports the conclusion that, in the absence of fecal contamination, there is no direct relationship between HPC values in ingested water and human health effects in the population at large." Therefore, the HPC bacteria found in natural bottled waters is considered to be part of the natural flora of the water, and does not pose a health risk in the absence of fecal indicators such as E. coli [12]. Although HPC is not an FDA-required test for bottled water, most bottled water companies currently, or will, under upcoming rules from the Food Safety Modernization Act (FSMA), monitor for HPC as part of their ongoing internal sanitation control and environmental monitoring programs.

In addition, as Messner, et.al. (2006) notes, pathogens have a wide range of resistance to public water system disinfection and *Cryptosporidium* is the most resistant. "Free chlorine, the most commonly used disinfectant, achieves virtually no inactivation of *Cryptosporidium* but appears very effective for inactivating most viruses [5]." The FDA permits only the use of ground water not under the direct influence of surface water, as defined in 21 C.F.R. §141.2, as source water for bottling. Exclusion of such source waters also precluded the need to regulate bottled water for surface water parasites like *Cryptosporidium parvum* and *Giardia lamblia*.

2.3. Monitoring

It is in the area of monitoring activities that tap water and bottled water truly diverge. One major reason for this divergence is the method of delivery. Tap water is delivered to consumers through systems of underground piping, while bottled water is packaged in a sealed container and delivered to consumers through retail outlets and home delivery.

2.4. EPA monitoring requirements — Microbiological testing frequencies

Testing frequency for total coliform at groundwater and surface water-sourced Community Water Systems (CWSs) is based primarily on the population served. The number of samples required is prescribed on a monthly schedule. Therefore, a CWS will collect a minimum of anywhere from 1 up to 480 samples per month. The following table, which lists the number of samples to be tested, is taken from 40 CFR 141:

CWS Monitoring schedule for total coliform (From the USEPA RTCR) [11]

Population served	
Minimum number of samples per month	
2,501 to 3,300	3
3,301 to 4,100	4
4,101 to 4,900	5
4,901 to 5,800	6
5,801 to 6,700	7
6,701 to 7,600	8
7,601 to 8,500	9
8,501 to 12,900	10
12,901 to 17,200	15
17,201 to 21,500	20
21,501 to 25,000	25
25,001 to 33,000	30
33,001 to 41,000	40
41,001 to 50,000	50
50,001 to 59,000	60
59,001 to 70,000	70
70,001 to 83,000	80
83,001 to 96,000	90
96,001 to 130,000	100
130,001 to 220,000	120
220,001 to 320,000	150
320,001 to 450,000	180
450,001 to 600,000	210
600,001 to 780,000	240

Population served	
780,001 to 970,000	270
970,001 to 1,230,000	300
1,230,001 to 1,520,000	330
1,520,001 to 1,850,000	360
1,850,001 to 2,270,000	390
2,270,001 to 3,020,000	420
3,020,001 to 3,960,000	450
3,960,001 or more	480

2.5. FDA monitoring requirements

Bottled water sources (other than municipal water sources) are required to be tested for total coliform weekly at each source used for bottling. If any source water sample is positive for total coliform, the FDA requires that it be evaluated for presence of E. coli. If a sample is confirmed to be contaminated with E. coli, the source is considered not suitable for bottling, and any product that contains water from that source is considered by the FDA to be adulterated.

Each bottled water finished product type (spring water, purified water, fluoridated water, etc.) is required to be tested for total coliform weekly. If any product sample is positive for total coliform, the FDA requires that it be evaluated for presence of E. coli. If a sample is confirmed to be contaminated with E. coli, the product type is considered by the FDA to be adulterated.

To fully understand a comparison of bottled water testing and public water system testing, one must look at the relative size of the operations and the amount of water processed by each. The FDA states in the preamble to their March 3, 2003 direct final rule for radionuclides that they base sample frequency on the following:

"According to EPA's per capita total water use estimates applied to bottled water, an average bottled water facility processes as much water as a municipal system serving between 42 and 72 households... serving between 100 and 500 people, which is the closest category EPA presents."

Applying this principle, a community water system serving between 100 and 500 people is required by the USEPA to test a minimum of one (1) total coliform sample per month. The FDA requires one (1) total coliform sample per week.

2.6. Comparisons of bottled water plant testing and PWS testing for total coliform

For more direct comparison of bottled water and public water testing, here are examples of each for total coliform.

In the table below, a large bottled water plant packaging approximately 250,000 gallons per day is compared to New York City, which, according to 2009 data, distributed approximately 1.086 billion gallons of water per day within its distribution system.

Bottled Water Plant (large bottler, 1) (product type)	New York City (large city)
250,000 gallons per day	1.086 billion gallons per day
7.5 million gallons per month	32.58 billion gallons per month
1 sample per week; 4 samples per month	480 samples per month (~16 samples per day)
1 sample per 1,875,000 gallons	**1 sample per 67,875,000 gallons**
Sample Ratio: 36:1	

Disclaimer: Both the bottled water plant and New York City likely test more than the minimum number of samples each month. Numbers above based on minimum regulatory requirements.

Table 2. Total coliform testing comparison – Large City

As the table above shows, even though New York City is required to collect a minimum of 480 samples per month, when those samples are viewed on a gallons of water produced basis, the bottled water plant tests 36 times more frequently than the New York City system. Of course, this assumes only the minimum number of samples required by the FDA and the EPA is collected. In all likelihood, both the bottled water plant and New York City are collecting more than the minimum number of samples.

Below is a comparison of large bottled water plant with a smaller public water system – the groundwater-based CWS serving 10,000 that was reviewed earlier in this paper:

Bottled Water Plant (large bottler, 1) product type	CWS Serving 10,000 (small city)
250,000 gallons per day	1.2 million gallons per day
7.5 million gallons per month	36 million gallons per month
1 sample per week; 4 samples per month	10 samples per month
1 sample per 1,875,000 gallons	**1 sample per 3,600,000 gallons**
Sample Ratio: 2:1	

Table 3. Total coliform testing comparison – Small City

The Table below compares a small home and office delivery (HOD) bottled water plant with the CWS serving 10,000 people.

Bottled Water Plant (small bottler, 1) product type	CWS Serving 10,000 (small city)
25,000 gallons per day	1.2 million gallons per day
750,000 gallons per month	36 million gallons per month
1 sample per week, 4 samples per month	10 samples per month
1 sample per 187,500 gallons	1 sample per 3,600,000 gallons
Sample Ratio: 19:1	

Table 4. Total coliform testing comparison – Small City, small Bottler

The ratio of bottled water samples tested versus the number of CWS samples tested is up to 19:1. Once again, this assumes both the bottled water plant and the community water system are collecting only the minimum number of samples required by their respective regulations.

3. Advisories

3.1. When public drinking water does not meet EPA standards — Advisories

Public water systems must notify the public when they violate EPA or state drinking water regulations (including monitoring requirements) in cases when the drinking water may pose a risk to consumer's health [13]. Under the EPA notification rule, there are three tiers of notification, depending on the seriousness of the violation. The table below shows how public system drinking water violations are assessed.

	Required Distribution Time	**Notification Delivery Method**
Immediate Notice (Tier 1)	Any time a situation occurs where there is the potential for human health to be immediately impacted, water suppliers have 24 hours to notify people who may drink the water of the situation.	Water suppliers must use media outlets such as television, radio, and newspapers, post their notice in public places, or personally deliver a notice to their customers in these situations.
Notice as soon as possible (Tier 2)	Any time a water system provides water with levels of a contaminant that exceed EPA or state standards or that hasn't been treated properly, but that doesn't pose an immediate risk to human health, the water system must notify its customers as soon as possible, but within 30 days of the violation.	Notice may be provided via the media, posting, or through the mail.
Annual Notice (Tier 3)	When water systems violate a drinking water standard that does not have a direct impact on human health (For Example, failing to take a required sample on time) the water supplier has up to a year to provide a notice of this situation to its customers.	The extra time gives water suppliers the opportunity to consolidate these notices and send them with Annual Water Quality Reports (Consumer Confidence Reports).

Source: EPA, "Water: Public Notification Rule"

Table 5. EPA'S 3 tiers of public notification

The EPA reports that in 2011, 93.2 percent of US public water systems met health-based standards for drinking water. Also in that year, the EPA reports US public water systems had 8,431 total coliform rule violations affecting 9,837,344 people [14].

3.2. When bottled water does not meet FDA standards — Advisories

Under FDA rule (21 C.F.R.§165.110), bottled water that "contains a substance at a level considered injurious to health under section 402(a)(1) of the Federal Food, Drug, and Cosmetic Act (the act), or that consists in whole or in part of any filthy, putrid or decomposed substance, or that is otherwise unfit for food under section 402(a)(3) of the act is deemed to be adulterated, regardless of whether or not the water bears a label statement of substandard quality prescribed by paragraph (c) of this section. If E. coli is present in bottled water, then the bottled water will be deemed adulterated under section 402(a)(3) of the act [15]." Adulterated food and beverages should not enter the food supply, and if they do, the manufacturer could face criminal or civil penalties and mandatory recalls. Criminal penalties could be assessed under the Park Doctrine, which places responsibility for adulterated product on company owners and/or senior management.

The FDA's website recall database indicates that in 2011 and 2012 there was one incidence of a bottled water Class II recall [16]. Mountain Pure, LLC voluntarily recalled 23,000 16.9 oz. bottles of its Mountain Pure bottled water in Clinton, AR on May 4, 2011 because of a biological contamination. In a FDA press release, the Arkansas Department of Health said it was unlikely that a healthy person would get sick from drinking the water, but people with a weakened immune system might be at higher risk [17]. In 2014, in Pittsburgh there was precautionary voluntary recall of bottled water because of a preliminary finding of E. coli in a finished product. All confirmatory tests performed in a number of certified laboratories were negative for both E. coli and total coliforms. These negative findings plus the high ozone concentration used in bottled waters in Pennsylvania (plus the bottling plan in additions uses ultraviolet light) makes this finding of E. coli without any merit.

3.3. People who have immune-compromised illnesses

Waterborne diseases can lead to serious acute, chronic and sometimes fatal health consequences, especially for people who have compromised immune systems. Both the CDC and the EPA advise people who have immune-compromised illnesses (such as people undergoing chemotherapy, living with HIV/AIDS, transplant patients, children and infants, elderly and pregnant women) to consider taking extra precautions with their drinking water [18]. An EPA video and accompanying booklet aimed at educating health care providers about drinking water tells providers to advise these patients to "to consider alternatives to tap water [19]."

4. Comparison of estimated incidences of public water system-borne and bottled waterborne diseases

4.1. EPA approach to a national estimate

Research into drinking water-related incidences of acute gastrointestinal illness (AGI) is sparse largely due to gaps in data caused by reporting uncertainties. However, the EPA has developed an analytical approach and model for generating a national estimate of AGI illness due to drinking water and using this model, it is estimated that public water systems cause 16.4 million cases of AGI per year in the United States [5].

A Messner, et al. (2006) study uses AGI to measure public water system health risk because AGI is the broadest indicator of health effects associated with most water-borne pathogens and allows for comparison to national data on AGI incidence due to all causes. His study focuses on public water systems because 94% of the US population lives in a community that is served by public water systems. He acknowledges that water-borne diseases caused by non-public water systems could be significant, but a lack of data makes it difficult to include non-public water systems in calculating a national estimate.

In his research, Messner, et al. (2006) cites a Laval household intervention study that shows significant differences in Highly Credible Gastrointestinal Illness (HCGI) incidences between tap water drinkers and bottled water drinkers. "The difference in incidence between the two groups of 0.26 cases of HCGI per person-year represents the estimated attributable risk to drinking tap water [5]."

Meanwhile, a much broader study by Reynolds, et al. (2008) calculated all possible water-borne infections and illnesses associated with exposure to pathogens in drinking water, not just AGI, and concluded the estimated number of water-borne illnesses per year in the US is 19.5 million cases [6].

5. Outbreaks associated with bottled water

The FDA testified before a United States House of Representatives Subcommittee on Oversight and Investigations in July 2009 that the agency was aware of no major outbreaks of illness or serious safety concerns associated with bottled water in the past decade [20]. And said: "Because FDA's experience over the years has shown that bottled water has a good safety record, bottled water plants generally are assigned a relatively low priority for inspection."

At that same hearing, the Government Accountability Office (GAO) made public its report on bottled water, which found that based on a survey of water quality or food and health protection officials in all 50 states and the District of Columbia, there was no evidence that bottled water caused any illnesses during the previous five years [21].

Meanwhile, the CDC attributes just five cases of AGI to bottled water in the past 10 years [22]. (One case of AGI in 2007 caused by an unidentified agent, one case of AGI in 2004 caused by gasoline byproducts, and three cases of AGI in 2003 caused by the chemical bromate, unidentified chemical cleaning product, and unidentified agent.)

5.1. Outbreak comparison

The following table summarizes the estimated incidences of Public Water System-borne and Bottled Waterborne diseases.

Drinking Water Sources & Estimated Cases of AGI 2003 - 2012										
Tap Water:	2003	2004	2005	2006	2007	2008	2009	2010	2011	2012	Total
EPA	16.4m	16.4m	16.4m	16.4m	16.4m	16.4m	16.4m	16.4m	16.4m	16.4m	164m
Reynolds	19.5m	19.5m	19.5m	19.5m	19.5m	19.5m	19.5m	19.5m	19.5m	19.5m	195m
Bottled Water:	2003	2004	2005	2006	2007	2008	2009	2010	2011	2012	Total
FDA	0	0	0	0	0	0	0	0	0	0	0
GAO	n/a	n/a	n/a	n/a	n/a	0	0	0	0	0	0
CDC	3	1	0	0	1	0	0	0	0	0	5

Table 6. Drinking water sources & estimated cases of AGI 2003-2012

6. Distribution system and contact surface comparisons

EPA-mandated protocols are designed to effectively eliminate pathogens from public water system drinking water, but treatment inadequacies and interruptions, as well as public drinking water distribution system failures, have been associated with waterborne disease outbreaks [6]. In fact, recent research indicates distribution system failures are increasingly the cause of waterborne outbreaks [23].

The pipes that connect treatment plants to consumers' taps span 1 billion miles in the United States [24]. Researchers studying public health risks associated with contamination occurring in public water supply distribution systems have found a list of probable causes including: cross connections and backflow, intrusion caused by pressure transients, nitrification, permeation and leaching, water main repair and replacement, aging infrastructure and microbial growth inside distribution pipes [25].

6.1. Number of outbreaks caused by public water supply distribution systems

Data from the CDC's passive drinking water surveillance system indicates the incidence of public water supply waterborne disease outbreaks has actually decreased since the 1980s, presumably due to the EPA's Surface Water Treatment Rule and the Total Coliform Rule. However, the number of outbreaks due to public water supply distribution system issues and failures has remained relatively consistent despite an apparent increase in the percentage of those outbreaks (see chart below). It is also the case that if contamination occurs but only affects a small number of people, it may not be reported and investigated as an outbreak. "Indeed, it has been acknowledged that a fairly sizable number of cases of cryptosporidiosis could be occurring in a large city such as New York City without detection of a possible outbreak [26]."

In a more recent update of the above data, CDC reports that in 2009-2010, there were 33 drinking water outbreaks. Of the 33 outbreaks, 25 (75.8%) occurred in community water systems.

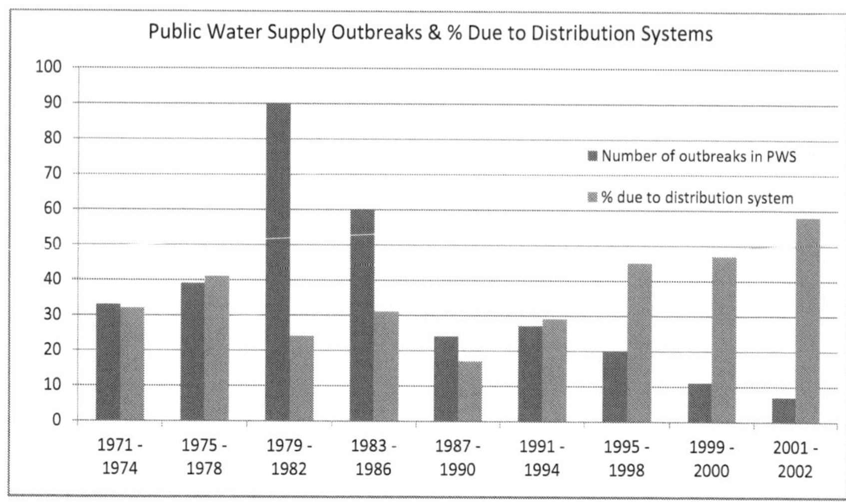

Source: "Public Water Supply Distribution Systems: Assessing and reducing risks," *National Academy of Sciences,* 2005.

Figure 1. Public water supply outbreaks and percentage due to distribution systems

6.2. Types of distribution deficiencies

Cross-connections and backflow issues pose serious public health threats. A backflow occurs when non-potable water flows directly into the drinking water supply through a cross connection, which occurs when the system has low water pressure or the non-potable system has backpressure [25]. A study that monitored public drinking supply distribution system failures from 1981 to 2002 found that 50% of waterborne outbreaks were the result of backflow [27]. A study by the University of Southern California examined the plumbing systems in 188 homes and found 9.6 percent had a direct cross connection that presented a health risk [28].

Water main breaks are another serious problem in the United States. Each day more than 700 water mains break, 36 exposing distribution system water and pipe interiors to external microbial and chemical contaminants, both during the break and the repair process. The EPA estimated in 2002 that 5 percent of all waterborne outbreaks due to distribution system deficiencies were caused by water main repairs or the installation of new pipes [29].

Issues with finished water storage (uncovered and reservoirs) is another cause of waterborne outbreaks as drinking water quality degrades over time and is susceptible to external contamination from wildlife, rain and algae [30]. Other public water supply distribution system risks include: biofilm build-up (the growth of bacteria on distribution system pipes and household plumbing), low-pressure intrusions [31] caused by leaks, permeation and leaching (in fact, 7 billion gallons leak from public water supply distribution pipes each day in the US [31] and the cost of water losses in 1994 was estimated $2.8 billion annually [32]).

Biofilm build-up, by itself, has been the subject of study by the EPA, which has concluded that: "Biofilms likely exist in all distribution systems, and are recognized as a normal part of the distribution system". Moreover, "...a wide range of primary and opportunistic pathogens have demonstrated the ability to survive, if not grow, in biofilms. These pathogens are of both fecal and non-fecal origin, and have a multitude of pathways through which they can enter the distribution system. Some of the pathogens identified as growing or potentially surviving in biofilms include Legionella, Mycobacterium avium complex, Pseudomonas aeruginosa, poliovirus 1, coxsackievirus B and several species of fungi. ...Once becoming established as part of the biofilm, pathogens can be protected from disinfection [33]."

6.3. Costs to address deficiencies in us public water supply distribution systems

According to the EPA's *Drinking Water Infrastructure Needs Survey and Assessment, 2009,* the national assessment of public water system infrastructure needs shows a total twenty-year capital improvement need of $334.8 billion, to repair or replace thousands of miles of pipe, thousands of treatment plants, storage tanks and other assets to protect the public health [34]. The pie chart below shows the majority of need is to address deficiencies with the public water supply distribution systems that include co-residency of leaking water pipes in the same trenches with leaking sewage lines [35].

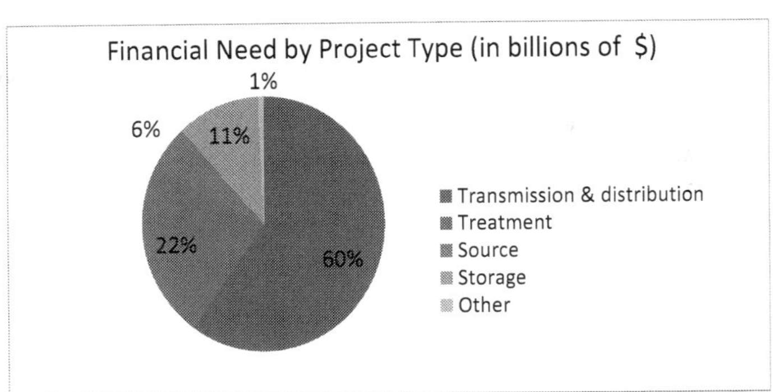

Source: EPA, "Drinking Water Infrastructure Needs Survey and Assessment," 2009

Figure 2. Financial requirement by repair type

In 2002, the EPA released a *Clean Water and Drinking Water Infrastructure Gap Analysis Report,* which calculated a "funding gap" of more than $500 billion dollars over the next 20 years. (Includes $122 billion for clean water capital costs, $102 billion for drinking water capital costs, $148 billion for clean water operation and maintenance and $161 billion for drinking water operation and maintenance [36]).

6.4. Water distribution

Under FDA rule (21 CFR Part 129), bottled water is: "required to be safe and that it be processed, bottled, held and transported under sanitary conditions. Processing practices addressed in the Current Good Manufacturing Practice (CGMP) regulations include protection of the water source from contamination, sanitation at the bottling facility, quality control to assure the bacteriological and chemical safety of the water, and sampling and testing of source water and the final product for microbiological, chemical, and radiological contaminants. Bottlers are required to maintain source approval and testing records to show to government inspectors [37]."

In addition, bottled water companies are required to conduct daily in-house total coliform monitoring on finished product of each product type and quarterly microbial rinse/swab tests which may be performed in-house by qualified plant personnel or by an approved laboratory on containers (incoming as well as those immediately from the washer) and closures as stipulated in 21 CFR Section 129.80 (f) [38]. This specific standard of sanitation for the interior of bottles and caps is: "No more than one of the four samples may exceed more than one bacterium per milliliter of capacity or one colony per square centimeter of surface area. All samples shall be free of coliform organisms." For example, not more than one of four 500 ml containers shall exceed 500 CFUs of bacteria. None of the containers are permitted to be positive for coliform bacteria. In comparison, there is an EPA guideline of 500 CFU/ml of heterotrophic plate count bacteria for public drinking water in the distribution system, beyond which the public water system must adjust disinfection levels to reduce the bacteria count. However, distribution pipes may still be lined with biofilms that may contribute to the bacteria load in the water.

Throughout the bottled water distribution system, each bottle is sealed and must remain sealed until it is opened by the consumer thus eliminating risk the of contamination during the distribution process. In addition, in the unlikely event that a problem with bottled water occurs, the product can be easily identified and recalled using a lot number printed on the bottled water container.

7. Conclusions

The quality of drinking water in the United States is extensively monitored and regulated by federal, state and local agencies, yet a close examination of both public system drinking water and bottled water processing and distribution procedures reveals striking differences that could explain why consumers have safety concerns regarding tap water. This paper has shown that on a gallon for gallon basis bottled water is tested more often than tap water. It is also the case that water quality breach notification differences means tap water drinkers would consume potentially hazardous drinking water before they are notified. Bottled water is tested before the water leaves the plant, and is withheld or withdrawn if the water does not meet FDA water quality standards.

A comparison of waterborne illness outbreaks reveals overwhelming evidence that the microbial health risks associated with drinking tap water are far greater than that of bottled water, with 195 million illnesses in the past 10 years for tap water compared to fewer than a dozen for bottled water.

In examining public water supply distribution systems, this paper highlights how deficiencies in these systems are key factors and causes of compromised tap water quality.

Overall, water is a precious resource. It has many uses for which there is no substitute and is therefore needed in many different ways for our survival and endurance. Thus, safe drinking water holds great value and to maintain its safety the public needs to stay educated and aware. Our government regulations are working to protect and produce our safe drinking water supply, but more needs to be done. And an informed consumer can help drive policies that will meet the needs of the American people—and ensure a safe drinking water supply.

Additional reading

J. Bartram, J. Cotruvo, M. Exner, C. Fricker, A. Glashmacher, eds., World Health Organization (2003). "Heterotrophic Plate Counts and Drinking-water Safety: The Significance of HPCs for Water Quality and Human Health".

F.A. Brigano, Ph.D. and Thomas A. Burke, "When is the Next *Boil Water Alert?*," *Water Conditioning & Purification*, August 2010, accessed October 2012, http://www.wcponline.com/pdf/August%20Flowing%20Issues.pdf

Centers for Disease Control and Prevention, "Reported Outbreaks Associated with Bottled Water", Commercially Bottled Water, accessed November 2012. http://www.cdc.gov/healthywater/drinking/bottled/

Centers for Disease Control and Prevention, "Waterborne Diseases Could Cost over $500 Million Annually in U.S.," press release, July 14, 2010, accessed October 2012, http://www.cdc.gov/media/pressrel/2010/r100714.htm

J. Cromwell, E. Speranza, and H. Reynolds. 2001a "Reinvesting in Drinking Water Infrastructure: Dawn of the Replacement Era." Denver, CO: AWWA.

Environmental Protection Agency, "Clean Water and Drinking Water Infrastructure Gap Analysis Report," 2002, accessed November 2012, http://water.epa.gov/infrastructure/sustain/infrastructureneeds.cfm

Environmental Protection Agency, "Drinking Water Infrastructure Needs Survey and Assessment," 2009, accessed November 2012, http://water.epa.gov/infrastructure/drinkingwater/dwns/upload/2009_03_26_needssurvey_2007_report_needssurvey_2007.pdf

Environmental Protection Agency, "Fiscal Year 2010 Drinking Water and Ground Water Statistics", June 2011, access December 2012, http://water.epa.gov/scitech/datait/databases/

drink/sdwisfed/upload/new_Fiscal-Year-2010-Drinking-Water-and-Ground-Water-Statistics-Report-Feb-2012.pdf

Environmental Protection Agency, "New or Repaired Water Mains," August 2002, accessed November 2012 http://water.epa.gov/lawsregs/rulesregs/sdwa/tcr/upload/neworrepairedwatermains.pdf

Environmental Protection Agency, Tap into Prevention, accessed December 2012, http://www.epa.gov/ogwdw/healthcare/pdfs/booklet_healthcarevideo_suppliement.pdf

Environmental Protection Agency, "Water: Public Notification Rule", accessed November 2012, http://water.epa.gov/lawsregs/rulesregs/sdwa/publicnotification/basicinformation.cfm

Environmental Protection Agency, Water on Tap: what you need to know, 2009, accessed December 2012, http://water.epa.gov/drink/guide/upload/book_waterontap_full.pdf

Food and Drug Administration, Safety – Recalls, accessed December 2012, http://www.fda.gov/Safety/Recalls/default.htm

Food and Drug Administration, Safety – Recalls, press release, May 4, 2011, accessed December 2012, http://www.fda.gov/Safety/Recalls/ucm254580.htm

Food and Drug Administration, Section 410, Federal Food, Drug & Cosmetic Act

Food and Drug Administration HHS, CFR-2010-title21-vol2, PART 165—BEVERAGES, accessed December 2012, http://www.gpo.gov/fdsys/pkg/CFR-2010-title21-vol2/pdf/CFR-2010-title21-vol2-sec165-110.pdf

Government Accountability Office, "Appendix III, Telephone survey administered to Officials from 50 States and the District of Columbia, and Summary of Responses," *United States Government Accountability Office Report on Bottled Water*, GAO-09-610, June 2009, accessed December 2012, http://www.gao.gov/new.items/d09861t.pdf

R. Hirst, "Bottled Water and Tap Water: Just the facts", Drinking Water Research Foundation, accessed October 2012). http://www.thefactsaboutwater.org/uploads/BW%20PWS%20Just%20the%20Facts%202011%20Final.pdf

International Bottled Water Association, *Model Code of Practice*, 2009, accessed November 2012, http://www.bottledwater.org/public/pdf/IBWA05ModelCode_Mar2.pdf

C.J. Kirmeyer, W. Richards, and C.D. Smith, "An Assessment of Water Distribution Systems and Associated Research Needs", *AWWA Research Foundation: Distribution Systems*, 1994.

M. LeChevallier, "Drinking Water: Challenges and Solutions for the Next Century," *Yale University Drinking Water Symposium*, 2009, accessed November 2012, http://www.yale-seas.com/watersymposium/

M. Messner, S. Shaw, S. Regli, K. Rotert, V. Blank and J. Soller, "An approach for developing a national estimate of waterborne disease due to drinking water and a national estimate model application," *Journal of Water and Health* 4(Suppl. 2).

National Academy of Sciences, "Public Water Supply Distribution Systems: Assessing and reducing risks," 2005, accessed October 2012, http://www.nap.edu/catalog.php?record_id=11262

National Research Council, "Watershed Management for Potable Water Supply: the New York City Strategy," The National Academies Press, page 249.

Natural Resources Defense Council, "Climate Change, Water and Risk: current water demands are not sustainable," accessed October 2012, http://www.nrdc.org/globalwarming/watersustainability/index.asp

M. Provost, "Evaluating the Potential Causes of Excess GI Illnesses Observed in the Payment's Distribution System," *Yale University Drinking Water Symposium*, 2009, accessed November 2012, http://www.yaleseas.com/watersymposium/

K.A. Reynolds, K.D. Mena, C.P. Gerba, "Risk of waterborne illness via drinking water in the United States," *Reviews of Environmental Contamination and Toxicology* 2008;192:117-58, accessed October 2012, http://www.ncbi.nlm.nih.gov/pubmed/18020305

Testimony of Joshua M. Sharfstein, M.D., Principal Deputy Commissioner of Food and Drugs, *FDA*, before an United States House of Representatives Oversight and Investigations Subcommittee hearing on bottled water, accessed November 2012. http://www.hhs.gov/asl/testify/2009/07/t20090708a.html

United States Code Statutes:
Federal Food, Drug, and Cosmetic Act:
§ 410, Bottled Drinking Water Standards, 21 U.S.C. § 349.
§ 414, Maintenance and Inspection of Records, 21 U.S.C. § 350c.
§ 709, Presumption of Interstate Commerce, 21 U.S.C. § 379a.
FDA Injunction against Distribution: 21 U.S.C. § 332.
FDA Criminal Penalties: 21 U.S.C. § 333.
FDA Product Seizure: 21 U.S.C. § 334(a).
FDA Administrative Detention: 21 U.S.C. § 334(g).
Food Safety Modernization Act: § 206, Mandatory Recall Authority, 42 U.S.C. § 247b-20.
Safe Drinking Water Act", §1412, 21 U.S.C. § 300g-1.
U.S. Food and Drug Administration Regulations:
Facility Registration: 21 CFR §§ 1.225-1.243.
Records Maintenance: 21 CFR §§ 1.326-1.368.
Recall Procedures: 21 CFR § 7.40-7.59.
Food Labeling: 21 CFR § 101.
Current Good Manufacturing Practices: 21 CFR § 110.
Bottled Water CGMPs: 21 CFR § 129.
Bottled Water Standards of Identity and Quality: 21 CFR § 165.110 (a) and (b).
Food Additive Regulations: 21 CFR § 177.

"Bottled Water Microbial Rule", 74 Fed. Reg. 25651 (May 29, 2009)

Rule on Radionuclides, 68 Fed. Reg. 9873 (March 3, 2003)

U.S. Food and Drug Administration Administrative Decisions:

70 Fed. Reg. 33694 (June 9, 2005)

66 Fed. Reg. 35439 (July 5, 2001)

63 Fed. Reg. 42199 (August 6, 1998)

U.S. Environmental Protection Agency Regulations:

Public Water System Quality Standards: 40 CFR 141, Subparts G and L.

Monitoring Requirements: 40 CFR 141, Subparts C, E, I, and L.

"Surface Water Treatment Rule", 54 Fed. Reg. 27486 (June 29, 1989)

"Interim Enhanced Surface Water Treatment Rule", 63 Fed. Reg. 69478 (December 16, 1998)

"Long Term 1 Enhanced Surface Water Treatment Rule", 67 Fed. Reg. 1812 (January 14, 2002)

"Long Term 2 Enhanced Surface Water Treatment Rule", 71 Fed. Reg. 654 (January 5, 2006)

"Ground Water Rule", 71 Fed. Reg. 65574 (November 8, 2006)

U.S. Environmental Protection Agency Resources:

"The Standardized Monitoring Framework: A Quick Reference Guide," EPA 816-F-04-010

www.epa.gov/safewater, March, 2004.

USEPA Public Water System Pivot Tables for FY 2010 (Data from July 1, 2009 through June 30, 2010).

Downloaded from http://water.epa.gov/scitech/datait/databases/drink/pivottables.cfm.

Yale University: The "Your Drinking Water: Challenges and Solutions for the 21st Century" Symposium was held at Yale University on April 20th & 21st, 2009. The purpose of the symposium was to bring together individuals who are leaders in their fields and discuss, given his/her area, the following:

- Introduction to his/her area

- Data regarding his/her area

- Analysis of the data

- Challenges faced

- Proposed solutions

The conference was conducted by Stephen Edberg, Professor in the Department of Laboratory Medicine at Yale's School of Medicine, Menachem Elimelech, Professor and Chair of the Chemical Engineering Department and Environmental Engineering Program at Yale's School of Engineering & Applied Science, and Dr. John Sinnott, Associate Dean and Professor at the Infectious Disease and International Medicine Department of the University of South Florida. It is the goal that policy makers and others will use the conference and its publications as the basis for decision making. The conference's publications are in the public domain and include: Full video presentations, supplementary papers, full transcripts, PowerPoint presentations, and speakers' biographies. Accessed January 2013, http://www.yaleseas.com/watersymposium.

Acknowledgements

The author acknowledges the Department of Chemical and Environmental Engineering, Environmental, Yale University for providing a forum from which much of this information was generated and Robert Hirst and Jill Culora of the International Bottled Water Association for their meticulous verification and generation of information. In addition Martin Allen of the American Water Works Association Research Foundation is thanked for review of this document. Lize-Mari Russo is thanked for her excellent technical assistance. http://www.yale-seas.com/watersymposium/

Author details

Stephen C. Edberg[1]

Address all correspondence to: stephen.edberg@Yale.edu

1 Mt. Sinai Health System, New York, New York, USA

2 Yale University School of Medicine, New Haven, Connecticut, USA

References

[1] Federal Food, Drug, and Cosmetic Act, Chapter IV, Section 410, § 349 (2010).

[2] Roberson, A., P. E. (2009). Your Drinking Water: A 21st Century Challenge and Solutions, slide #4. Yale Drinking Water Symposium. Retrieved January 2013 from http://www.yaleseas.com/watersymposium/powerpoints.html

[3] Brigano F. A., Ph.D. and Burke T. A. (August 2010). When is the Next Boil Water Alert? Water Conditioning & Purification. Retrieved October 2012 from http://www.wcponline.com/pdf/August%20Flowing%20Issues.pdf

[4] Centers for Disease Control and Prevention. (July 14, 2010). Waterborne Diseases Could Cost over $500 Million Annually in U.S. (press release). Retrieved October 2012 from http://www.cdc.gov/media/pressrel/2010/r100714.htm

[5] Messner, M., Shaw, S., Regli, S., Rotert, K., & Soller, J. (2006). An approach for developing a national estimate of waterborne disease due to drinking water and a national estimate model application. Journal of Water and Health 4 (Supp. 2), 201.

[6] Reynolds, K. A., Mena, K. D., & Gerba, C. P. (2008). Risk of waterborne illness via drinking water in the United States. Reviews of Environmental Contamination and Toxicology, 192,117-58. Retrieved October 2012 from http://www.ncbi.nlm.nih.gov/pubmed/18020305

[7] House Committee on Energy and Commerce, Subcommittee on Oversight and Investigations. Regulation of Bottled Water, Hearing. (July 8, 2009). Statement of Joshua M. Sharfstein, M.D., Principal Deputy Commissioner of Food and Drugs, Food and Drug Administration, Department of Health and Human Services. Retrieved January 2013 from http://www.fda.gov/NewsEvents/Testimony/ucm170932.htm

[8] National Research Council Division on Earth and Life Studies, Water Science and Technology Board Committee on Public Water Supply Distribution Systems. (2005). Public Water Supply Distribution Systems: Assessing and Reducing Risks, National Research Council of the National Academies. Retrieved October 2012 from http://www.nap.edu/catalog.php?record_id=11262

[9] Hirst, R. (2011). Bottled Water and Tap Water: Just the Facts. Drinking Water Research Foundation. Retrieved October 2012 from http://www.thefactsaboutwater.org.

[10] FDA Regulatory Procedures Manual. (2011). Chapter 6, 49. Retrieved January 2013 from http://www.fda.gov/downloads/ICECI/ComplianceManuals/RegulatoryProceduresManual/UCM074317.pdf

[11] USEPA Revised Total Coliform Rule – Final Rule, published in the Federal Register on February 13, 2013, requires an MCL for E. coli in source water.

[12] Allen, M., Edberg, S., & Reasoner, D. (2004). HPC Bacteria in Drinking Water: Public Health Implications Heterotrophic plate count bacteria—what is their significance in drinking water? International Journal of Food Microbiology, 92(3). Retrieved January 2013 from http://www.sciencedirect.com/science/article/pii/S0168160503004537

[13] EPA website (n.d.). Water: Public Notification Rule. Retrieved November 2012 from http://water.epa.gov/lawsregs/rulesregs/sdwa/publicnotification/basicinformation.cfm

[14] EPA. (2011). Fiscal Year 2010 Drinking Water and Ground Water Statistics. Retrieved December 2012 from http://water.epa.gov/scitech/datait/databases/drink/sdwisfed/upload/new_Fiscal-Year-2010-Drinking-Water-and-Ground-Water-Statistics-Report-Feb-2012.pdf

[15] FDA. (2010). CFR-2010-title21-vol2, PART 165—BEVERAGES. Retrieved December 2012 from http://www.gpo.gov/fdsys/pkg/CFR-2010-title21-vol2/pdf/CFR-2010-title21-vol2-sec165-110.pdf

[16] FDA. (n.d.). Safety – Recalls. Retrieved December 2012 from http://www.fda.gov/Safety/Recalls/default.htm

[17] FDA. (2011). Safety – Recalls (press release). Retrieved December 2012 from http://www.fda.gov/Safety/Recalls/ucm254580.htm

[18] EPA. (2009). Water on Tap: what you need to know. Retrieved December 2012 from http://water.epa.gov/drink/guide/upload/book_waterontap_full.pdf

[19] EPA. (2004). Tap into Prevention. Retrieved December 2012 from http://www.epa.gov/ogwdw/healthcare/pdfs/booklet_healthcarevideo_suppliement.pdf

[20] House Committee on Energy and Commerce, Subcommittee on Oversight and Investigations. Regulation of Bottled Water, Hearing. (July 8, 2009). Statement of Joshua M. Sharfstein, M.D., Principal Deputy Commissioner of Food and Drugs, Food and Drug Administration, Department of Health and Human Services. Retrieved January 2013 from http://www.fda.gov/NewsEvents/Testimony/ucm170932.htm

[21] United States Government Accountability Office (2009) Report on Bottled Water, "Appenix III, Telephone survey administered to Officials from 50 States and the District of Columbia, and Summary of Responses". GAO-09-610. Retrieved December 2012 from http://www.gao.gov/new.items/d09861t.pdf

[22] CDC. (n.d.). Reported Outbreaks Associated with Bottled Water, Commercially Bottled Water. Retrieved November 2012 from http://www.cdc.gov/healthywater/drinking/bottled/

[23] Allen, M. (2009). Integrity of Distribution Systems: Role of Microbial Monitoring, supplemental paper, 16-19. Yale Symposium. Retrieved January 2013 from http://www.yaleseas.com/watersymposium/pdfs/allen1.pdf

[24] Kirmeyer, C.J., Richards, W., & Smith, C.D. (1994). An Assessment of Water Distribution Systems and Associated Research Needs, AWWA Research Foundation: Distribution Systems.

[25] National Research Council Division on Earth and Life Studies, Water Science and Technology Board Committee on Public Water Supply Distribution Systems. (2005).

[26] National Research Council. (1999). Watershed Management for Potable Water Supply: the New York City Strategy. The National Academies Press. 249.

[27] Prevost, M. (2009). Evaluating the Potential Causes of Excess GI Illnesses Observed in the Payment's Distribution System, Yale University Drinking Water Symposium. Retrieved November 2012 from http://www.yaleseas.com/watersymposium/

[28] Cromwell, J., Speranza, E., & Reynolds, H. (2001). Reinvesting in Drinking Water Infrastructure: Dawn of the Replacement Era. Denver, CO. American Water Works Association.

[29] EPA. (2002). New or Repaired Water Mains. Retrieved November 2012 http:// water.epa.gov/lawsregs/rulesregs/sdwa/tcr/upload/neworrepairedwatermains.pdf

[30] National Research Council Division on Earth and Life Studies, Water Science and Technology Board Committee on Public Water Supply Distribution Systems. (2005).

[31] Le Chevallier, M. (2009). Water Quality Risk Modeling, slides 27-29. Yale Drinking Water Symposium. Retrieved January 2013 from http://www.yaleseas.com/water-symposium/powerpoints.html

[32] EPA. (2002). New or Repaired Water Mains. Retrieved November 2012 from http:// water.epa.gov/lawsregs/rulesregs/sdwa/tcr/upload/neworrepairedwatermains.pdf

[33] EPA. (2002). Health Risks from Microbial Growth and Biofilms in Drinking Water Distribution Systems, Office of Ground Water and Drinking Water Distribution System White Paper. 2 & 36. Retrieved January 2013 from http://www.epa.gov/ogwdw/ disinfection/tcr/pdfs/whitepaper_tcr_biofilms.pdf

[34] EPA. (2009). Drinking Water Infrastructure Needs Survey and Assessment. Retrieved November 2012 from http://water.epa.gov/infrastructure/drinkingwater/dwns/ upload/2009_03_26_needssurvey_2007_report_needssurvey_2007.pdf

[35] Le Chevallier, M. (2009). Separation from Sewer Lines, slide 16. Yale Drinking Water Symposium. Retrieved January 2013 from http://www.yaleseas.com/watersymposi-um/powerpoints.html

[36] EPA. (2002). Clean Water and Drinking Water Infrastructure Gap Analysis Report. Retrieved November 2012 from http://water.epa.gov/infrastructure/sustain/infra-structureneeds.cfm

[37] FDA. (n.d.). For Consumers – Bottled water and carbonated soft drinks guidance documents and regulatory information.Retrieved November 2012 from http:// www.fda.gov/ForConsumers/ConsumerUpdates/ucm077065.htm

[38] International Bottled Water Association. (2012). Bottled Water Model Code of Practice. Retrieved November 2012 from http://www.bottledwater.org/files/ IBWA_MODEL_CODE_2012_1212_FINAL_0.pdf

Accelerated Detection of Microbes Utilizing an Organic Particle Catalyst in the Total Coliforms and *Escherichia coli* MMO-MUG (Colilert®) test

Stephen C. Edberg

Additional information is available at the end of the chapter

http://dx.doi.org/10.5772/59128

1. Introduction

In 1992, the United States Environmental Protection Agency (EPA) approved the first dual total coliform and *Escherichia coli* (*E. coli*) direct detection test for public drinking water [1]. The MMO-MUG test, commercially known as Colilert® (Idexx Laboratories Inc., Westbrook, ME), could detect 1 total coliform or 1*E. coli* in a 100 mL sample in 24 hours of incubation [2]. Over the next decades, the original MMO-MUG and variants have achieved worldwide use with consistently robust accuracy. Recently one form of the MMO-MUG, Colilert-18®, achieved European Union recognition as an ISO standard for total coliforms and *E. coli* [3].

One barrier to the utilization of new methods has been the need for an 18 to 24 hour incubation time. One form of the MMO-MUG, Colilert-18®, has a shorter incubation time than the original but requires an inconvenient and time consuming pre-heating step. Employing a new strategy that fosters the development of biofilm by incorporation of inert natural particles in the sample was reported to significantly reduce the incubation time of the MMO-MUG drinking water tests and other microbiological analyses.

The natural particles (see Figure 1) are made as a dried hydrophilic colloid extract obtained from *Gelidium cartilagineum*, *Gracilaria confervoides*, *Pterocladia lucida* and related algae of the class *Rhodophyceae*. These particles (Colloidands®, Pilots Point LLC, Sarasota, FL) have no innate significant nutritive value with the following composition: total fat 0%, saturated fat 0%, polyunsaturated fat 0%, monounsaturated fat 0%, cholesterol 0% sodium <1 mg/L, potassium 23 mg/L; total carbohydrate 0.7 g/L, fiber 0.1 g/L, sugar 0 g/L, protein 0 g/L, iron 10 g/L.

The particles are a heterogeneous natural mixture:

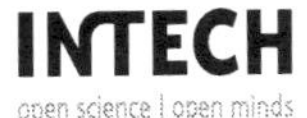

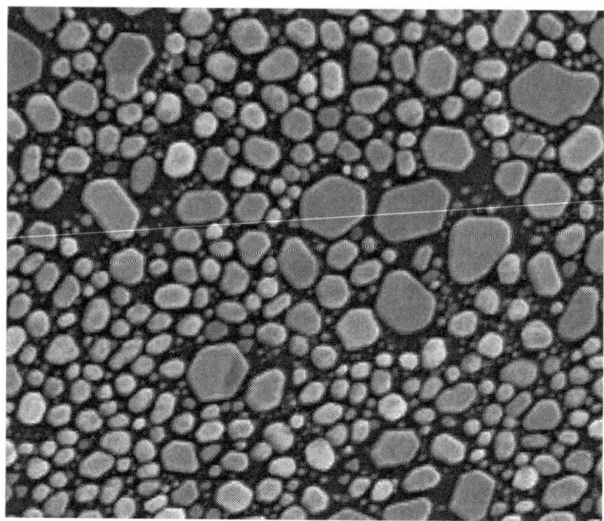

Figure 1. High resolution photomicrograph of the phycocolloid particles (Colloidands®, Pilots Point LLC, Sarasota, FL)

A study was conducted with the original MMO-MUG (Colilert®) to determine if from cold water < 8°C the incorporation of the particles could significantly reduce detection time of total coliforms and *E. coli*

2. Materials and methods

2.1. Activity of the particles

In order to establish that the particles were acting as a physical catalyst, the Colisure® variation of the MMO-MUG test was used. This test uses a yellow/gold beta-galactosidase substrate that becomes red/magenta when positive. Accordingly, the exact physical location of the beginning of the development of color could be directly determined photographically.

Colloidands® particles (Pilots Point LLC, Sarasota, FL) were added to the Colisure® test at 10 grams per liter. Both the standard Idexx *Klebsiella pneumoniae* (*K. pneumoniae*) and *Escherichia coli* (*E. coli*) quality control bacteria were utilized. Photographic records were taken each hour of incubation at 35°C for 20 hours at a concentration of 10 bacteria per mL.

2.2. Level of sensitivity

2.2.1. Quality control Klebsiella and Escherichia coli (Idexx Laboratories Inc., Westbrook, Maine)

Figure 2 and Figure 3 describe the complete protocol by which the MMO-MUG (Colilert®) was examined for its ability to detect 1 total coliform and 1 *E. coli* in 16 hours. For the purpose of studying universally available bacteria, the standard quality control strains available from the manufacturer of Colilert® (Idexx Laboratories Inc., Westbrook, ME) were utilized. Virtually all water testing laboratories use these for quality control or have access to them.

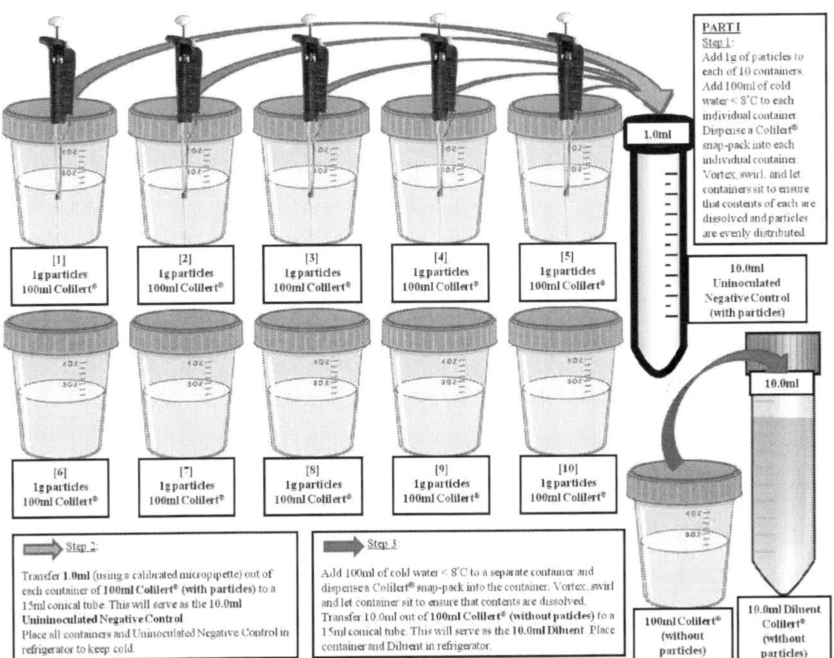

Figure 2. Test Protocol Part I for the detection of 1 total coliform *Klebsiella* and 1 *E. coli* in 16 hours

Analysis was made both by visual observation and also by an instrument. Visual observation: Yellow color development (for total coliforms and *E. coli*) and fluorescence (*E. coli*) was determined each hour while there was a person in the laboratory. The observations were structured to best represent the optimum work pattern in the standard drinking water laboratory: inoculation no later than 4 pm (1600 hours) and the reading of results at 8 am (0800 hours) the next day.

Instrumented Analysis: Figure 4 presents the Pilots Point Monitor (Pilots Point LLC, Sarasota, FL) that was used. This instrument utilizes white light sent through a sample and determines the change in three parameters: Luminosity, or white to black (a measure of turbidity), called the "L" value; a change from red to green (called the "a" value), and a change from blue to yellow (called the "b" value). See Figure 5. Measurements are made every 15 minutes. The instrument can measure light changes from 365 nm through the visible spectrum therefore it can detect both the color change produced by total coliforms and the fluorescence produced by *E. coli*.

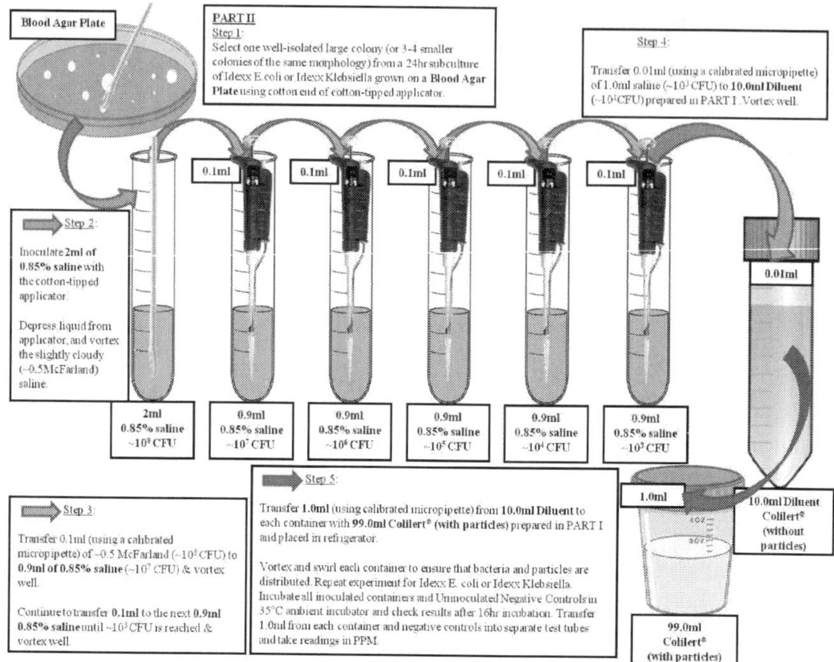

Figure 3. Test Protocol Part II for the detection of 1 total coliform *Klebsiella* and 1 *E. coli* in 16 hours

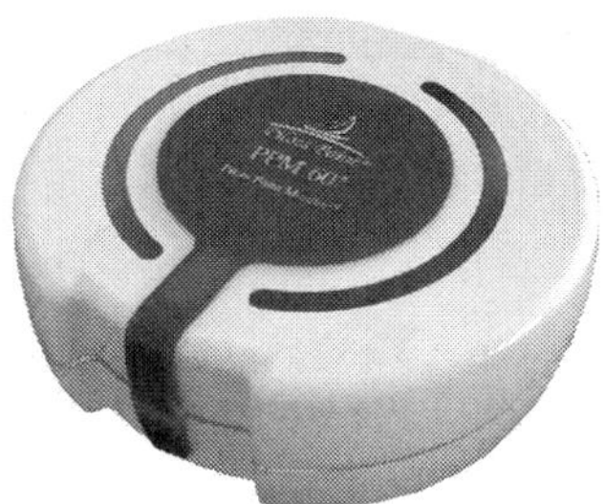

Figure 4. Pilots Point Monitor® (PPM60®)

2.3. Isolates from source water

Lake source water from the supply to the Regional Water Authority (New Haven, CT) was obtained. While protected from human intrusion, there are abundant animal life, particular deer, rabbit, and small animals. This is the same water source that was used in the original certification of the MMO-MUG test [4].

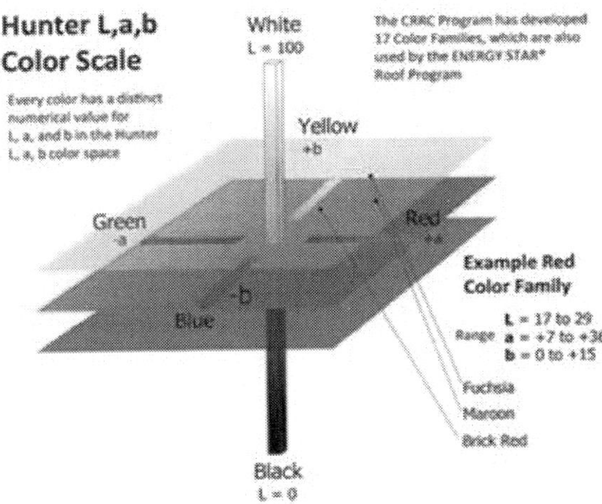

Figure 5. Principle of Pilots Point Instrument

The same protocol as for the quality control bacteria described in the protocol (see Figure 2 and Figure 3) was used. To avoid possible enhancement of enzyme stimulation by the substrates present in the MMO-MUG formula, the source water samples were processed by the classical membrane filtration method as described in Standard Methods [5]. Bacteria consistent with total coliforms and *E. coli* were identified to species (API® ID strip range, bioMérieux, Durham, NC).

3. Results

3.1. Activity of the particles

Figure 6 presents the results of the Colloidands® particle analysis. The top tube is inoculated with Idexx *Klebsiella*, the bottom tube with Idexx *E. coli*. The original color of the Colisure® is yellow/gold; a positive occurs when the hydrolysable substrate is cleaved during growth and multiplication. The particles have largely sunk to the bottom of the tube. It is clearly shown that the red/magenta color is overwhelmingly seen in the particle layer at the bottom of the test tube. Over time, the positive color spreads fully into the liquid layer. The observation that the particle layer consistently is where the color develops first substantiates the ability of the particles to accelerate the growth and multiplication of the target bacteria.

3.2. Level of sensitivity

Table 1 and Graph 1 present the visual observation of the Colilert® test with and without phycocolloid particles at low numbers of *E. coli*, Table 2 and Graph 2 present the visual

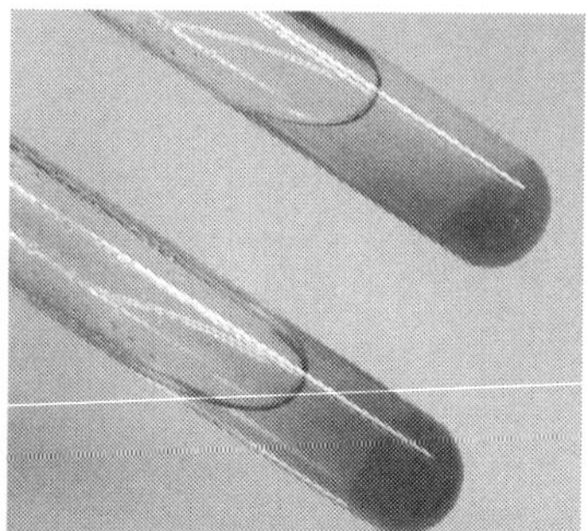

Figure 6. Growth of total coliform *Klebsiella* and *E. coli* utilizing phycocolloids as catalysts

observation of Colilert® with *Enterobacter cloacae* (*E. cloacae*) added, Table 3 and Graph 3 present the observation with *K. pneumoniae* added, and Table 4 and Graph 4 present the observation with *E. coli* added. The water was < 8°C and there were 7 grams of Colloidands® particles per liter of Colilert®. Overall the presence of the particles decreases the time to a positive, both for *K. pneumoniae* and *E. coli* demonstrating the efficacy of the particles. Specifically both for the Idexx *Klebsiella* and Idexx *E. coli*, Colilert® is able to detect 1 bacterium in 100 mL of water in 16 hours or less as seen in Figure 7.

E. coli added count	Hours to Yellow (no particles)	Hours to Fluorescence (no particles)	Hours to Yellow (7g particles)	Hours to Fluorescence (7g particles)
10 CFU (test a)	16	16	10	10
10 CFU (test b)	19	22	11	15
10 CFU + NTO (test a)	13	13	11	11
10 CFU + NTO (test b)	13	13	10	10
1 CFU + NTO (test a)	14	16	11	11
1 CFU + NTO (test b)	14	15	11	10

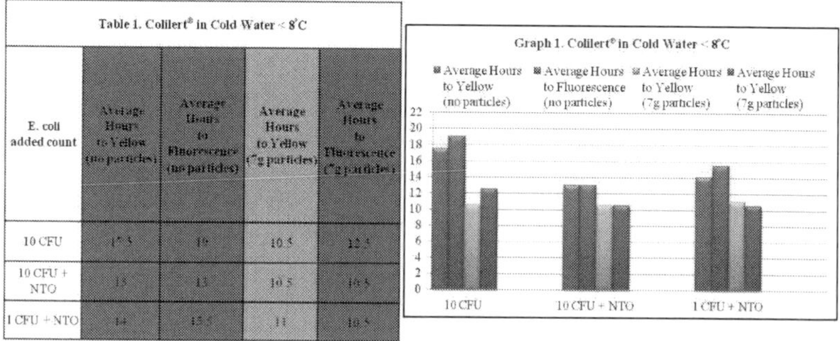

Table 1. Colilert® in Cold Water < 8°C

E. coli added count	Average Hours to Yellow (no particles)	Average Hours to Fluorescence (no particles)	Average Hours to Yellow (7g particles)	Average Hours to Fluorescence (7g particles)
10 CFU	17.5	19	10.5	12.5
10 CFU + NTO	13	13	10.5	10.5
1 CFU + NTO	14	15.5	11	10.5

Graph 1. Comparison of Time to Detection of MMO-MUG (Colilert®) with and without phycoccolloids. CFU (colony forming units), NTO (non-target organisms), Neg (negative)

E. cloacae (24 isolates)	Hours to Yellow (no particles)	Hours to Fluorescence (no particles)	Hours to Yellow (7g particles)	Hours to Fluorescence (7g particles)
10 CFU (test a)	16	Neg	12	Neg
10 CFU (test b)	18	Neg	11	Neg
10 CFU + NTO (test a)	13	Neg	12	Neg
10 CFU + NTO (test b)	13	Neg	12	Neg
1 CFU + NTO (test a)	21	Neg	15	Neg
1 CFU + NTO (test b)	20	Neg	15	Neg

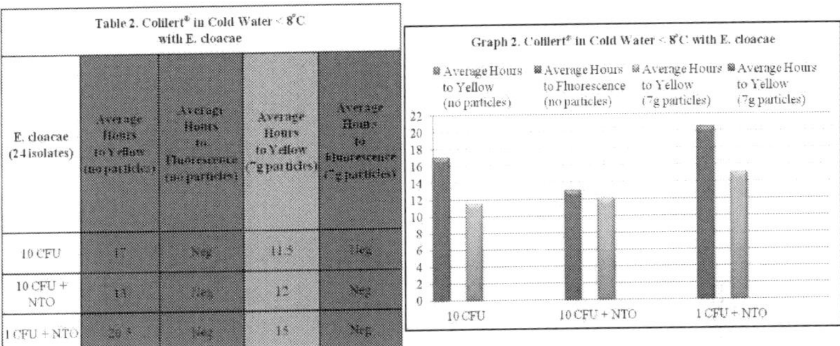

Graph 2. Comparison of Time to Detection of MMO-MUG (Colilert®) with and without phycoccolloids with *E. cloacae* added. CFU (colony forming units), NTO (non-target organisms), Neg (negative)

K. pneumoniae (31 isolates)	Hours to Yellow (no particles)	Hours to Fluorescence (no particles)	Hours to Yellow (7g particles)	Hours to Fluorescence (7g particles)
10 CFU (test a)	16	Neg	10	Neg
10 CFU (test b)	19	Neg	11	Neg
10 CFU + NTO (test a)	13	Neg	11	Neg
10 CFU + NTO (test b)	13	Neg	10	Neg
1 CFU + NTO (test a)	21	Neg	15	Neg
1 CFU + NTO (test b)	20	Neg	14	Neg

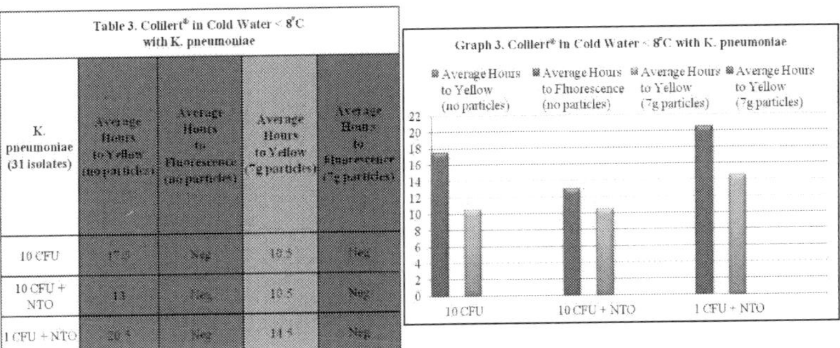

Graph 3. Comparison of Time to Detection of MMO-MUG (Colilert®) with and without phycoccolloids with *K. pneumoniae* added. CFU (colony forming units), NTO (non-target organisms), Neg (negative)

E. coli (8 isolates)	Hours to Yellow (no particles)	Hours to Fluorescence (no particles)	Hours to Yellow (7g particles)	Hours to Fluorescence (7g particles)
10 CFU (test a)	16	16	10	10
10 CFU (test b)	19	22	11	14
10 CFU + NTO (test a)	13	14	11	11
10 CFU + NTO (test b)	13	13	10	11
1 CFU + NTO (test a)	21	21	15	14
1 CFU + NTO (test b)	20	21	15	15

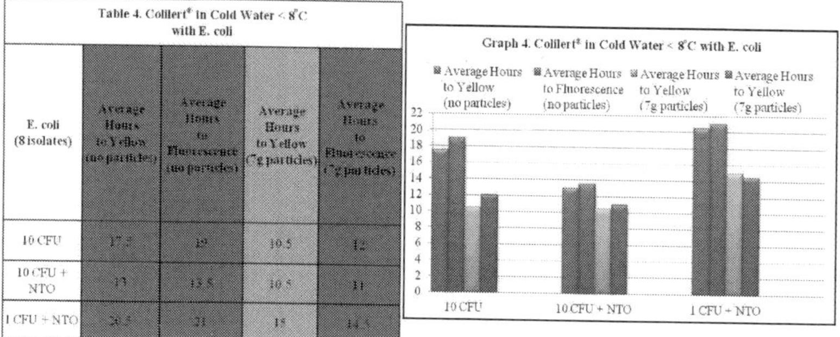

Table 4. Colilert® in Cold Water < 8°C with E. coli

E. coli (8 isolates)	Average Hours to Yellow (no particles)	Average Hours to Fluorescence (no particles)	Average Hours to Yellow (7g particles)	Average Hours to Fluorescence (7g particles)
10 CFU	17.5	19	10.5	12
10 CFU + NTO	13	13.5	10.5	11
1 CFU + NTO	20.5	21	18	14.5

Graph 4. Colilert® in Cold Water < 8°C with E. coli

Graph 4. Comparison of Time to Detection of MMO-MUG (Colilert®) with and without phycoccolloids with *E. coli* added. CFU (colony forming units), NTO (non-target organisms), Neg (negative)

Figure 7 presents the actual pictures of the replicates of the analysis of the Colilert® test to detect 1 bacterium per 100 mL. As can be seen, each of the 100 mL samples was clearly positive. As shown in Figure 6, the particle layer at the bottom of the water collection vessel is densely colored. The liquid is also clearly positive.

Figure 8 and Figure 9 present the results of the testing shown in Figure 7 as follows: from the 100 mL samples in Figure 7, 1 mL of supernatant was added to a 13 x 100 mm polystyrene test tube and placed in the PPM instrument. Readings in the PPM instrument were taken and a definite change in the "L", "a", and "b" values can be seen which indicate positive results for both quality control Idexx *E. coli* and Idexx total coliform *Klebsiella*. Because the light path in the test tube is much smaller than in the 100 mL vessel, the time required for a positive in a 100 mL sample is longer.

In all configurations – 1 mL in a test tube and 100 mL in a water collection vessel – the phycocolloids significantly decreases the time to detect the quality control Idexx total coliform *Klebsiella* and the Idexx quality control *E. coli*. In addition, the phycocolloids decreases the time to detect 1 bacterium in 100 mL of cold water < 8°C to within 16 hours.

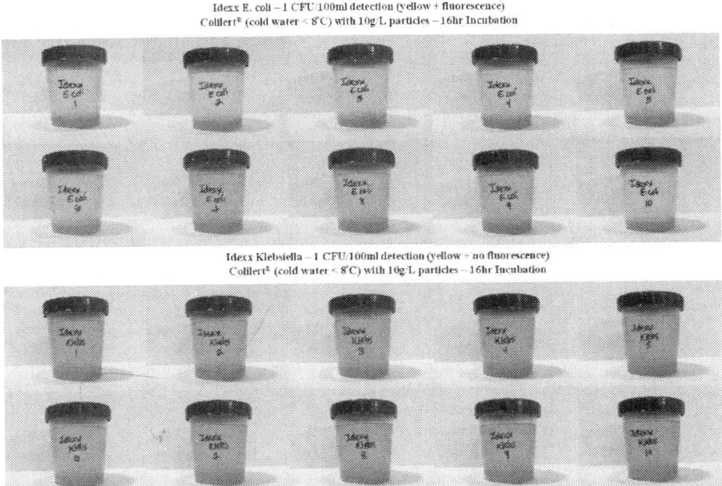

Figure 7. Replicate Testing with Idexx Quality Control *E. coli* and *Klebsiella* showing the ability of Colilert® to detect 1 bacterium per 100 mL within 16 hours in a cold water <8°C sample with phycocolloids added

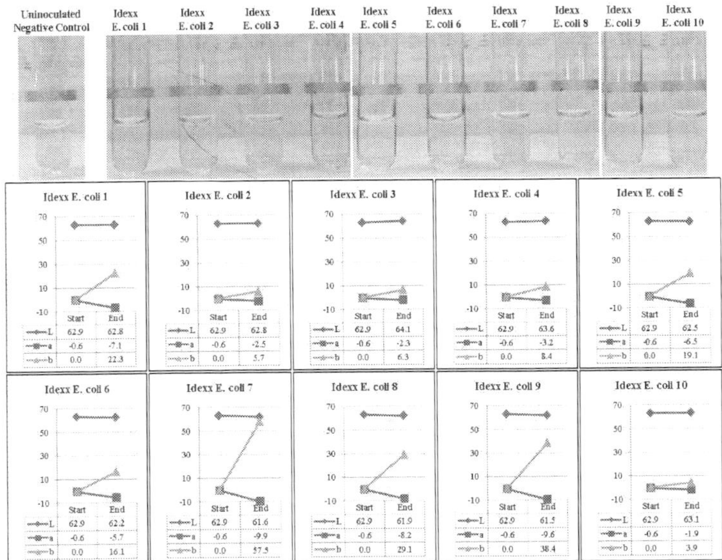

Figure 8. PPM Readings of 10 Quality Control *E. coli* at the 1 CFU/100 mL level

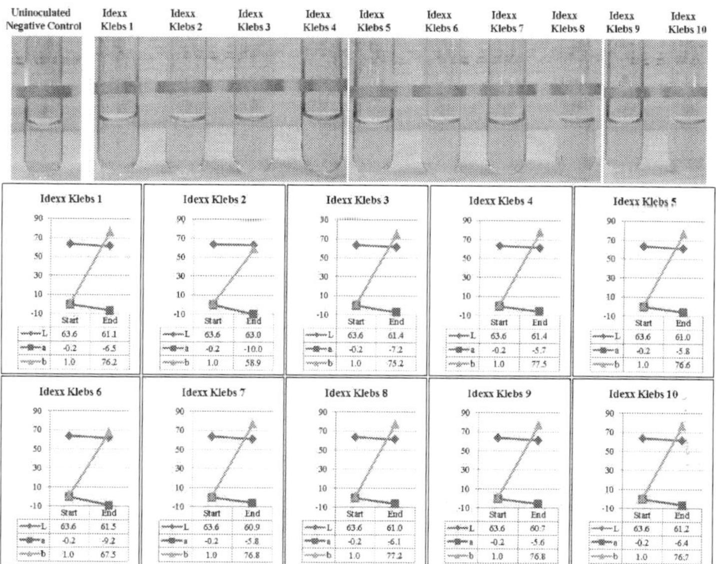

Figure 9. PPM Readings of 10 Quality Control *Klebsiella* at the 1 CFU/100 mL level

Figure 10 and Figure 11 present 1 mL duplicate data from the PPM instrument on detection of 10 bacteria per mL of Idexx *E. coli* in Colilert® with the addition of phycocolloids in cold water <8°C. The "b" value on the graph indicates the color change from colorless (Colilert® negative) to yellow (Colilert® positive). Once the yellow color starts to develop, a strong yellow color is observed in a two hour time period. In the experiment shown in Figure 10, the time to detection was 8.5 hours. In the experiment shown in Figure 11, the time to detection was 9.5 hours. The phycocolloid particles not only reduces the time to positive detection but also reduces the time bacteria spend in lag phase and increases the multiplication of bacteria in log phase as seen in the graphs.

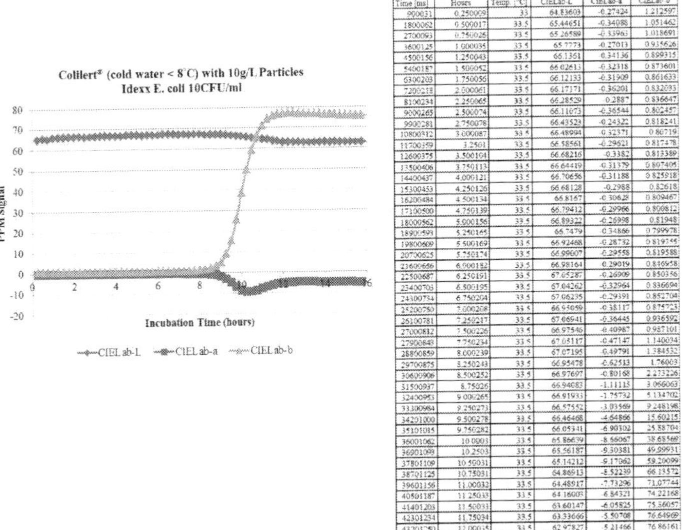

Time [ms]	Hours	Temp. [°C]	CIELab-L	CIELab-a	CIELab-b
900031	0.250009	33	64.83603	-0.27424	1.212597
1800062	0.500017	33.5	65.44651	-0.34088	1.051462
2700093	0.750026	33.5	65.26589	-0.33963	1.018691
3600125	1.000035	33.5	65.7773	-0.27013	0.935626
4500156	1.250043	33.5	66.1361	-0.34136	0.899315
5400187	1.500052	33.5	66.02613	-0.32318	0.873601
6300203	1.750056	33.5	66.12133	-0.31909	0.861633
7200218	2.000061	33.5	66.17171	-0.36201	0.832093
8100234	2.250065	33.5	66.28529	0.2887	0.836647
9000265	2.500074	33.5	66.11073	-0.36544	0.802457
9900281	2.750078	33.5	66.43523	-0.24322	0.818241
10800312	3.000087	33.5	66.48994	-0.32371	0.80719
11700359	3.2501	33.5	66.58561	-0.29621	0.817478
12600375	3.500104	33.5	66.68216	-0.3382	0.813389
13500406	3.750113	33.5	66.64419	-0.31379	0.807405
14400437	4.000121	33.5	66.70656	-0.31188	0.825918
15300453	4.250126	33.5	66.68128	-0.2988	0.82618
16200484	4.500134	33.5	66.8167	-0.30628	0.809467
17100500	4.750139	33.5	66.79412	-0.29966	0.808812
18000562	5.000156	33.5	66.89322	-0.26998	0.81948
18900599	5.250165	33.5	66.7479	-0.34866	0.799978
19800609	5.500169	33.5	66.92468	-0.28732	0.819755
20700625	5.750174	33.5	66.99007	-0.29558	0.819588
23600656	6.000182	33.5	66.98164	0.29019	0.846958
22500687	6.250191	33.5	67.05287	-0.26909	0.850356
23400703	6.500195	33.5	67.04262	-0.32964	0.836694
24300734	6.750204	33.5	67.06235	-0.29393	0.852704
25200750	7.000208	33.5	66.95059	-0.38117	0.875723
26100781	7.250217	33.5	67.06941	-0.36445	0.936592
27000812	7.500226	33.5	66.97546	-0.40987	0.987101
27900843	7.750234	33.5	67.05117	-0.47147	1.140034
28800859	8.000239	33.5	67.07195	-0.49791	1.384522
29700875	8.250243	33.5	66.95478	-0.62513	1.76003
30600906	8.500252	33.5	66.97697	-0.80168	2.273226
31500937	8.75026	33.5	66.94083	-1.11115	3.066063
32400953	9.000265	33.5	66.91933	-1.75732	5.134702
33300984	9.250273	33.5	66.57552	-3.03569	9.248198
34201000	9.500278	33.5	66.46468	-4.64866	15.60215
35101015	9.750282	33.5	66.05341	-6.90302	25.83704
36001062	10.0003	33.5	65.86639	-8.56067	38.68569
36901099	10.2503	33.5	65.56187	-9.30381	49.99931
37801109	10.59031	33.5	65.14212	-9.17062	59.20099
38701125	10.75031	33.5	64.86913	-8.52239	66.13572
39601156	11.00032	33.5	64.48917	-7.73296	71.07744
40501187	11.25033	33.5	64.16003	-6.84321	74.22168
41401203	11.50033	33.5	63.60147	-6.05825	75.56057
42301234	11.75034	33.5	63.33666	-5.50708	76.64969
43201250	12.00035	33.5	62.97827	-5.21466	76.86161

Figure 10. Actual PPM Data for detection of Idexx *E. coli* at 10 CFU/mL. Positive detection at 8.5hr incubation.

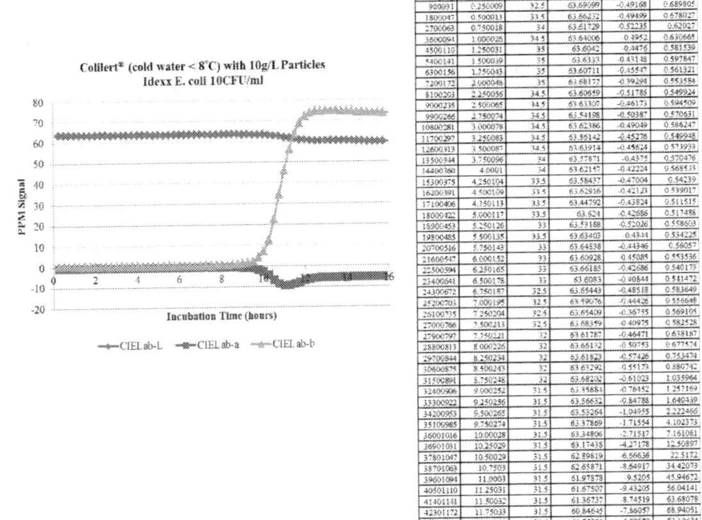

Time [ms]	Hours	Temp. [°C]	CIELab-L	CIELab-a	CIELab-b
900031	0.250009	32.5	63.69699	-0.49168	0.689805
1800047	0.500013	33.5	63.66232	-0.49499	0.678027
2700063	0.750018	34	63.61729	-0.52235	0.62027
3600094	1.000025	34.5	63.64806	0.4952	0.630665
4500110	1.250031	35	63.6042	-0.3476	0.581539
5400141	1.500039	35	63.6333	-0.43148	0.597847
6300156	1.750043	35	63.60711	-0.45547	0.561321
7200172	2.000048	35	63.68177	-0.39298	0.553584
8100203	2.250056	34.5	63.60659	-0.51785	0.549924
9000235	2.500065	34.5	63.63307	-0.46173	0.594509
9900266	2.750074	34.5	63.54198	-0.50387	0.570631
10800281	3.000078	34.5	63.62386	-0.49049	0.586247
11700297	3.250083	34.5	63.55142	-0.45276	0.549948
12600313	3.500087	34.5	63.63914	-0.45824	0.573933
13500344	3.750096	34	63.57871	-0.4375	0.570476
14400360	4.0001	34	63.62157	-0.42224	0.568533
15300375	4.250104	33.5	63.58437	-0.47004	0.54239
16200391	4.500109	33.5	63.62916	-0.42123	0.539017
17100406	4.750113	33.5	63.44792	-0.43824	0.511515
18000422	5.000117	33.5	63.624	-0.42686	0.517488
18900453	5.250126	33	63.53168	-0.52026	0.558608
19800485	5.500135	33.5	63.63403	0.4344	0.534225
20700516	5.750143	33	63.64538	-0.44346	0.56057
21600547	6.000152	33	63.60928	0.45085	0.553536
22500594	6.250165	33	63.66185	-0.42686	0.540173
23400641	6.500178	33	63.6083	-0.40844	0.541472
24300672	6.750187	32.5	63.65443	-0.48518	0.583649
25200703	7.000195	32.5	63.59076	-0.44426	0.556648
26100735	7.250204	32.5	63.65409	-0.36735	0.569105
27000766	7.500213	32.5	63.68359	-0.40975	0.582528
27900797	7.750221	32	63.61187	-0.46471	0.638187
28800813	8.000225	32	63.66132	-0.50753	0.675574
29700844	8.250234	32	63.61823	-0.57426	0.753474
30600875	8.500243	32	63.63292	-0.55173	0.880742
31500906	8.750248	32	63.68202	-0.61023	1.035964
32400906	9.000252	31.5	63.35884	-0.76452	1.257169
33300922	9.250256	31.5	63.56632	-0.84788	1.640439
34200953	9.500265	31.5	63.53264	-1.04955	2.222466
35100985	9.750274	31.5	63.37869	-1.71554	4.102373
36001016	10.00028	31.5	63.34806	-2.71517	7.161081
36901031	10.25029	31.5	63.17438	-4.27178	12.50897
37801047	10.50029	31.5	62.89819	-6.56636	22.5172
38701063	10.7503	31.5	62.65871	-8.64917	34.42073
39601094	11.0003	31.5	61.97878	9.5205	45.94672
40501110	11.25031	31.5	61.67507	-9.43205	56.04141
41401141	11.50032	31.5	61.36737	-8.74519	63.68078
42301172	11.75033	31.5	60.84645	-7.86057	68.94051
43201203	12.00033	31.5	60.75281	-6.99872	72.19634

Figure 11. Actual PPM Data for detection of Idexx *E. coli* at 10 CFU/mL. Positive detection at 9.5hr incubation.

4. Discussion

Since the introduction of the MMO-MUG (Colilert®) test in 1989 for the simultaneous detection of total coliforms and *E. coli* from drinking water, wastewater, bathing water, and other uses, attempts to decrease the time to a positive have been met with limited success. A variation of the Colilert® test, Colilert-18®, reduced the time from 24 hours to 18 hours incubation but requires the heating of the water sample adding an additional hour or two. Water samples are transported to the laboratory chilled by regulation. However, because many water samples arrive and are processed at the end of the work day after collection, the time to a result is often in the middle of the work day, thus delaying remediation and response and adversely affecting the public's health protection.

The two types of bacteria that generally exist are describes as either sessile (a unit that attaches to a surface or exist in a biofilm) or planktonic (existing freely in bulk solution). Antonie van Leuwenhoek described biofilms in 1674 as "animalcules" through observation of material scraped from human tooth surfaces with his microscope, but with advances in technology, biofilms can more accurately be described [6]. Biofilms can be described as microbial communities that are sessile and grow on surfaces surrounded by a matrix of extracellular polymeric substances; microcolonies are distinct communities of bacterial cells of one or many different species that are surrounded by a matrix. The advantages of biofilm formation by bacteria is that it provides protection against antibiotics, disinfectants, and environments that are constantly changing [7]. The key to the catalyst activity of the phycocolloids is their ability to interact with the bacteria and the attendant production of microcolonies. The bacteria multiply much faster when attached to the particles as microcolony biofilm.

The micro particles increase the surface area in the liquid broth and allow microbes that multiply in vitro to establish a biofilm. In effect, the micro particles act in an analogous way as a catalyst does in a chemical reaction. In the microbiology area, the micro particles provide multiple attachment surfaces for the microbes to "establish residence". Microbes prefer surfaces on which to grow and multiply rather than being free in a liquid environment. For example, the microbes may experience quorum sensing, which accelerates the generation of a biofilm. The biofilm is produced when the microbes multiply, and it yields colonies of microbes that are held together by external capsules, pili, and glycocalyxes of the microbes which, in the broad context, are surface components, such as polysaccharides, proteins and/or mixtures thereof. The micro particles are static, in that they are not consumed but serve as a physical structure that provides shelter and attachment and promotes the multiplication and expression of the target microbe. There may be attached nutritive elements on the micro particles that serve to stimulate the development of the bacterial nidus. The micro particles may be colloidal, in suspension, or a combination. Any materials or structures that encourage the growth of microbes on a biofilm are highly preferred for use in this invention. Supporting the catalytic activity of the phycocolloids is the observation that growth starts first at the bottom of the test tubes, where particles have gravitationally settled and microbial biofilms have developed, attached to the particles. Additional particles are distributed with the remainder of the admixture, but have not yet been associated with metabolizable substrate creating a color change. The image of the test tubes illustrates well how the particles expedite the detection of the bacteria (i.e., *E. coli*) targeted by the metabolizable substrate of the test mixture, and the increased sensitivity associated therewith; i.e., the micro particles provide surface area or attachment surfaces for the *E. coli* microbes to establish residence, grow, and multiply (e.g., creating biofilms), which growth is indicated by the color change created when the nutrient portions of the metabolizable substrate are metabolized by the microbes.

This report demonstrates that phycocolloids introduced into the classical Colilert® formula significantly decreases the time to a positive. By visual observation with both standard quality control *Klebsiella* and *E. coli*, plus with total coliforms and *E. coli* isolated from source water, it was demonstrated that Colilert® could detect 1 target bacterium in 100 mL of cold water < 8°C in repetitive experiments. The detection in cold water < 8°C is particularly important because the Colilert-18® variation, while rated positive in 18 hours, requires the pre-heating of the water sample before the test is started, thus effectively increase the time to approximately 20 hours.

The 16 hour benchmark is particularly important for laboratory work flow. It provides the ability to perform a 4 to 8 test – in by 4 pm, finished by 8 am, the optimum for the work flow. Further enhancing the time to detection is the use of the PPM instrument. With it, detection of 1 total coliform and 1 *E. coli* in cold water < 8°C was decreased by several hours; furthermore the instrument signals a positive at the time it is positive.

Author details

Stephen C. Edberg[1,2*]

Address all correspondence to: stephen.edberg@yale.edu

1 Mt. Sinai Health System, New York City, New York, USA

2 Yale University and Yale University School of Medicine, New Haven, Connecticut, USA

References

[1] International Organization for Standardization (ISO). (2012). *ISO 9308-2:* Water quality--Enumeration of *Escherichia coli* and coliform bacteria--Part 2: Most probable number method. ISO, Geneva Switzerland.

[2] Environmental Protection Agency (EPA). (1992) National Primary Drinking Water Regulations, Analytical Techniques: Coliform Bacteria: Final Rule. *Federal Register* 57(112):24744-24747.

[3] Edberg, S.C., M.J. Allen, D.B. Smith, and the National Collaborative Study. (1989) National field evaluation of a defined substrate method for the simultaneous detec-

tion of total coliforms and *Escherichia coli* from drinking water: Comparison with presence-absence techniques. *Applied and Environmental Microbiology* 55(4):1003-1008.

[4] Edberg, S.C., M.J. Allen, D.B. Smith, and N.J. Kriz. (1990) Enumeration of total coliforms and *Escherichia coli* from source water by the defined substrate technology. *Applied and Environmental Microbiology* 56(2):366-369.

[5] American Public Health Association (APHA). (1992) Standard Methods of Water and Wastewater. 22nd ed. American Public Health Association, American Water Works Association, Water Environment Federation publication. APHA, Washington D.C.

[6] Costerton, J.W. Introduction to biofilm. (1999) *International Journal of Antimicrobial Agents,* 11(3-4):217–221.

[7] Garret T.R., A. Bhakoo, and Z. Zhang. Bacterial adhesion and biofilms on surfaces. (2008) *Progress in Natural Science,* 18:1049–1056.

Chapter 7

A New Direct Detection System for Antibiotic Resistant Bacteria

Stephen C. Edberg and J. Michael Miller

Additional information is available at the end of the chapter

http://dx.doi.org/10.5772/59345

1. Introduction

A new system based on the phenotypic expression of antibiotic resistance has been developed. The system, the Defined Substrate Utilization® (DSU®) process, enhances the metabolism of the target microbe while providing inadequate nutrients for the non-target microbes. Accordingly, the target microbe multiples to a much greater extent than the non-target microbes and this differential allows for the specific detection of the target microbe. The non-target microbes multiply insufficiently to be noticed. Incorporated in the DSU® screening tools are substrates, that when metabolized, produces a sensible signal such as color or luminescence. In addition, specific inhibitors to the non-target microbes are included in the formulas. This format allows a more sensitive screen than parallel agar-based methods. In terms of time to positive, the liquid (once the powder is hydrated with sterile water), coupled with the optimization of nutrients generates results in the same time frame as genetic amplification tests. The mixing of the ingredients in powder form permits a much less expensive individual screen than either conventional agar-based or genetic amplification methods. In addition, the format permits utilization of the DSU® tools both in the remote field environment or the clinical microbiology laboratory.

There are two basic protocols utilized for the epidemiological screening of microbes. The first is the conventional agar-based culture technique. Here a specimen is plated on one or more selective agars and incubated 24 to 48 hours. A trained medical technologist examines the colonies and those compatible with the target microbe are subjected to specific biochemical and/or immunochemical testing, and antibiotic susceptibility procedures. These may require from 24 to 72 hours incubation [1]. In an attempt to facilitate the culture protocol, chromogenic substrate media have been introduced for some, but not all, bacteria of epidemiological interest. Chromogenic substrate agars have a short shelf life, must be stored cold and often in

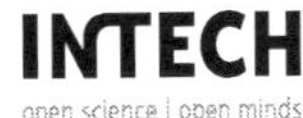

the dark, and the colors differentiating the positive and negative colonies may not always be distinct, necessitating confirmatory testing [2]. They are generally held 48 hours before calling a negative, although 48 hours can result in false-positives [3, 4].

The second technique utilizes genetic amplification (GA) to detect the target microbe. A number of companies make different types of GA. However, in common to them all are: each requires an expensive instrument, utilizes reagents which are expensive, requires highly skilled labor in a centralized laboratory, and does not recover living bacteria [5]. In addition, each is subject to false-positives and false-negatives because of unexpected mutations [6, 7].

A new and novel, one-step, direct epidemiology screening method based on classical phenotypic parameters was developed as an alternative to conventional agar-based methods for a variety of antibiotic resistant bacteria. For example, for *Staphylococcus aureus* (S. aureus), the key enzyme is coagulase and specificity is achieved equal to that of conventional identification schemes [8]. The method of Defined Substrate Utilization® (DSU®) optimizes specific, selective, and differential biochemicals in powder form. Hence, it overcomes the observation by Selepak and Witebsky that the lot-to-lot variation of commercial plasma was too variable to be used directly from patient specimens [9]. For each target microbe, an optimum background of nutrients and inhibitors was generated tailored to the biochemical physiology of that bacterium. Accordingly, the target microbes are preferentially fed while the non-target microbes are in a nutrient deficit.

The powder format allows optimization of ingredients much more precisely than an agar gel. Moreover, the overall sensitivity of the DSU® method is enhanced since liquid culture (once the powder is hydrated with sterile water) detects a lower number of colony forming units (CFU) than on the surface of agar [10, 11]. The DSU® tools are generally positive from a colony within 4 to 5 hours and from a human or animal sample in 6-9 hours on average. The bacteria remain viable in the screens and thus provide the opportunity to further evaluate the target microbe.

In addition to be able to be done manually by visual observation, an inexpensive instrument was developed to read and analyze results of all the screens (Pilots Point Monitor 60®, Pilots Point LLC, Sarasota, FL). One may add any combination of any of the DSU® screening tools into the instrument and results are generated by an algorithm controlling the analysis. Results can be sent to cell phones, via Wi-Fi, or in any format to any location. For example, the instruments may be stationed at various clinics.

This paper shall describe in detail four of the epidemiological screens: methicillin-resistant S. aureus (MRSA), all S. aureus including MRSA and methicillin-susceptible S. aureus (MSSA), vancomycin-resistant enterococci (VRE), and carbapenemase-resistant Enterobacteriaceae (CRE). Screens for vancomycin-intermediate resistant S. aureus (VISA), and ciprofloxacin-resistant (cipR) bacteria will be described briefly as subsets of the above. In addition, the principles and function of the instrument will be presented.

While this paper presents six of the DSU® epidemiology screens, the format and phenotypic expression in the presence of defined nutrients, allows for the rapid development of others.

2. The Defined Substrate Utilization® Method

2.1. Screening Method for S. aureus: Both Methicillin-susceptible (MSSA) and Methicillin-resistant (MRSA)

2.1.1. EPI-M® and aureusAlert® — Quantitative analysis with pure and anterior nares cultures

[EPI-M® is the DSU® epidemiology screen for MRSA, aureusAlert® is the DSU® epidemiology screen for all S. aureus – both MSSA and MRSA (Pilots Point LLC, Sarasota, FL)]

2.1.1.1. Pure cultures

S. aureus ATCC 43300 (MRSA), S. aureus ATCC 34591 (MRSA), S. aureus ATCC 25923 (MSSA), S. aureus ATCC 29213 (MSSA), S. epidermidis ATCC 12228, the MRSA USA 600 (6 isolates), MRSA USA 300 (2 isolates), and MRSA USA 100 (2 isolates), plus 5 clinical patient laboratory isolates of MRSA and 5 of MSSA were utilized.

A suspension of each of the bacterial isolates was made in normal physiological saline to a 0.5 McFarland standard. From this suspension, 0.1 mL was transferred to 9.9 mL of sterile normal saline and vortexed well. Using a quantitative pipette (Rainin, Rainin Instrument LLC, Oakland, CA) 1 and 10 microliters of the suspension was transferred to aureusAlert® and EPI-M® and a dilution series generated. Colony counts were made from the 0.5 McFarland standard and the 9.9 mL normal saline [8].

2.1.1.2. Human surveillance study

Nasal swabs (Culturette™ II, Becton, Dickinson and Company, Cockeysville, MD) were obtained from people entering or leaving a building at the following locations: Yale-New Haven Hospital (New Haven, CT, USA); Walter E. Washington Convention Center (Washington, D.C., DC, USA), George Washington University Hospital (Washington, D.C., DC, USA) and Tampa General Hospital (Tampa, FL, USA). Two swabs were obtained from the same nostril.

2.1.1.3. Conventional procedure

S. aureus: Volunteer nasal swab specimens were aseptically transferred to Trypticase Soy Broth (TSB) containing 6.5% NaCl for 24 hours enrichment at 33°C-35°C. The enrichment samples were subcultured on to Tryptic Soy Sheep Blood Agar (TSBA) plates, and the plates were incubated aerobically for 24 hours at 35°C. Suspicious colonies of S. aureus were identified by using standard laboratory methods including catalase, tube or slide coagulase, Gram staining, and mannitol salt agar. Confirmed S. aureus colonies were tested for methicillin resistance using the CLSI recommended reference method (e.g., 30 mcg cefoxitin disk) [12]. In addition, an assay for PBP-2 (Remel, Lenexa, KS) was performed.

MRSA: Cultures were inoculated into TSB with 6.5% NaCl and incubated for 18-24 hours. A subculture was made to blood agar (BA) plates and a Staphaurex® (Remel, Lenexa, KS) test performed. In addition, an assay for PBP-2 (Remel, Lenexa, KS) was performed. Antibiotic susceptibility test (AST) was performed by both an agar dilution method (Mueller-Hinton agar with 4 mcg/mL oxacillin, Becton, Dickinson and Company, Cockeysville, MD) and also by the Sensititre™ (Trek Diagnostic Systems, Oakwood Village, OH) microdilution method.

2.1.1.4. Defined Substrate Utilization® screens

All ingredients of the Defined Substrate Utilization® screens are optimized in powder form in a tube and are performed in the same way. Each tube is labelled with the name of the screen, and a specific amount of water is transferred to the tube to hydrate the powder. The sample is added to the tube and incubated at 35°C. A positive result, which can occur any time after the initiation of incubation, is seen as follows:

Interpretation: aureusAlert® – a clot or coalescence forms in the liquid; no observable clot or coalescence is a negative result. EPI-M® – the liquid changes color from straw-colored to amethyst with an increase in coalescence; no change from straw-colored is a negative result. Tubes are held a maximum of 24 hours before calling them negative.

Control S. aureus standards ATCC 25923 (MSSA) and ATCC 43300 (MRSA) plus 5 MSSA and 5 MRSA isolates from patients were tested. MSSA and MRSA isolates were diluted from 7 log10 to 1 log10 and incubated at 35° and 23°C.

Based on quantitative analysis of pure cultures, the Defined Substrate Utilization® screens were able to detect as low as 20 CFU (18 hours of incubation) with both MSSA and MRSA (Table 1; Table 3). Tables 2A and 2B, and Tables 4A and 4B, present the results of the nasal screening of normal subject volunteers. For both the detection of S. aureus and MRSA there was no difference between the Defined Substrate Utilization® screens and conventional methods. aureusAlert® and EPI-M® showed a specificity of 100%.

2.1.2. aureusAlert® for all S. aureus (MSSA & MRSA)

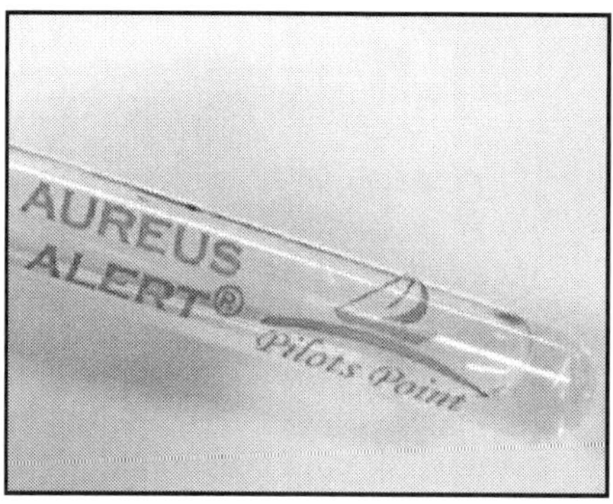

Figure 1. S. aureus Negative – Liquid

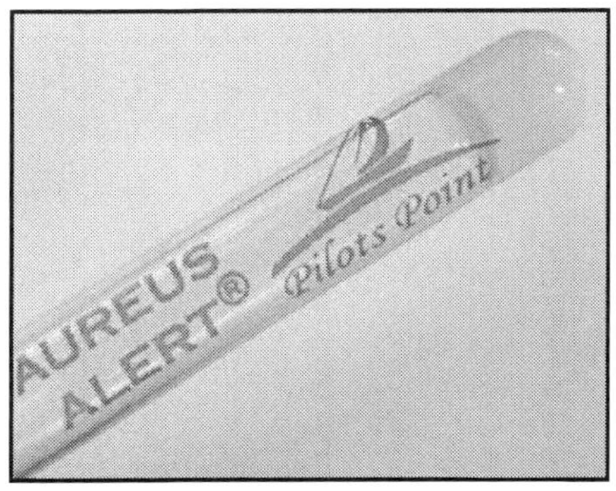

Figure 2. S. aureus Positive – Clot

MSSA ATCC 25923 (CFU/mL)	Detection Time at 35°C
7 log10	2.0 h
6 log10	3.0 h
5 log10	4.0 h
4 log10	7.0 h
3 log10	10.0 h
2 log10	15.0 h

Table 1. Detection time of Quality Control Clone ATCC 25923 in aureusAlert®

	Conventional Positive	Conventional Negative	Total
aureusAlert® Positive	450	20	470
aureusAlert® Negative	10	1787	1797
Total	460	1807	2267
(A)			

Site	aureusAlert® (Positive / Negative)	Conventional (Positive / Negative)
Tampa General Hospital	69 / 322	72 / 322
Yale-New Haven Hospital	63 / 289	58 / 289
(B)		

Table 2. A&B. Detection comparison of S. aureus nasal swabs in aureusAlert® and conventional methods

2.1.3. EPI-M® (MRSA)

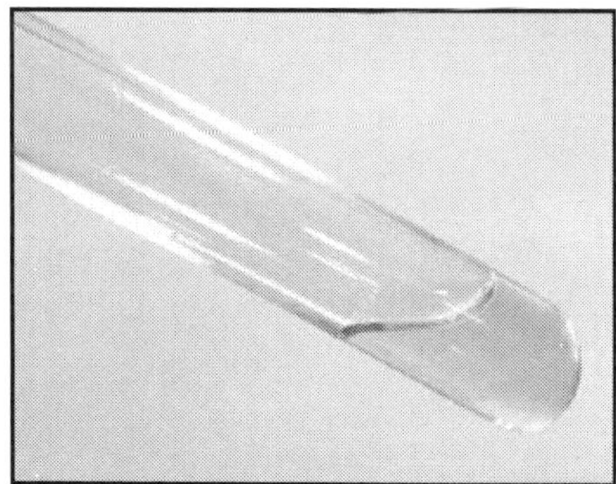

Figure 3. MRSA Negative – Straw-colored

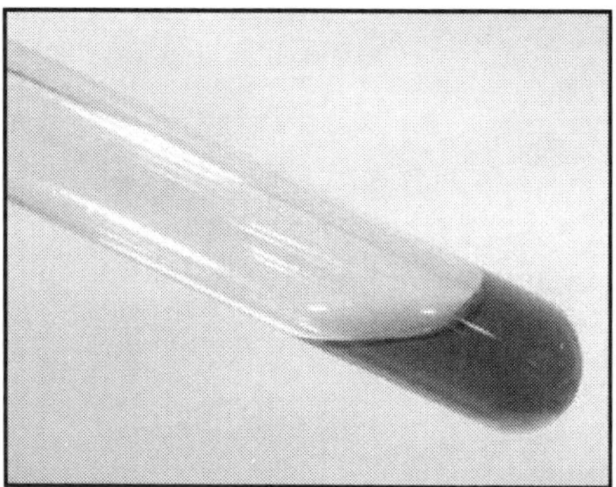

Figure 4. MRSA Positive – Amethyst

MRSA ATCC 43300 (CFU/mL)	Detection Time at 35°C
7 log10	2.0 h
6 log10	3.0 h
5 log10	4.0 h
4 log10	6.5 h
3 log10	14.0 h
2 log10	18.0 h

Table 3. Detection time of Quality Control Clone ATCC 43300 in EPI-M®

	Conventional Positive	Conventional Negative	Total
EPI-M® Positive	49	2	51
EPI-M® Negative	1	480	481
Total	50	482	532
	(A)		
Site	EPI-M® (Positive / Negative)	Conventional (Positive / Negative)	
Tampa General Hospital	33 / 317	32 / 317	
Yale-New Haven Hospital	19 / 217	18 / 217	
	(B)		

Table 4. A & B. Detection comparison of MRSA nasal swabs in EPI-M® and conventional methods

Described here is a method to detect S. aureus, both MSSA and MRSA, directly from a human, animal, or environmental sample. The key innovation was to optimize all ingredients and generate a stable, ready-to-use powder. The system's central ingredient is an enhanced coagulase substrate. The enhanced coagulase reaction overcame the observation by Selepak and Witebsky that rabbit plasma variability precluded the ability to directly detect S. aureus directly from samples. In one form, aureusAlert®, all S. aureus are detected. Using the aureusAlert® as a base, the addition of a mecA inducer specifically distinguishes MRSA (EPI-M®). By employing the definitive tests in the right milieu, as low as 20 CFU of MSSA and MRSA could be detected.

This study demonstrated that the sensitivity was equivalent to conventional methods by direct comparison and molecular methods from literature references. The time to detection was in the clinically useful range for the epidemiological screening of anterior nares (Table 1; Table 3). Because coagulase was chosen as the core detection system, a specificity of 49/49 for EPI-M® was seen from sampled subjects. Likewise, aureusAlert® being an enhanced coagulase test also showed complete agreement with conventional identifications.

The bacteria remain viable in the aureusAlert® and EPI-M® epidemiology screening tools. The tubes can be transported, as is, from the field for further analysis (e.g., antibiotic susceptibility testing, molecular fingerprinting). The powder format offers great flexibility of use. It has the ability to gather information from a broad spectrum of sampling: in the field, in satellite facilities, in clinics, and in large volume central laboratories. It requires no skilled labor. Because it is a stable powder, it can be inexpensively transported. Its cost is 20% of genetic amplification and 75% of conventional processing surveillance samples.

2.1.4. Additional S. aureus screen: EPI-VISA®

The screen for vancomycin-intermediate resistant S. aureus (VISA) utilizes the EPI-M® base with the substitution of 3 mcg/mL (3 mg/L) of vancomycin for cefoxitin. The colors produced are the same as the EPI-M®.

2.2. Screening Method for Vancomycin-resistant Enterococci (VRE)

Both asymptomatically colonized and infected patients serve as reservoirs for transmission of VRE, as well as contaminated surfaces and patient care equipment. European Union and United States public health agencies have developed recommendations for preventing the transmission of vancomycin resistance within and among hospitals and nursing homes. Current surveillance methods require a number of sequential steps and needs a special series of culture media and identification tests. A highly skilled and trained medical technologist is needed to perform the analysis. Molecular tests are expensive and require special equipment.

A new, simple, and one-step screening method for the detection of VRE (as defined as a minimum inhibitory concentration (MIC) to vancomycin of 6 mcg/mL) directly from rectal/ perirectal specimens was compared to the Food and Drug Administration (FDA) reference or predicate method. The screening tool (EPI-V®, Pilots Point LLC, Sarasota, FL) contains all the required ingredients in a stable powder form, in a standard test tube. The presence of VRE in a rectal swab is denoted by the production of a two sequential biochemical reactions inside the test tube: substrate hydrolysis representing bile-esculin followed by pyrrolidonyl arylamidase (PYR) substrate hydrolysis. Bile-esculin plus PYR is the generally accepted identification of the genus *Enterococcus* [13].

2.2.1. Standard culture method

The FDA predicate VRE culture method is Bile Esculin Azide agar with 6 mcg/mL vancomycin (BEAV) (Remel, Lenexa, KS) [14]. Specimens consisted of 400 sequential human rectal/ perirectal surveillance swabs obtained as part of the ongoing surveillance program. The collection device was a Culturette™ II (Becton Dickinson and Company, Cockeysville, MD). There was no prior notification of individuals collecting the specimens. The Culturette™ II swab was twirled vigorously in 1 mL of pH 7.0, 50 mM HEPES (Sigma-Aldrich, St. Louis, MO) buffer so that each of the two methods would be challenged with the same inoculum. From the HEPES buffer, 0.1 mL of the extracted patient specimen was plated on the surface of the BEAV agar plate. After incubation for 24 hours at 35°C in ambient air, colonies that were brown-black were gram-stained. Colonies showing gram-positive cocci in chains were then tested by the PYR reaction (Becton-Dickinson, Cockeysville, MD). The MIC to vancomycin from PYR positive colonies was performed by the Etest® method (bioMérieux, Durham, NC).

2.2.2. EPI-V®

The EPI-V® screening tool is in a powder format, in a flange-capped test tube, and stored at room temperature. To use, 3 mL of sterile water was added to dissolve the powder. To this solution, 0.1 mL of the extracted patient's specimen was added. EPI-V® test tubes were incubated for a maximum of 24 hours at 35°C in ambient air to call a specimen negative. However, color development at any time, denoted a positive result. Test tubes demonstrating a brown-black color (bile-esculin positive) were tilted to coat the disk present in the EPI-V® cap. This cap contains an enhanced reagent for the detection of PYR hydrolysis [15]. The development of a bright fuchsia color within 15 seconds is a positive reaction for PYR. Positive bile-esculin and PYR results demonstrated the presence of VRE.

In order to determine if a false-positive or false-negative reaction had occurred from the EPI-V®, approximately 0.1 mL was subcultured from all tests tubes to the surface of a Bile Esculin Azide agar plate containing 6 mcg/mL vancomycin. Plates were incubated at 35°C for 24 hours in ambient air. All colonies compatible with *Enterococcus* were then identified to species. If an *Enterococcus* species was isolated, an Etest® MIC to vancomycin was performed. All isolates were identified to species using the Vitek 2 system (bioMérieux, Durham, NC).

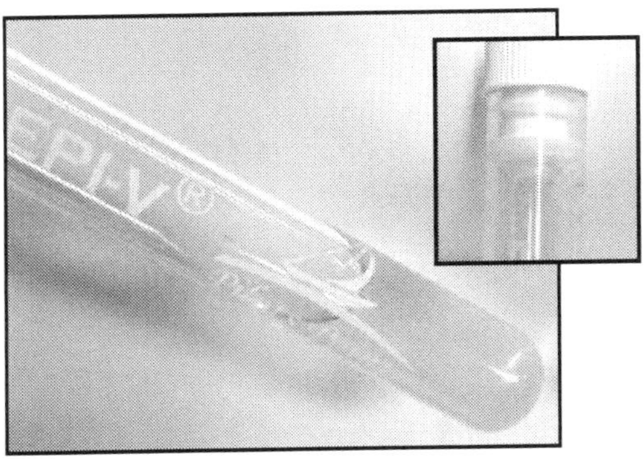

Figure 5. VRE Negative – Straw-colored with white disk

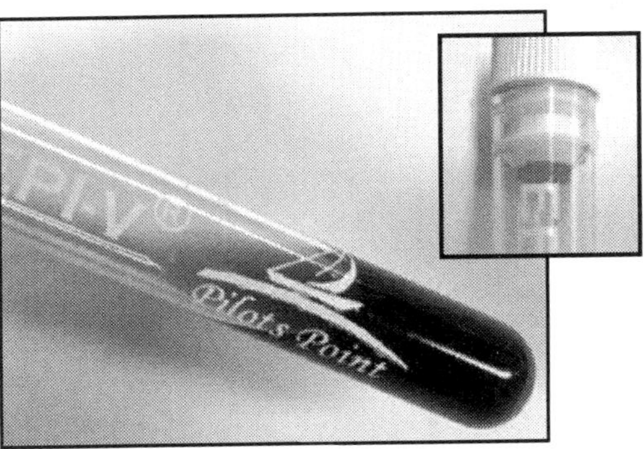

Figure 6. VRE Positive – Dark brown/black with bright fuchsia disk

The EPI-V® tool, from a diluted specimen, demonstrated a sensitivity of 107% and a specificity of 98.4%. Table 5 presents the comparison of the EPI-V® results versus the Bile Esculin Azide (BEAV) culture method. Table 6 presents the time course of the 120 positive analyses by the EPI-V® tool.

	BEAV Positive	BEAV Negative
EPI-V® Positive	111	9
EPI-V® Negative	0	280

Table 5. Comparison of EPI-V® and Bile Esculin Azide Media for the recovery of VRE from stool samples

Time	Number of Specimens Positive	Cumulative
5 h	12	12
6 h	6	18
7 h	5	23
8 h	11	34
9 h	3	37
10 h	7	44
16 h	73	107
18 h	8	115
20 h	5	120

Table 6 EPI-V® Time to Positive from 120 positive stool samples

The EPI-V® screening tool consists of both a substrate in the liquid (a bile-esculin substrate) and a detection disk for a second biochemical reaction (PYR).

The EPI-V® tool showed excellent sensitivity and specificity relative to the Bile Esculin Azide FDA referenced method and required only a maximum of 20 hours. In addition, the EPI-V® tool offered several significant advantages over the FDA referenced method. These included: no skilled technologist time required, simple quality control, highly conserved incubator and refrigerator space, and approximately 1/4-1/3 the cost of agar-based methods. The simplicity and ease of use of the EPI-V® epidemiology screen allows for more efficient and timely processing of large numbers of patient surveillance specimens for VRE. This new screen offers the clinical microbiologist, hospital epidemiologist, or infection control practitioner, flexibility as to the timing of collection and number of rectal or perirectal patient surveillance cultures.

2.3. Screening Methods for Antibiotic Resistant Enterobacteriaceae

Carbapenems are a class of antibiotics made by modifying penicillin. This chemical modification keeps part of the penicillin molecule, called the beta-lactam structure, and makes the rest artificial. Therefore, carbapenems are referred to, with other classes of penicillin modified antibiotics, as semi-synthetic penicillins. The modifications were made because bacteria rapidly became resistant to penicillin. Chemists added bits and pieces of chemical structures to penicillin to avoid this resistance. The bacteria figured out how to make enzymes to chemically destroy these new modifications. After 70+ years of this war between chemists and bacteria, the bacteria have topped the chemists by making a class of enzymes called carbapenemases [16].

The original carbapenem was first used in the U.S. in 1976. Since then better forms of this class have been made chemically. Currently, the most common carbapenem antibiotic used is meropenem. In the fight between chemists and bacteria, meropenem is the last antibiotic standing. If a bacterium is resistant to meropenem, there are no good alternatives [16].

2.3.1. What is CRE?

The clinical microbiology laboratory, where infections are diagnosed, divides bacteria into various shapes (spheres are cocci, cylinders are rods) and armor (gram-positive or gram-negative). A particular class of antibiotic generally has activity against either gram-negative or gram-positive bacteria, but not both. Carbapenems were developed to treat the gram-negative bacteria found in hospitals. Gram-negative bacteria in hospitals are associated with a very large morbidity and mortality, plus tremendous cost.

The gram-negative bacteria that have become resistant to carbapenems are known as CRE, or carbapenem-resistant enterics. Until a short time ago carbapenem resistance was only in one type of enteric, called *Klebsiella pneumoniae* (K. pneumoniae); therefore resistant bacteria were called *K. pneumoniae carbapenemase* (KPC). Unfortunately resistance has spread to bacteria related to Klebsiella and we now use the term CRE. These enteric bacteria normally live in the intestines of humans [16].

2.3.2. What is the CRE problem?

CRE is primarily a nosocomial associated problem. The likely reasons include the following: the use of large amounts of various antibiotics that select for the CRE bacteria; the transport from patient to patient of CRE on the hands of health care workers, including doctors and nurses; an environment such as a hospital room in which the bacteria can be deposited to infect new residents. For example, the CRE bacteria can remain alive in hospital rooms for a very long time period. In one study, after 30 days significant numbers of CRE could be found in a hospital room, and even after 100 days CRE were recovered. Death rates of up to 50% can be seen in patients with CRE isolated from the blood. The CDC has identified CRE as one of the prime problems for hospitalized patients [16].

2.3.3. Impediments to the control of CRE

Lack of funding: There is no billing code for CRE under Medicare and Medicaid. Therefore, reimbursement for the actual laboratory testing is not available. While there would be a huge financial benefit to the prevention of infections (in addition to the obvious benefit to the patient) hospitals do not balance costs and benefits between departments.

Lack of a systems approach: Many hospitals are now actually networks of hospitals. It has been difficult to achieve uniformity of action across the networks.

Lack of a diagnostic test: The IDSA says "New, rapid accurate diagnostic tests are sorely needed. Unfortunately, there is little impetus for companies…"

Need for highly skilled labor: Current methods require several days and utilize highly skilled and costly labor [16].

2.3.4. Methods for the detection of Carbapenemase-producing Enterobacteriaceae

2.3.4.1. Centers for Disease Control Method

The CDC method utilizes a series of sequential steps and can require up to 4 days to determine either positive of negative [17].

Procedure:

Step 1. *Day One*

1.   Aseptically, place one 10-µg ertapenem or meropenem disc in 5 mL trypticase soy broth (TSB).

2.   Immediately inoculate the broth with the rectal culture swab.

3.   Incubate overnight at 35 ± 2°C, ambient air.

Step 2. *Day Two*

1.   Vortex and subculture 100 µl of the incubated broth culture onto a MacConkey agar plate.

2.   Streak for isolation.

3.   Incubate overnight at 35 ± 2°C, ambient air.

Step 3. *Day Three*

1.   Examine the MacConkey agar for lactose-fermenting (pink-red) colonies.

2.   More than one colony morphology may represent different species of Enterobacteriaceae.

NOTE: Carbapenemases are known to exist in several different species of gram-negative bacilli including species of Enterobacteriaceae and *Pseudomonas aeruginosa* (P. aeruginosa). However, carbapenemases are more common in lactose-fermenting species of Enterobacteriaceae (e.g. K. pneumoniae and E. coli) than in non-lactose fermenting Enterobacteriaceae (e.g. *Serratia marcescens* and some *Enterobacter* spp.) and P. aeruginosa. In this procedure, it is suggested that laboratories focus their efforts on detection of resistant lactose-fermenting bacteria to reduce workload. Healthcare facilities that have identified clinical infections with carbapenemase-producing non-lactose fermenting gram-negative species should consider altering this procedure to include characterization of colonies with a morphology that is consistent with those species.

It may be necessary to subculture representative colonies of each morphology type to a non-selective media for isolation and/or for susceptibility testing. Screen representative isolated colonies using a phenotypic test for carbapenemase production, such as the Modified Hodge Test (MHT) or test for carbapenem susceptibility using a standardized method and follow the CLSI guidelines for identification of carbapenemase-producing Enterobacteriaceae [12].

Step 4. *Day Four*

1.   For CRE and/or MHT-positive isolates, perform species-level identification.

2.3.4.2. Hydrolysis of Carbapenem Methods

Rapid Detection of Carbapenemase-producing Enterobacteriaceae

This method takes advantages of the observation that the hydrolysis of imipenem results in an acid molecule. Therefore, the authors incorporate a pH indicator that changes from red to yellow when acid is produced in sufficient amounts. One advantage of the method is that by using a pH change, a broad spectrum of carbapenemases can be detected. A significant disadvantage is that imipenem is not stable and the whole formula must be made fresh each time it is used. This aspect seriously inhibits the method's use [18].

Detection of Carbapenemase Producers in Enterobacteriaceae by Use of a Novel Screening Medium

Different concentrations of several carbapenem molecules were tested, and finally, ertapenem was added to Drigalski agar medium at a concentration of 0.25 mg/mL. $ZnSO_4$ (70 mg/mL) was added to improve expression of metallo-beta-lactamases (MBLs) by MBL producers. Cloxacillin (250 mg/mL), which is a cephalosporinase (AmpC-type beta-lactamase) inhibitor, was used to prevent growth of isolates expressing high levels of cephalosporinases, such as *Enterobacter cloacae* (E. cloacae), *Enterobacter aerogenes* (E. aerogenes), *Morganella morgannii* (M. morgannii), and *Serratia marcescens* (S. marcescens). These isolates are clinically significant sources of carbapenem resistance associated with an outer membrane permeability defect [19].

2.4. Screening Method for Carbapenem-resistant Enterobacteriaceae (CRE)

EPI-CRE® is a selective and differential medium containing 2 mcg/mL of meropenem, intended for use in the qualitative detection of gastrointestinal colonization with carbapenem-resistant Enterobacteriaceae (CRE) to provide epidemiological data. It is based on classical biochemicals in an optimized form. EPI-CRE® is performed with rectal swabs and fecal specimens from patients to screen for CRE colonization. The presence of CRE is established when the color of the medium changes from red to yellow. In addition, a violet precipitate may also be observed.

Specimens should be collected, handled and disposed of in compliance with accepted guidelines and in accordance with all regulations. Cotton swabs should be avoided with preference to synthetic fibers such as Dacron or rayon. A generally available reference is the Manual of Clinical Microbiology [8]. EPI-CRE® is performed with rectal swabs and fecal specimens which should be collected and handled following recommended guidelines [13].

2.4.1. EPI-CRE®

2.4.1.1. Procedure

1.   Inoculate the sample into the medium. If a swab is used, twirl the swab in the medium for 10 seconds and express excess fluid from the swab before removing and discarding into disinfectant. Do not use a cotton swab.

2.   Incubate the tube(s) at 34-36°C.

3.   The tube(s) may be examined any time up to 24 hours for a color change from red to yellow. If the medium has not become yellow in 24 hours, it is negative.

4.   At any time after the start of incubation, if a yellow color is observed, EPI-CRE® is positive. In addition, a violet precipitate may be observed.

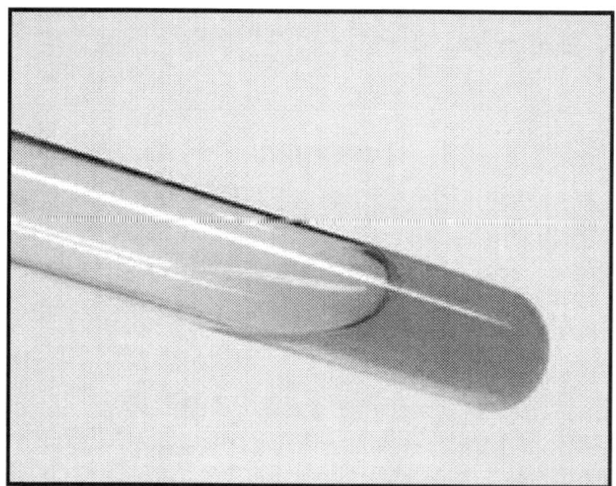

Figure 7. CRE Negative – Red

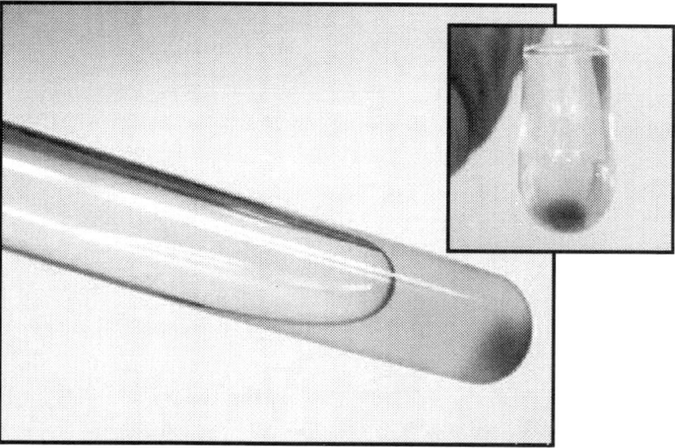

Figure 8. CRE Positive – Yellow with violet precipitate

2.4.1.2. Note on the biology of EPI-CRE®

EPI-CRE® detects ONLY living bacteria. It is 100% specific (based on Bergy's Manual and the Manual of Clinical Microbiology).

PCR positive and EPI-CRE®negative: Genetic amplification is not to be used as a "test of cure". The reason is that PCR and other genetic amplification methods will detect dead bacteria. Therefore, if a patient is treated intra-nasally or systemically with an effective antibiotic, the bacteria may be killed but their genetic material still is present. EPI-CRE® only detects living bacteria so this situation is not a limitation with this method.

2.5. Screening Method for Ciprofloxacin-resistant (cipR) Bacteria

EPI-FLOX® is a selective medium that allows the differentiation of ciprofloxacin-resistant from ciprofloxacin-susceptible bacteria. EPI-FLOX® contains 2 mcg/mL of ciprofloxacin, intended for use in the qualitative detection of ciprofloxacin-resistant (cipR) bacteria to provide epidemiological data. It is based on classical biochemicals in an optimized form. EPI-FLOX® is performed with urethral swabs and specimens, or rectal swabs and fecal specimens from patients to screen for cipR bacterial colonization. The presence of cipR bacteria is established when the color of the medium changes from red to yellow. In addition, a violet precipitate may also be observed.

The base formula of the EPI-FLOX® is the same as that of EPI-CRE® with the substitution of ciprofloxacin for meropenem. Therefore the procedure for use and the color changes are the same.

2.5.1. Note on the utility of the antibiotic resistant Enterobacteriaceae format

Because the base formula is designed to select for lactose positive Enterobacteriaceae, changes in the antibiotic can easily produce tailored screens. For example, by decreasing the concentration of meropenem to 0.25 mcg/mL, an epidemiological screen for OXA-48 can be produced.

3. Instrument: Pilots Point Monitor 60® (PPM 60®)

As described above, each of the DSU® epidemiology screens can be done manually. However, there are advantages to be able to place the screens in an instrument. Among these are:

Standardization: the instrument will read and interpret the screens in a completely uniform manner.

Positives reported when detected: the instrument monitors the color change of each screen every 15 minutes. Once the algorithm determines that a significant change has occurred compared to a control the results are reported at that time. Therefore there is continuous monitoring and reporting. Another benefit is that response time will be shortened.

Satellite screening: Because results are available from the instrument via Wi-Fi, internet, and intranet, screening at various locations can be controlled from a central location.

Epidemiological pattern analysis: Either from a central location or from satellite laboratories, data can be analyzed to determine if any increase of any of the epidemiological threats from any location is occurring.

Inexpensive cost: the instrument is designed to minimize cost. As shall be discussed below the instrument's function is to produce light and measure a change. Data are transferred to a computer – either a personal computer (PC) or an information technology (IT) system – for analysis. This format lowers the cost of the instrument.

Single instrument for all screens: Because of the light source chosen (see below) all of the screens, regardless of color, can be performed in one instrument. Moreover, wavelengths from 360nm through the entire visible light can be accurately measured, which allowed both fluorescent (366nm) and visible light measurements. The ability to use both ultraviolet and visible wavelengths permits the development of two separate biochemical identification systems. The separation of two biochemicals can allow for the detection of two separate target microbes (if each is specific for each microbe) of an enhanced specificity for a single target microbe (if the two together provide enhance specificity over one alone).

3.1. Principle of the instrument

The choice of the light source is critical to the generation of a functioning inexpensive instrument. Instead of using laser, fluorescence polarization, light scattering, reflectance spectrophotometry that are expensive and functionally limited, an inexpensive instrument that uses a white light generator that passes through the sample was generated. Absorption of one or more of the colors allows other to pass through. In addition an overall measure of turbidity, called luminosity, is also measured. For EPI-M® the coagulase coalescence change enhances the process.

The principal of the instrument is based on the way the human eye sees color.

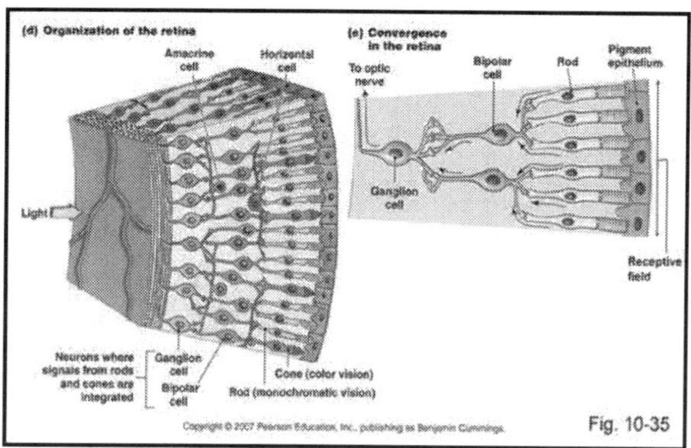

There are three primary colors that the cones see, which translate into the full range of colors.

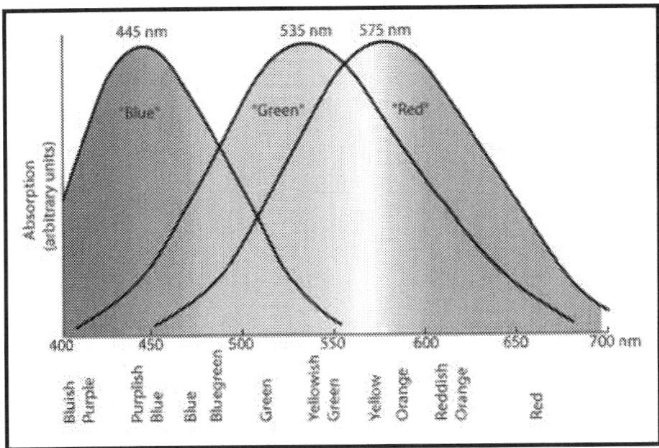

In the analysis program the light coming out of the sample is broken down as shown below. The first measure, which is called the "L" value, is essentially luminosity. It determines a scale from black to white. The second measure is the "a" value, which measures a change from green to red. The third measure is the "b" value, which measures a change from blue (and effectively includes as shown below yellow). Any particular reading can be determined exactly on the graph below by knowing the "L", "a", and "b" values. The sensitivity of the analysis program is enhanced because it can relate the changes of any combination of "L", "a", and "b" values.

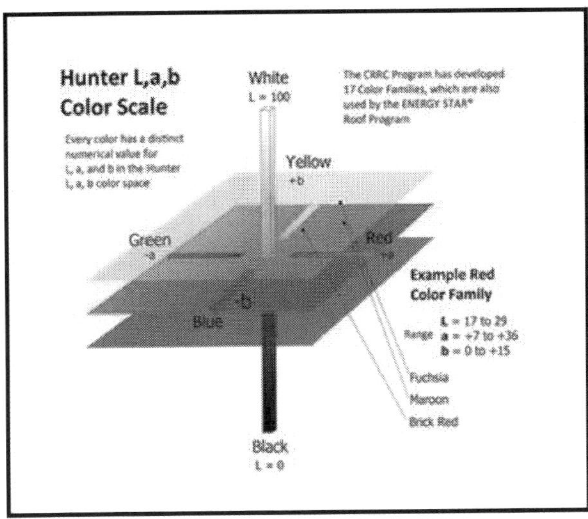

An example of a typical analysis is shown below for an EPI-M® MRSA analysis with standard ATCC MRSA 43300. The tube is scanned every 15 minutes and "L", "a", and "b" values generated (see the spreadsheet below for the individual values). The analysis program then translates the values into graphical form, which are shown above the spreadsheet. The analysis program then determines by a combination of "L", "a", or "b", or any combination thereof, if there is a significant change compared to a control. In this analysis 3 log10 of ATCC 43300 was detected in 14.5 hours.

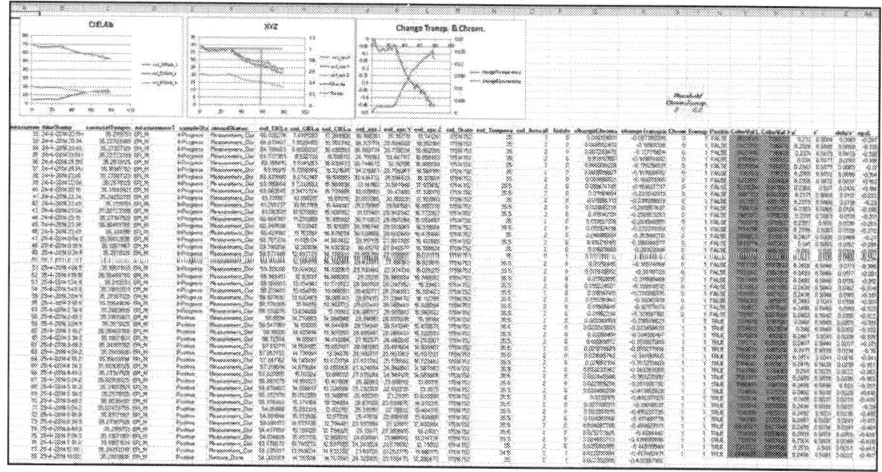

3.2. The instrument

The inside of the Pilots Point Monitor 60® is shown below. It is designed to accept the largest number of screens with the smallest footprint. It is approximately 0.8 meters in diameter. In the current configuration, 6 instruments can be connected to one PC. In practice the instrument cannot be opened. The tube (as shown in the opened instrument below) in practice is added to the instrument by sliding the blue plastic bar below the PPM 60® logo so as to expose only one slot. The instrument via a barcode on the test tube recognizes the name of the screen and all the demographics of the patient. The carrousel moves past the light generator with each shift of position every 15 minutes. There is an incubator in the instrument that can be adjusted +/-0.2°C.

Below is a diagram of the working aspects of the instrument: 46 is the carrousel block, 28 is the wall of the carrousel. 50 are the holes in the carrousel into which the tubes are place, 34 is the white light source, and 32 is the detector which reads the amount and quality of light ("L", "a", and "b") that is represented by 54.

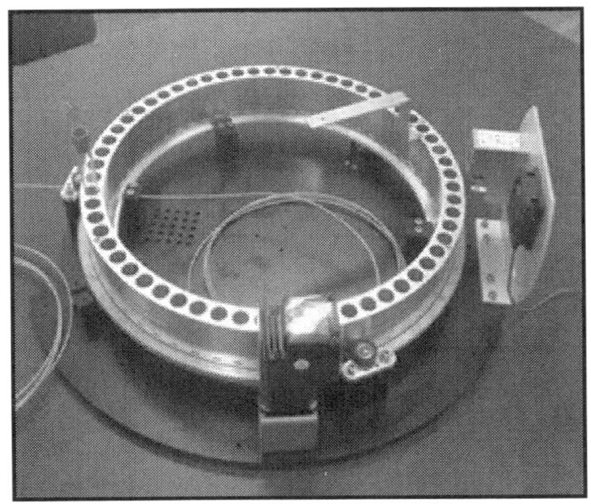

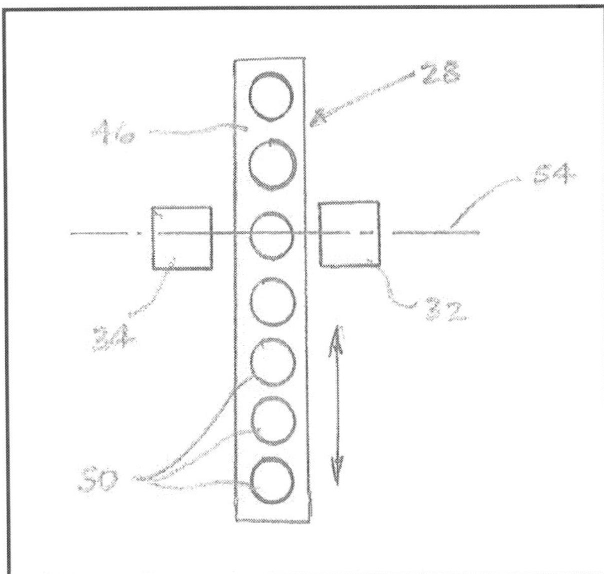

Below is the instrument as it would be used.

As the scanning of the tubes progresses, the information is sent to a PC or to a central IT station. This flexibility allows both large and small laboratories, epidemiologists in the field, researchers studying the prevalence of antibiotic resistant bacteria in animals, people, and even surfaces to use one system.

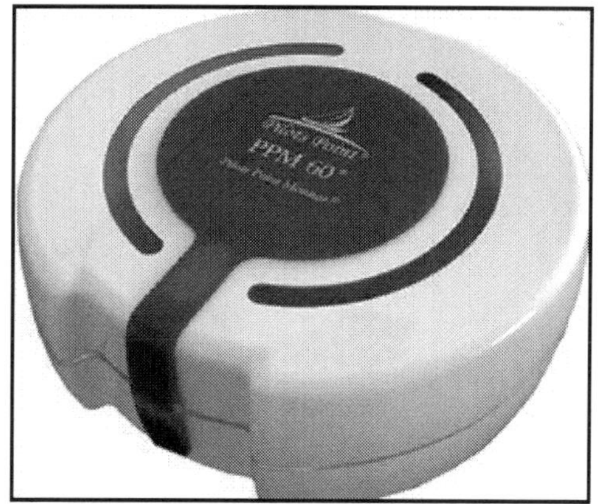

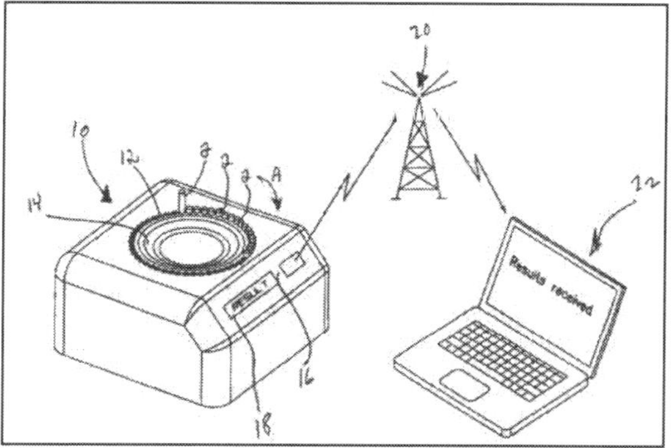

3.3. Enhanced sensitivity of the Defined Substrate Utilization® tools

3.3.1. Agar compared to liquid

Compared to agar-based microbial detection systems, liquid with the same formulas are always more sensitive, meaning liquid has the ability to detect a smaller number of bacteria than agar and in shorter period of time [10]. The reasons for this difference are based first on the fact that on the surface of agar, bacteria must make colonies to be observed. A visible colony requires a minimum number of bacteria. The surface of agar has a surface tension that inhibits the spreading of the bacterial colony. By comparison in liquid, the bacteria are free to divide in three dimensions.

In addition, the nutrients from the agar must enter the colony from only one direction – from the agar vertically into the colony. Likewise the waste products, which are inhibitory to the growth of the microbial colony, diffuse in close proximity to the developing colony thus inhibiting the colony's lateral development. The production of a colony can be thought to reach development when the nutrients below the colony (all that is available to it) combined with the production of waste products cause the bacteria to stop multiplying and expanding. By contrast, a bacterium in liquid suffers no such inhibitions. Nutrients, including the metabolizable substrate, are available from all directions. Therefore, there is no inhibition for the development of the bacteria. Likewise any waste products diffuse away from the developing bacteria nidus into the liquid, away from the nidus.

3.3.2. Optical parameters

Microbiological optical systems have over the years moved to a microtiter format. The microtiter structures are either the classical 96 well microtiter tray, or a variation, or a microtiter format in a vertical series of cupules, as exemplified by the Vitek 2 system (bioMérieux, Durham, NC). The decrease in the light path has significant negative effects on both sensitivity and the time to detection. The reason for this is that the optics of light absorbance is governed by the Beer-Lambert law. As shall be discussed below, the intensity of light is logarithmically related to the length of the light path. This means that a decrease in the light path results in a log decrease in the amount of measurable light that reaches the detector. This relationship was presented as the linear relationship between absorbance and concentration of an absorbing species.

The general Beer-Lambert law is usually written as:

A=a (lambda) * b * c

where A is the measured absorbance, a (lambda) is a wavelength-dependent absorptivity coefficient, b is the path length, and c is the analyte concentration.

When working in concentration units of molarity, the Beer-Lambert law is written as:

A=*epsilon* * b * c

where *epsilon* is the wavelength-dependent molar absorptivity coefficient with units of M^{-1} cm^{-1}

Regarding instruments, measurements are usually made in terms of transmittance (T), which is defined as:

T=I / I_o

where I is the light intensity after it passes through the sample and I_o is the initial light intensity.

The relation between A and T is:

A=-log T=-log (I / I_o)

and this formula is the one that is generally associated with the Beer-Lambert law.

The PPM 60® instrument uses traditional 1 centimeter (cm) light path test tubes. By comparison, the light path of the well formatted microtiter trays is 0.1 cm and the light path of the Vitek 2 system even less. Therefore, the differences in the light paths inherently make the PPM 60® instrument on the order of 100 times more sensitive. In terms of number of bacteria per mL, 6

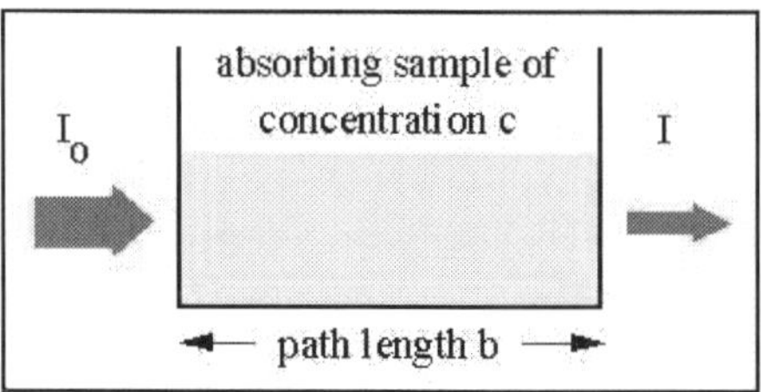

log10/mL of bacteria is the lowest limit of detection in a 0.1 cm light path (based on turbidity, without a chemical signal, such as the release of a chromophore from a hydrolysable substrate or change in a pH indicator) and in a 1 cm pathway, the limit increases to 8 log10/mL.

Practically, because bacteria in log phase have a generation time of 15-20 minutes, the time to detection in the PPM 60® instrument is much less than other methods, and significantly less than the observation of colonies on agar.

3.3.3. Example of data produced by the PPM 60® and analysis of a positive

Below are the results from the PPM 60® from a patient isolate of MRSA from the Mt. Sinai Hospital, New York City, NY, USA (courtesy of Dr. Camille Hamula). The initial inoculum was less than that found in the nose at 6.0 x 10⁴ CFU.

A Time [s]	B Hours	C Temp [°C]	D Gain	E Averaging Cycles	F X	G Y	H Z	I CIE Lab L	J CIE Lab a	K CIE Lab b
[illegible]	[illegible]	[illegible]	[illegible]	[illegible]	[illegible]	[illegible]	[illegible]	[illegible]	[illegible]	[illegible]

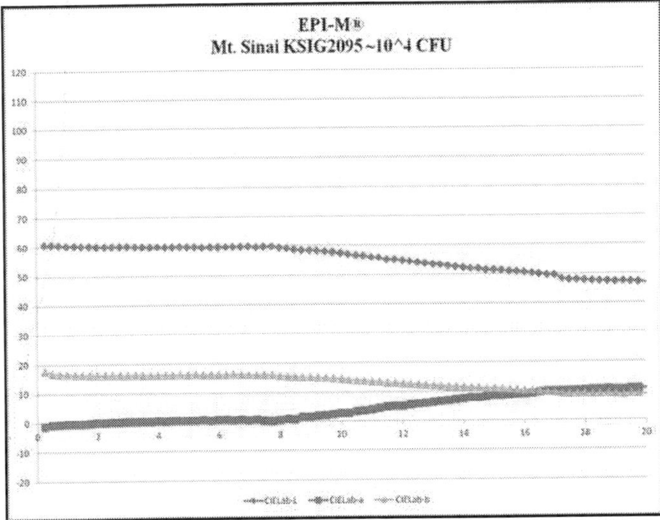

There was a significant change beginning at 9 hours and the positive was called at 11.25 hours.

3.3.4. Quantification of CFU/mL by the PPM 60® instrument

The time to a positive is proportional to the number of bacteria in the sample. Bacteria go through four stages of growth in liquid (but not agar): lag phase, log phase, stationery phase, and decline phase.

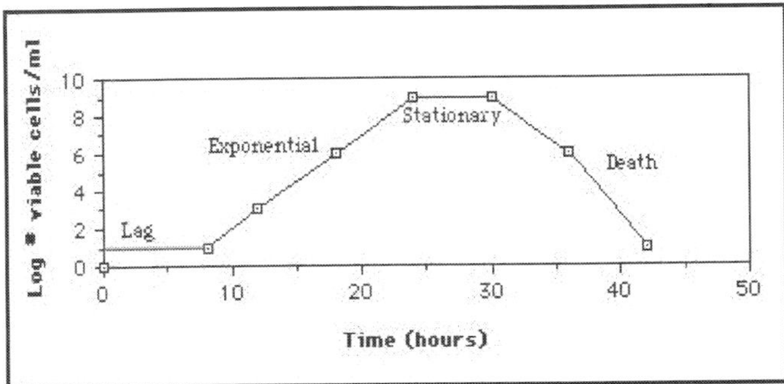

It is well known that the greater the number of bacteria in a sample, the shorter the lag phase. Lag phase is the time that the bacteria acclimate to a new environment. When bacteria enter a new environment, there is a heterogeneous population in terms of physiological health. Each of the cells acclimates to the new environment and leave lag phase and enter log phase at different times. By analogy it is similar to a kettle of popcorn kernels; one adds the kernels and all are in the same oil at the same temperature. The "healthier" ones pop first, the number of pops increase, and then there are a very large number of pops. Then there is a declining number of pops. Likewise with bacteria, some leave lag phase and enter log phase before others. The greater the number of bacteria, the shorter is the overall time the population goes from lag phase to log phase. In the PPM 60® instrument as discussed above, once the bacteria enter log phase they are dividing every 15-20 minutes. Therefore, the more bacteria in a population that leaves lag phase and enters log phase, the shorter the time to a positive since each bacteria multiplying produces a signal.

Below are examples of the ability of the PPM 60® to provide quantitative information with a variety of target bacteria.

3.3.4.1. MRSA

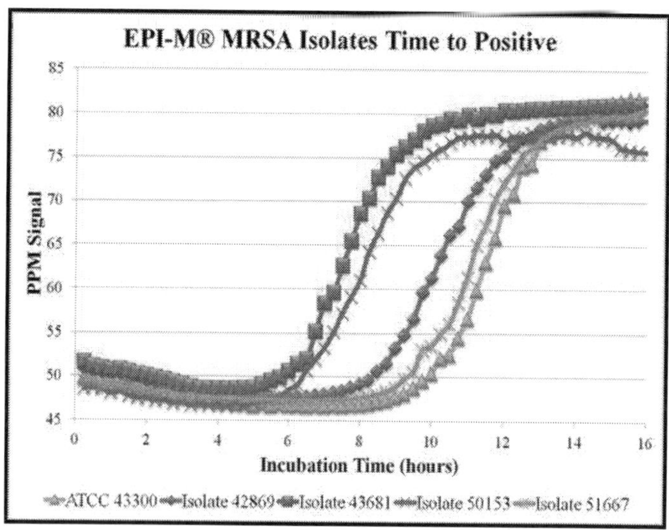

Isolate	Positive Result	Total CFU
Clinical Isolate 50153	6.25 hrs	24,000
Clinical Isolate 43681	6.0 hrs	14,800
Clinical Isolate 42869	8.5 hrs	10,400
Clinical Isolate 51667	9.0 hrs	4,800
ATCC 43300	9.75 hrs	4,000

3.3.4.2. VRE

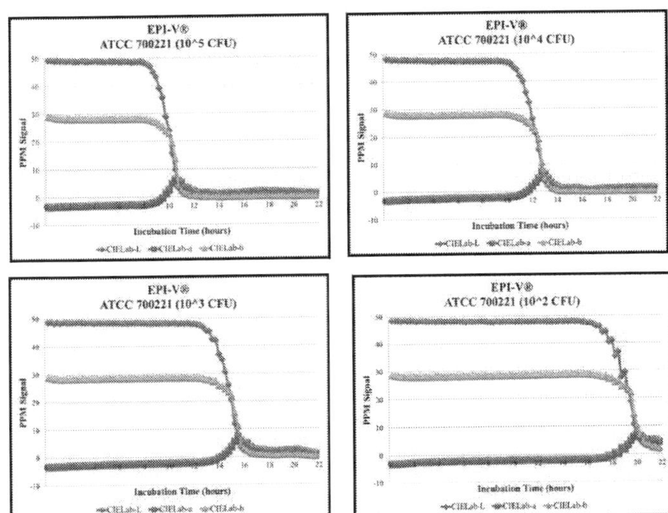

3.3.4.3. CRE

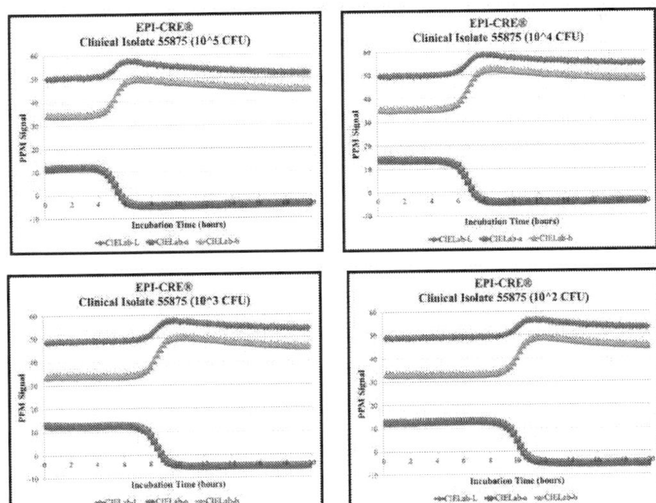

Acknowledgements

Lize-Mari Russo is thanked for excellent technical assistance with this project. SCE is the developer and patent holder of the DSU® epidemiology screens including EPI-M®, aureusAlert®, EPI-VISA®, EPI-V®, EPI-CRE® and EPI-FLOX®.

Author details

Stephen C. Edberg[1*] and J. Michael Miller[2]

*Address all correspondence to: stephen.edberg@yale.edu

1 Mt. Sinai Health System, New York City, New York and Yale University School of Medicine, New Haven, Connecticut, USA

2 Microbiology Technical Services, Dunwoody, Georgia, USA

References

[1]   Health Protection Agency (2012) Investigation of Specimens for Screening for MRSA. UK Standards for Microbiology Investigations. B 29: Issue 5.2.

[2]   Flayhart D, Hindler J.F, Bruckner D.A, Hall G, Shrestha R.K, Vogel S.A, Richter S.S, Howard W, Walther R, Carroll K.C (2005) Multicenter evaluation of BBL CHROMagar MRSA medium for direct detection of methicillin-resistant *Staphylococcus aureus* from surveillance cultures of the anterior nares. J. Clin. Microbiol. 43:5536-5540.

[3]   Kluytmans J, Van Belkum A, Verbrugh H (1997) Nasal carriage of *Staphylococcus aureus*: Epidemiology, underlying mechanisms, and associated risks. Clin. Microbiol. Rev. 10:505-520.

[4]   CHROMagar™ MRSA [package insert]. Sparks, M.D. Becton, Dickinson and Company. 2008:1-2.

[5]   Yang S, Rothman R.E (2004) PCR-based diagnostics for infectious diseases: uses, limitations, and future applications in acute-care settings. Lancet Infect. Dis. 4:347-348.

[6]   Garcia-Alvarez L, Holden M.T.G, Lindsay H, Webb C.R, Brown D.F.J, Curran M.D, et al. (2011) Methicillin-resistant *Staphylococcus aureus* with a novel mecA homologue in human and bovine populations in the UK and Denmark: a descriptive study. Lancet Infect. Dis. 11:595-560.

[7]   Shore A.C, Deasy E.C, Slickers P, Brennan G, O'Connell B, Monecke S, Ehricht R, Coleman D.C (2011) Detection of Staphylococcal Cassette Chromosome mec Type XI

Carrying Highly Divergent mecA, mecI, mecRI, blaZ, and ccr Genes in Human Clinical Isolates of Clonal Complex 130 Methicillin-Resistant *Staphylococcus aureus*. Antimicrob. Agents Chemoth. 55:3765-3773.

[8] Bannerman, T.L (2003) *Staphylococcus, Micrococcus,* and other catalase-positive cocci that grow aerobically. In: Murray P.R, Baron E.J, Jorgensen J.H, Pfaller M.A, Yolken R.H, editors. Manual of Clinical Microbiology. 8th edn. Washington, DC: American Society for Microbiology. pp. 384-404.

[9] Selepak S.T, Witebsky F.G (1985) Inoculum size and lot-to-lot variation as significant variables in the tube coagulase test for *Staphylococcus aureus*. J. Clin. Microbiol. 22:835-837.

[10] Rice E.W, Fox K.R, Nash H.D, Read E.J, Smith A.P (1987) Comparison of media for recovery of total coliform bacteria from chemically treated water. Appl. Environ. Microbiol. 53:1571-1573.

[11] Pipes W.O, Minnigh H.A, Moyer B, Troy M.A (1986) Comparison of Clark's presence-absence test and the membrane filter method for coliform detection in potable water samples. Appl. Environ. Microbiol. 52:439-443.

[12] CLSI (2009) Performance standards for antimicrobial susceptibility testing; nineteenth informational supplement. M100-S19. Wayne, PA: Clinical Laboratory Standards Institute.

[13] Murray P.R, Baron E.J, Jorgensen J.H, Landry M.L, Pfaller M.A (2007) Manual of Clinical Microbiology. 9th edn. Washington, D.C: American Society for Microbiology.

[14] FDA (2009) 510(k) Substantial Equivalence Determination Decision Summary, Assay Only Template. K091025. Silver Spring, MD: United States Food and Drug Administration. http://www.accessdata.fda.gov/cdrh_docs/reviews/K091025.pdf

[15] Edberg S.C (2013) Enhanced Reagent for the Detection of L-pyrrolidonyl-β-naphthalyamide (PYR) Hydrolysis. 23rd European Congress on Clinical Microbiology and Infectious Diseases, Berlin, 27-30 April 2013.

[16] Edberg, S. C. "CRE and a New CRE Test." Innovated Products Newsletter (Oct. 2013): 6-7. Committee to Reduce Infection Deaths. http://www.hospitalinfection.org/PDF/RID%20Fall%20Newsletter.pdf

[17] Centers for Disease Control and Prevention. 2009. Laboratory protocol for detection of carbapenem-resistant or carbapenemase-producing *Klebsiella* spp. and *E. coli* from rectal swabs. Centers for Disease Control and Prevention, Atlanta, GA. http://www.cdc.gov/NCIDOD/DHQP/pdf/ar/Klebsiella_or_Ecoli.pdf

[18] Nordmann P, Poirel L, Dortet L (2012) Rapid Detection of Carbapenemase-producing *Enterobacteriaceae*. Emerg. Infect. Dis. 1503-1507.

[19] Nordmann P, Girlich D, Poirel L (2012) Detection of Carbapenemase Producers in *Enterobacteriaceae* by Use of a Novel Screening Medium. J. Clin. Microbiol. 50(8):2761.

Developments in Diagnosis and Treatment of Diseases of Public Health Importnace

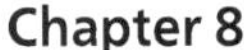

Chapter 8

Review of Iron Supplementation and Fortification

Lauren C. Ramsay and Christopher V. Charles

Additional information is available at the end of the chapter

http://dx.doi.org/10.5772/58987

1. Introduction

Iron deficiency anemia (IDA) is the most prevalent micronutrient condition globally, with nearly 50% of anemia cases being caused by iron deficiency according to the World Health Organization (WHO) [1]. While it is a condition that does not discriminate between the developed and developing world, the incidence is still higher in developing countries. In South-East Asia the WHO reported that 65.5% of preschool-age children suffer from anemia, and 48.2% and 45.7% of pregnant and non-pregnant women, respectively, also suffer from anemia, which represents the highest prevalence in the world [1].

As the most prevalent micronutrient condition in the world it is critical that there is a strong understanding of how to improve iron intake. In many cases this may involve taking iron supplement pills, however this is by no means the only approach that is currently being used. This chapter seeks to provide background information on iron deficiency and iron deficiency anemia (IDA), and review a number of current strategies currently being used to address these conditions around the world. This review is by no means exhaustive, but aims to cover a number of studies in each of the major iron deficiency intervention strategies.

2. Iron deficiency and iron deficiency anemia

The word anemia is derived from the Greek word ἀναιμία *anaimia*, meaning "without blood," [2]. Anemia is a deficiency of red blood cells and/or hemoglobin resulting in a reduction of the oxygen-carrying capacity of blood [3]. An individual with a circulating hemoglobin concentration less than 120g/L is considered to be anemic, but this varies across age and sex based on iron requirement and hemoglobin thresholds, which can be seen in Figure 1 [1, 4].

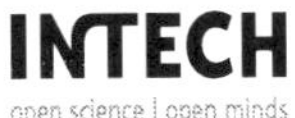

Hemoglobin thresholds used to define anemia	
Age or Gender	**Hemoglobin Threshold (g/L)**
Children (0.5-4.99 yrs)	110
Children (5-11.99 yrs)	115
Children (12-14.99 yrs)	120
Non-pregnant Women (≥15.00 yrs)	120
Pregnant Women (≥15.00 yrs)	110
Men (≥15.00 yrs)	130

Figure 1. Hemoglobin concentration thresholds below which anemia is present

Anemia is caused by a long-term iron imbalance resulting in the depletion of bodily iron stores over time [2, 5]. Iron is a necessary component in the production of red blood cells, and so the absence of sufficient supplies results in decreased hemoglobin production and subsequently red blood cell production [2, 5, 6]. The focus of this chapter is on IDA, and this is typically a result of inadequate dietary intake, but could also be a result of excessive blood loss from trauma or post-partum hemorrhage, or other diseases such as parasitic infections, malaria, and inherited hemoglobin disorders [5, 6].

There are several risk factors of IDA, which have resulted in uneven distribution of prevalence around the world, with the highest concentration in developing countries in Africa and Asia [4]. The most commonly reported risk factors of IDA include: poverty [4, 7]; local dietary staples such as rice which have low bio-availability of iron [8]; genetic hemoglobinopathies [9]; consumption of untreated water [10]; sex where typically females are more likely to experience IDA than males [11]; low parental educational attainment [10-12]; maternal anemia [13]; and food insecurity [13]. Based on the information presented above, it is clear that the determinants of IDA are complex and a number of social, ecological, biological and socioeconomic factors are at play. Across each study, however, poverty is the most salient predictor.

2.1. Signs and symptoms of iron deficiency anemia

The signs and symptoms vary among individuals but there are always adverse effects of IDA. Pregnant and postpartum women and young children are most susceptible to iron deficiency and IDA because of the high demands for iron that growth and pregnancy have [14]. These groups also experience some of the most severe symptoms [14].

Symptoms of IDA may include diminished work capacity, immune system dysfunction, neurocognitive impairment, dizziness, fatigue, and pallor [2, 6, 7]. Severe anemia can reduce significantly a woman's ability to survive giving birth due to bleeding during and after childbirth [14, 15]. Additionally, pregnant women are at higher risk of preterm delivery when anemic [8]. For these reasons, anemia is considered to be a major contributor to maternal mortality in the developing world. The WHO reports that anemia is a factor in 20% of maternal deaths [16].

Children are also highly susceptible to adverse effects of IDA and experience additional signs and symptoms if left untreated. Anemic children may experience height and weight disturbances, slowing of learning and behavior development, and interruptions in physical or mental growth [12]. IDA can affect neurocognitive development, resulting in reduced psychomotor and cognitive abilities in children [2, 17]. These are most often measured on standardized measures of mental development, cognitive function tests, psychomotor scales, and educational achievement tests [18]. The impaired cognitive and psychomotor development that children affected by iron deficiency or IDA experience is speculated to have a causal relationship to future earning potential, though study terms have not yet been long enough to quantify this [17]. This is thought to occur because of the direct relationship between iron and oxygen delivery to the brain and muscles [14].

3. Iron in the body

Iron is a critical component in many metabolic functions, particularly in delivering oxygen throughout the body as an essential component of red blood cells. The majority of human iron stores are found in hemoglobin [19]. Iron is a component of every human cell and plays a critical role in many biochemical reactions in the body. It is involved in oxygen transportation, energy production, cellular respiration, DNA synthesis and the production of dopamine and serotonin, which are essential to neurotransmission [7, 14, 20, 21]. The storage and transportation of iron are highly dependent on red blood cells morphology and the presence of sufficient amounts of hemoglobin. Iron is toxic when too much is stored in the body and may cause tissue damage when the iron capacity has been exceeded [5, 19]. This problem can be compounded by the very slow rate at which humans naturally lose iron [22].

3.1. Dietary iron

Dietary iron comes in two forms: heme and non-heme. Heme iron, which is more easily absorbed, comes from meat, poultry and fish. This source of iron is easily absorbed because it is delivered as the stable prophyrin complex and is unaffected by other food components [21]. Contrary to this, non-heme iron is more difficult to absorb and comes from cereals, legumes and some vegetables [21].

Non-heme iron from food comes in several different chemical forms and the elemental iron is dependent on this and the body's ability to recognize and absorb the iron. For example, the chemistry of ferric (Fe^{3+}) is much more dependent on pH levels in the stomach relative to ferrous (Fe^{2+}) iron; ferric iron requires a more acidic environment to be absorbed [21]. Thus, consuming vitamin C with dietary iron or iron supplementation can be a critical step to absorbing the maximum amount of elemental iron possible [5, 23]. Non-heme iron is further complicated in the presence of tannins (e.g. in tea) or phytate (e.g. in whole grains), as these are known to inhibit the absorption of non-heme iron [5, 21].

4. Implications of parasitic infections and malaria

4.1. Helminths

Infection with soil-transmitted intestinal helminths is a common problem among populations living primarily in rural areas of low-income countries. These parasites are a large, polyphyletic grouping of multicellular organisms that can generally be seen with the naked eye in their mature stages. Helminths typically include roundworm (*Ascaris lumbricoides*), whipworm (*Trichuris trichiura*) and the hookworms (*Necator americanus* and *Ancylostoma duodenale*) [24]. Some estimates suggest that more than 2 billion people on the planet are infected with one, or multiple helminths, with the highest prevalence occurring where sanitation is poor and water supplies are compromised [24].

Soil-transmitted helminths live in the intestine of an infected person, and are easily spread when a person comes into contact with the feces of an infected individual. This contact might result from the use of gardens, bushes or fields as an open latrine, or could result from the use of human feces as fertilizer that is intentionally sprayed onto crops and deposited into the soil. A new host is established when an uninfected person then unknowingly ingests the eggs of these parasites [25].

The association between parasite infection and anemia is well known and has been widely documented [26]. Primarily, the organisms cause gastrointestinal bleeding resulting in blood loss, lowered hemoglobin values, and resultant anemia. Further, some organisms disrupt nutrient absorption by damaging the mucosal surface of gut, leading to poor absorption of micronutrients. For example, the two significant hookworm species *Ancylostoma duodenale* and *Necator americanus*, produce 5000-10,000 and 10,000-25,000 eggs per day, resulting in 0.03 mL and 0.15-0.23 mL blood loss per day, respectively [27]. In addition, some hookworms release anti clotting factors that ensures continuous blood flow and thereby further leads to poor health outcomes [27].

4.2. Malaria

Malaria is a well-known cause of morbidity and mortality in the developing world, initiated by infection by parasites of the genus *Plasmodium*. Estimates of the burden of disease suggest that more than 515 million episodes occur annually, representing 18% of all childhood deaths in Sub-Saharan Africa [28, 29]. Anemia caused by malaria has a multi-factorial pathophysiology with unknown molecular mechanisms [30]. Research has shown that malaria is implicated in both the destruction of red blood cells through hemolysis of both infected and uninfected erythrocytes, but also through the decreased production of erythrocytes in the bone marrow [30]. Malarial anemia is therefore typically normocytic and normochromic with a distinct absence of reticulocytes.

Severe malarial anemia is of great public health concern because of the widespread prevalence of malaria in the developing world where access to appropriate healthcare is limited, and because children and pregnant women are the hardest hit by the condition [31]. Malarial anemia is most often observed in areas where high malarial transmission occurs [31]. Severe anemia caused by *P falciparum*, one species of malarial infection, is responsible for approximately one-third deaths associated with the disease [30].

5. Treating iron deficiency anemia

Treating iron deficiency and iron deficiency anemia must continue to be a priority of governments, non-governmental organizations and international aid agencies alike. The ideal approach to addressing iron deficiency is a nutritious and well balanced diet that naturally provides adequate iron intake. However, this is not a reality in much of the developing world where subsistence comes from cereals with low iron bioavailability. This generates the need for a cost-effective, simple and easy to administer solution that may be found in supplementation and fortification. Food fortification is widely considered to be the most cost-effective approach to treating IDA, but this is not without its challenges [8]. While in the developed world fortified products are rampant, and often there are government regulations to ensure fortification of common food items (e.g. milk, breakfast cereals, and salt) this strategy can be less effective in the developing world. Even the smallest price increase in staple products in developing countries may be a deterrent to purchase and use them [8]. With escalating food prices, which peaked in the 2008 food crisis, households in developing countries were spending large shares of their incomes on food and commonly had to switch to cheaper but less nutritious foods to combat hunger [32]. In this case, the likelihood of households purchasing fortified foods may be a more difficult intervention to implement.

Currently several fortification approaches are being implemented; reference [33] describes three methods; 1) fortified products added during food processing (e.g. wheat flour); 2) fortification added at home during food preparation (e.g. multiple micronutrient powders); and 3) genetically engineered foods with enhanced nutrition (e.g. genetically engineered cereals). In general, iron fortification has been found to be very successful around the world; in a meta-analysis of randomized controlled trials for iron deficiency alleviation, 13 studies on iron fortification for women and 41 for children were assessed [34]. These studies included fortification via sodium iron ethylenediaminetetraacetic acid (NaFeEDTA), ferrous sulfate, fortified candies, fortified curry powder and ferrous pyrophosphate [34]. In these studies, efficaciousness of iron fortificants all showed significant results in improving hemoglobin concentration and reducing anemia in study populations [34]. A separate meta-analysis of 60 studies showed similar results: iron-fortified foods are efficacious in increasing hemoglobin concentrations and reducing IDA in study populations [35].

6. Iron supplements

The Lancet Series (2013) on maternal and child nutrition reported that during a trial of iron supplements in pregnant women they found a 67% reduction of iron deficiency anemia [36]. Additionally, in non-pregnant women a review of studies showed that intermittent iron supplementation was effective in reducing the risk of anemia by 27% [36]. This review also indicated that daily iron supplementation reduced the incidence of low birth weight by 19% [36]. Despite the high success rates of iron supplementation, distribution and cost become major concerns and make compliance in iron deficiency reduction strategies very difficult to navigate. Iron supplementation, often in the form of a pill or liquid, is an expensive option for treating iron deficiency and IDA, though the elemental iron present is much higher [8].

Apart from the difficulties of program implementation, a cost-effectiveness analysis was conducted in four subregions of the world (African subregion, South American subregion, European subregion and South-East Asian subregion) in order to compare the cost-effectiveness (in $USD) of iron supplementation versus fortification. This study showed that in the developed world supplementation was more cost-effective due to well-developed distribution chains already in place [18]. But despite the higher overall impact of iron supplementation on a population's health, fortification is more cost-effective in rural and developing communities [18].

7. Case study: Iron fortified candies for children

The use of micronutrient fortified candies and lozenges have been tested in some countries, including India and Indonesia. There are relatively few randomized controlled trials (RCTs) that assess the efficaciousness of this intervention compared to many of the other programs reviewed in this chapter.

Nutri-candy was developed as a strategy to alleviate iron deficiency and other micronutrient deficiencies in children aged 2-6 years, pregnant and lactating women and adolescent girls in the developing world [37].

Nutritional content of nutri-candy	
Nutrients	**Levels per 3 gram lozenge**
Vitamin A	500 IU
Vitamin C	10 mg
Folic acid	50 mcg
Iron	7 mg

Figure 2. Nutri-candy nutritional content [37]

In India, where various manufacturers produce nutri-candy, more than five million people in four states take a fortified candy every day at a cost of US $1.33 per person per year which includes the cost of transportation [38]. In West Bengal a study showed that while using nutri-candy the prevalence of iron deficiency anemia reduced by 15%. In Haryana another study took place that found the prevalence anemia changed from 50% at baseline to 9.6% in the group receiving a daily nutri-candy [39].

In Indonesia a similar study took place to test the impact of Vitella, a chewy fruit candy fortified with multiple micronutrients, on iron levels in children aged 4-6 years [40]. This study found that the hemoglobin concentration of children receiving the candies increased by 10.2g/L, and anemia prevalence decreased by 42.1% after 12 weeks of intervention [40].

Based on these few studies in India and Indonesia the use of fortified candies should be further researched and incorporated into national strategies to alleviate iron deficiency. All studies reported high acceptability of the product both from caregivers and children [38-40]. If incorporated into school programs or other national strategies it may be very effective in reducing the burden of iron deficiency in low-income countries.

8. Fortified staples

Certain foods can be fortified after harvesting in order to deliver more iron during consumption and some can be genetically modified and bred to include more iron. The universal fortification of foods has been promoted as a strategy to address micronutrient deficiencies around the world. For example, in Canada and the United States it is a legal requirement to fortify milk during processing with Vitamins A, C and D [41, 42]. Universal food fortification is viewed to be an efficacious and cost-effective strategy to address IDA [43].

To use rice as an example, there are some strains of rice that have been genetically modified to have greater amounts of iron but the research in this area is still relatively new [44]. This can be achieved by introducing other genes to rice breeds that increase the storage of iron on polished white rice [45]. One way that this is done is by adding a gene from soybeans that adds the protein ferritin to rice, and studies have shown that this source of iron is bioavailable [45].

When rice is polished it loses much of its natural iron during this process and so a method of fortifying rice by applying an edible coating that improves the available iron in the rice [46]. A third way to fortify rice is by using a product called Ultra Rice which is a high-iron simulated rice grain that can be mixed in with regular rice and is highly accepted with no reports of bad texture or taste [43, 47].

During a randomized controlled trial in the Philippines iron fortified rice was proportionately mixed with regular rice to provide more available iron in a serving of rice. Hemoglobin concentrations of children in the study sites significantly increased from baseline to endline, and prevalence of anemia significantly decreased by 4.7% [48]. In Mexico when female factory workers were given fortified rice five days a week for six months iron status improved significantly, and the prevalence of anemia was reduced by 80% [43]. However, a study in Brazil found that the use of fortified rice only once weekly in child-care centres brought about similar results [47]. In addition to improved iron status, another study in Brazil found that study participants and their families exhibited a very high rate of acceptance of the fortified rice as part of their diet with no adverse effects or undesirable taste, colour or smell [49]. Iron fortified rice, with proven effectiveness in improving iron status as well as high acceptability of the product, may be an important part of national nutrition strategies.

Wheat flour and maize flour can also be fortified to be more iron rich, and may be a useful tool in addressing iron deficiency in communities where large amounts of wheat flour and its products are consumed [50]. The WHO supports the fortification of wheat and maize flour but suspects that it will be the most effective in reducing iron deficiency when it is mandated at the national level [51].

In a trial that assessed the efficacy of fortified wheat flour it was found that there was a lower prevalence of iron deficiency in women who consumed the fortified flour more regularly [50]. In a study conducted with Indian school children, iron fortified whole wheat flour, after seven months the prevalence of iron deficiency significantly declined from 62% to 21% [52].

Iron biofortified pearl millet has also been tested as an approach to address iron deficiency in communities of developing countries. A study in Benin found that consuming iron fortified pearl millet can double the absorption of iron in women and may be a highly effective approach to combatting iron deficiency in millet-eating communities [53].

Despite the improvement in hemoglobin concentration in trial communities, there were challenges and limitations to this approach for addressing iron deficiency and IDA. Primarily, the cost to households associated with switching to fortified products proved to be a challenge. For example, in the Philippines when the market was flooded with unfortified rice by the government, the population began purchasing the cheaper, unfortified variety rather than the iron-fortified rice that was slightly more expensive, despite the added benefit [48]. The other studies reviewed did not test the possibility of selling fortified products in markets so it is uncertain how this would work in different countries. It is likely that higher costs of fortified rice could be a barrier to the sale of the fortified rice, and this strategy may be difficult to sustain within a competitive market environment.

9. Food fortification involving sodium ferritin

It is possible to fortify condiments such as fish sauce and soy sauce, which are commonly consumed in Asian countries. A study conducted using iron fortified Thai fish sauce showed that iron absorption from ferric sulfate fortified fish sauce added to a meal of rice and vegetables showed positive results [54]. This suggests that fortified fish sauce may be an effective solution to combat iron deficiency in countries with high fish sauce use. A similar study conducted in Switzerland assessed NaFeEDTA fortified fish sauce and found that it is a potential fortification method to address iron deficiency and iron deficiency anemia [55]. In Cambodia fortified fish sauce and soy sauce are becoming more salient in the iron deficiency discussion and the government intends to legislate fortifying these condiments by 2015 [56]. In Vietnam, where fish sauce is consumed as part of the regular diet and produced locally, a study was conducted and found that women using iron fortified fish sauce for six months had an average higher hemoglobin concentrations by 8.7g/L than women who used regular fish sauce [57]. However, there are still challenges associated with fortifying condiments which include a changing of the colour of the sauce due to the addition of fortificants as well as political challenges to monitoring and rolling out this type of initiative [54, 56].

While the cost-effectiveness ratio of this type of fortification has been positive, these analyses do not include the costs of potential health implications of high sodium diets [58]. Sodium is known to cause many adverse health problems including hypertension, increased risk of cardiovascular disease and increased risk of stroke [59]. It is possible that this type of intervention may promote excessive salt intake and the negative health impacts may outweigh the benefit of increased iron intake [60]. In fact, the WHO recommends that "the use of salt as the vehicle for new fortification initiatives other than iodine and fluoride should be discouraged," [60].

10. Micronutrient Powders (MNPs)

Micronutrient powders include any fortified powders that have at least two micronutrients in their composition. These powders are added to food being prepared in the home and then consumed, providing the benefits of the micronutrients they contain. This fortification method has received a great amount of attention in the nutrition world, as many micronutrient deficiencies are so prevalent around the world in both developed and developing countries and this strategy has the potential to address multiple deficiencies at once.

Sprinkles, a brand of MNP, were developed as a fortification method by creating a powder with iron and various micronutrients that can be 'sprinkled' on complementary foods before being fed to children [61, 62]. Various studies have shown that this is an effective method of increasing hemoglobin concentration and treating iron deficiency anemia in children [62-66]. In Cambodia two studies were conducted that demonstrated a significant decline in iron deficiency anemia among groups of children who were on a daily regiment of sprinkles versus a control group with no intervention [67, 68]. A study in Kenya assessed Sprinkles in a more real world setting by selling the product in local markets and found that in this situation they remained efficacious in reducing iron deficiency [69]. In India, where IDA is incredibly prevalent, the use of MNPs resulted in significantly reduced levels of IDA in children after 24 weeks of treatment [70]. In a meta-analysis conducted on 17 studies, micronutrient powders showed to significantly reduce the prevalence of anemia by 34%, iron deficiency anemia by 57%, and improves hemoglobin concentration [71]. These results were from studies that occurred in various countries including Ghana, India, Bangladesh, Kenya, Pakistan and Haiti, which represents a number of regions in the world [71].

While the randomized clinical trials that have been conducted to test various MNPs have been successful, these are all in highly controlled situations. Studies have consistently showed success in improving biomarkers such as hemoglobin concentration and a reduction in anemia prevalence, however the adherence to such programs in a less-controlled environment may differ. Distribution, cultural cooking practices, and cultural perceptions of MNPs may impact the effectiveness of such programs, though in the case of MNPs there is potential for this intervention to remain efficacious. Micronutrient powders were accepted in many communities by caregivers around the world because they can be incorporated into the regular feeding practices [64, 68]. In a study conducted in Bangladesh on sprinkle adherence [63] it showed that adherence was higher and hematological improvements were greater in groups who received more flexible instructions for use of 60 Sprinkles packets, rather than being told to use them daily. Further research into adherence and acceptability would be useful in order to develop a strong implementation strategy for different regions of the world.

11. Taking advantage of adventitious sources of dietary iron

11.1. Cast iron pots

Early studies demonstrated that cooking food in cast iron pots increases the iron content of certain foods and that this iron is bioavailable [72]. In the face of the global iron deficiency endemic, researchers believed that promoting the use of cast iron pots could be efficacious in reducing the incidence of iron deficiency and iron deficiency anemia. Studies have taken place that assess the effectiveness, cost effectiveness and acceptability of this approach.

A laboratory study was conducted in order to assess the impact on the iron contents of green leafy vegetables when cooked in different pots. This study demonstrated that the material of the pot plays a significant role in the bioavailable iron in green leafy vegetables, and those cooked in iron utensils had 9% more available iron than those cooked in non-iron pots [73]. There is still some debate whether or not the iron that leaches into the food is bioavailable, and the need for more extensive analysis into improving iron availability in more types of food such as maize and rice [74].

The main limitations of using cast iron pots to improve iron status are that there was low acceptability during randomized controlled trials [75-77]. Cast-iron pots were reported to be heavy, rust easily, and required more attention for cooking due being prone to higher cooking temperatures [75]. In one study it was found that participants were selling the cast iron pots in the market in order to supplement low family incomes [78]. On the other hand, cast iron pots required less wood for stoves since cooking times were faster, and the pots were considered to be very durable [75].

Despite increases in hemoglobin concentrations and a reduction in anemia in the trial communities, the use of cast iron pots is not an effective strategy for addressing iron deficiency and IDA in most cases. It is possible that in communities where the use of cast iron pots is already prevalent then promoting continued or increased use has potential to be a part of a larger strategy to eliminate iron deficiency and IDA because the communities already accept the use of these pots [79].

11.2. The Lucky Iron Fish

The Lucky Iron Fish, an intervention based on the same principles of cooking with a cast iron pot, has shown in a randomized controlled trial to be effective in increasing hemoglobin concentrations by 11.6g/L, and reducing anemia by half in the study population, compared to the control group after 12 months [80]. This method involves boiling water or cooking soup with the Lucky Iron Fish (an iron ingot shaped like a common Cambodian fish) for 10 minutes and adding some form of ascorbic acid (citrus juice, most commonly) [80, 81].

While this has potential to be effective in addressing iron deficiency it has only been tested on women of reproductive age, and thus it is not certain that the Lucky Iron Fish will provide the right amount of iron for children. The clinical trial included only 6 pregnant women, and future research could seek out larger numbers of pregnant and lactating women to test the efficaciousness in these times of high iron demand. Furthermore, gaining a better understanding of the type of iron that leaches into water and foods would be beneficial, as would further testing of fortifiable foods. Additional challenges associated with this approach are predominantly surrounding acceptability and education, as this intervention requires significant behavior change in home practices. Research regarding the acceptability, adherence and cost-effectiveness of this strategy should take place in order to carefully compare it with alternate interventions to be included in a national nutrition strategy.

12. Case study: Treating IDA in Cambodia in pregnant and post-partum women

In Cambodia, it is reported that in 2006 63% infants and young children suffer from anemia [67]. Current projects addressing iron deficiency in Cambodia include: the government supported supplementation for pregnant and post-partum women; Sprinkles; weekly iron folic acid supplements for women of reproductive age; helminth control; fortified foods such as rice and fish sauce; and the Lucky Iron Fish [82-84]. However, the official government stance, as advised by the World Health Organization (WHO) is for a supplementation program, and thus no official fortification program is currently in place or widely accepted by the numerous government and non-government groups working to address nutrition issues in Cambodia [84]. Recent research assessing the possibility of iron-fortified condiments has put fortification on the government's radar and is speculated to result in a change in government legislation [56]. Iron deficiency and its associated anemia remains a salient health issue in Cambodia and looking ahead a more multi-faceted approach may be necessary to successfully combat this challenge.

12.1. Government supplementation program

The following guidelines are followed by Health Centres in Cambodia: First contact during pregnancy: 60 iron/folic acid tablets provided; Second contact during pregnancy: 30 iron/folic acid tablets provided; Post-partum: 42 iron/folic acid tablets provided [84].

Iron supplementation is known to be incredibly effective due to the high bioavailability of iron [85-87]. This is especially important to ensure during pregnancy when iron demands of women are greater, and the risks can be more severe [1, 87]. Daily iron supplementation is the most effective strategy at protecting iron stores in women during pregnancy but large doses of iron are also associated with negative side effects [87]. The negative side effects may cause problems with compliance, thus damaging the effectiveness of these programs [86]. Currently an urgent need for evaluation on the government's supplementation program exists – as no studies have reported the effectiveness in at-need populations and monitoring the changes in iron deficiency and IDA.

In two focus groups held in February 2014 in the remote Preah Vihear province in northern Cambodia, women (approximately 30 in each village; Koh Ker and Ker) reported that less than 5% of participants visited a health centre during their pregnancy [88]. Collectively, the women reported that they were aware that at their community health centre they would have received free iron supplements for during pregnancy and after delivering their child. Despite this, women chose (by personal preference or circumstances dictated this) to deliver in their homes with a local midwife from their village. The health centres can be expensive to travel to and are far away from their villages, in the case of the two villages that were visited. The roads used to travel are barely passable, which only becomes more difficult during the rainy season (June – November) [88]. This suggests that in some parts of Cambodia the government initiatives may not be reaching marginalized populations, the population that demonstrates the greatest need.

13. Discussion

There is a significant difference between fortification and supplementation with regards to economic feasibility, government involvement and effectiveness in improving health. Fortification has an opportunity to be a more cost-effective and efficacious treatment for iron deficiency and iron-deficiency anemia than supplementation in many developing countries. While iron supplements should continue to be a critical component of a national strategy to alleviate iron deficiency and its associated anemia, particularly in times of high iron demands such as pregnancy, a multifaceted approach should be developed to more effectively combat this micronutrient deficiency.

Each of the fortification strategies reviewed in this chapter were efficacious in improving iron status in a controlled environment. However in many cases this does not provide assurance that adopting these strategies will be effective in every community. Adherence and acceptability are critical to the success of these interventions, but most RCTs do not assess these conditions, as it can be difficult with the need for controlled settings to conduct trials. As with many other development strategies, the approach will vary across, and even within countries, which makes developing guidelines for the treatment of ID and IDA difficult. What works in one country will likely not work in the exact same way in a neighbouring country, and the same can be said from one village to the next. However, some of the interventions that were reviewed in this chapter demonstrated greater success in different regions of the world than others. The use of cast-iron pots did not prove to be an acceptable strategy in most countries due to the preference for lighter, easier to clean aluminum pots.

Multi-micronutrient powders have proven to be consistently effective in RCTs in alleviating iron deficiency in children. Both government distribution channels and selling sachets of MNPs in a market setting have been successful. A limitation of this approach is that few studies have tested the efficaciousness of MNPs in treating ID and IDA in groups other than children. The few studies conducted testing the effectiveness of MMPs in pregnant women the results are modest, and has been suggested that alone they are not adequate to address maternal iron deficiency [89]. There are still challenges being addressed with this approach but it has the potential to be efficacious as part of a national strategy. Since women of reproductive age are in great need of iron fortification programs multi-micronutrient powders should not be the sole component of a national approach, but could be included as part of a strategy to improve children's iron status.

Similarly, biofortified staples such as rice and wheat flour were highly acceptable and effective in decreasing ID and IDA. Future research could focus on cereals beyond rice and wheat flour and the possibility of enriching them with iron either during the breeding and growing of a crop, or during processing. Further research surrounding genetically modifying rice to contain more iron is required, otherwise the iron must always be added during processing and risks being rinsed off when the rice is washed. Biofortified staples can be very sensitive to market prices, which could be a serious limitation in competitive market settings. This approach would work if governments are able to pass legislation that mandates all of the main staple product in a region be fortified with iron. The challenges associated with this are difficult, but the positive health outcomes have the potential to be vast.

Ultimately, for any of these fortification strategies to be successfully implemented extensive education and health behavior campaigns must take place. Properly planned education materials and outreach can promote adherence and acceptability at a community level. Iron deficiency can sometimes not be felt immediately by an individual, especially when compared to hunger, which is why it is often called "hidden hunger," along with other micronutrient deficiencies. This is relevant to education and behavior change because certain behaviours that aren't routine (such as washing your hands, or taking an iron supplement) may not seem credible or urgent because there are no immediately visible health concerns [90]. This may pose a challenge to communicate the future implications and the less tangible impacts of these things on their health in order to promote healthier behaviours.

One of the largest and most difficult questions is then: who is responsible? At this point in the battle to alleviate iron deficiency and IDA the most dangerous thing that can be done is nothing. Inaction in the face of this epidemic will benefit no one, and the negative health consequences of iron deficiency will persist. The cognitive and physical development consequences and threat to maternal health that iron deficiency poses are severe and will only continue to be the most prevalent nutrition issue in the world without the combined support of governments, aid agencies and non-government agencies alike.

Author details

Lauren C. Ramsay[1*] and Christopher V. Charles[2]

*Address all correspondence to: lauren@lauren-ramsay.com

1 Department of Biomedical Sciences, University of Guelph, Guelph, Canada

2 Michael G. DeGroote School of Medicine, McMaster University, Hamilton, Canada

References

[1] de Benoist, B., McLean, E., Egli, I., Cogswell, M. Worldwide prevalence of anaemia 1993-2005. WHO Global Database on Anaemia 2008

[2] Clark, S. F. Iron deficiency anemia. Nutrition in Clinical Practice 2008; 23(2) 128-41. doi:10.1177/0884533608314536

[3] Loney, M., Chernecky, C. Anemia. Continuing Education 2000; 27(6) 951-962.

[4] Balarajan, Y., Ramakrishnan, U., Ozaltin, E., Shankar, A. H., Subramanian, S. V. Anemia in low-income and middle-income countries. The Lancet 2011; 378 2123-35. doi: 10.1016/S0140-6736(10)62304-5

[5] the 21st century. Therapeutic Advances in Gastroenterology 2011; 4(3) 177-84. doi: 10.1177/1756283X11398736

[6] Means, R. T. Iron deficiency anemia. Hematology 2013 18(5), 305-6. doi: 10.1179/1024533213Z.000000000197

[7] Charles, C. V. Iron Deficiency Anemia: A Public Health Problem of Global Proportions, Public Health-Methodology, Environmental and Systems Issues, Prof. Jay Maddock (Ed.), ISBN: 978-953-51-0641-8, InTech; 2012 p109-130. Available from: http://www.intechopen.com/books/public-health-methodology-environmental-and-systems-issues/iron-deficiency-anemia-a-public-health-problem-of-global-proportions (Accessed 20 July, 2013)

[8] Lynch, S. R. Why nutritional iron deficiency persists as a worldwide problem. The Journal of Nutrition 2011; 141(4) 763S-768S. doi:10.3945/jn.110.130609

[9] George, J., Yiannakis, M., Main, B., Devenish, R., Anderson, C., An, U. S., Williams, S. M., Gibson, R. S. Genetic hemoglobin disorders, infection, and deficiencies of iron and vitamin A determine anemia in young Cambodian children. The Journal of Nutrition 2012; 142(4) 781-7. doi:10.3945/jn.111.148189

[10] Cotta, R. M., Oliveira, F. C., Magalhães, K. A., Ribeiro, A. Q., Sant'Ana, L. F., Priore, S. E., Franceschini, S. C. Social and biological determinants of iron deficiency anemia. Cadernos De Saúde Pública 2011; 27(2) S309-20.

[11] Tengco, L. W., Rayco-Solon, P., Solon, J. A., Sarol, J. N., Solon, F. S. Determinants of anemia among preschool children in the Philippines. Journal of the American College of Nutrition 2008; 27(2) 229-43.

[12] Choi, H. J., Lee, H. J., Jang, H. B., Park, J. Y., Kang, J. H., Park, K. H., Song, J. Effects of maternal education on diet, anemia, and iron deficiency in Korean school-aged children. BMC Public Health 2011; 11 870-878. doi:10.1186/1471-2458-11-870

[13] Pasricha, S. R., Black, J., Muthayya, S., Shet, A., Bhat, V., Nagaraj, S., Prashanth, N. S., Sudarshan, H., Biggs, B., & Shet, A. S. Determinants of anemia among young children in rural India. Pediatrics 2010; 126(1) e140-9. doi:10.1542/peds.2009-3108

[14] Stoltzfus, R. J., Mullany, L., Black, R. E. Iron deficiency anemia. Comparative quantification of health risks 2004; 1 164-209.

[15] Brabin, B., Hakimi, M., Pelletier, D. An analysis of anemia and pregnancy-related maternal mortality. The Journal of Nutrition 2001; 131(2) 604S-615S.

[16] World Health Organization. Micronutrient Deficiencies: Iron Deficiency Anemia. Available from http://www.who.int/nutrition/topics/ida/en/ (Accessed 5 July 2014).

[17] Horton, S., Ross, J. The economics of iron deficiency. Food Policy 2003; 28 51-75.

[18] Baltussen, R., Knai, C., Sharan, M. Iron fortification and iron supplementation are cost-effective interventions to reduce iron deficiency in four subregions of the world. The Journal of Nutrition 2004; 134(10) 2678-2684

[19] McLaren, G. D., Muir, W. A., Kellermeyer, R. W. Iron overload disorders: Natural history, pathogenesis, diagnosis, and therapy. Critical Reviews in Clinical Laboratory Sciences 1983; 19(3) 205-266.

[20] Singh, M. Role of micronutrients for physical growth and mental development. Indian Journal of Pediatrics 2004; 71(1) 59-62.

[21] Theil, E. C. Iron, ferritin, and nutrition. Annual Review of Nutrition 2004; 24 327-43. doi:10.1146/annurev.nutr.24.012003.132212

[22] Conrad, M. E., Umbreit, J. N. Iron absorption and transport-an update. American Journal of Hematology 2000; 64(4) 287-98.

[23] Sobieraj, D. Heme or non-heme? An overview of iron supplements. Available from https://www.cedrugstorenews.com/userapp/lessons/page_view_ui.cfm?lessonuid=&pageid=86975F921481E289FB3858040268C2A0 (Accessed 3 July 2014)

[24] World Health Organization. Soil transmitted helminthiases. World Health Organization, Geneva, Switzerland 2012. Available from http://whqlibdoc.who.int/publications/2012/9789241503129_eng.pdf?ua=1 (Accessed 15 July 2014).

[25] Centres for Disease Control and Prevention. Parasites: Soil transmitted helminthes. http://www.cdc.gov/parasites/sth/ (Accessed 15 July 2014).

[26] World Health Organization. Working to overcome the global impact of neglected tropical diseases. World Health Organization 2010, Geneva, Switzerland. Available from http://whqlibdoc.who.int/publications/2010/9789241564090_eng.pdf (Accessed 15 July 2014).

[27] Shetty, P. S. Nutrition, Immunity and Infection. Cambridge: Cambridge University Press; 2010

[28] Rowe A. K., Rowe S. Y., Snow R. W. The burden of malaria mortality among African children in the year 2000. Int J Epidemiol 2006; 35 691-704.

[29] Snow R. W., Guerra C. A., Noor A. M., Myint H. Y., Hay S. I. The global distribution of clinical episodes of Plasmodium falciparum malaria. Nature 2005; 434 214-217.

[30] Haldar K., Mohandas, N. Malaria, erythrocytic infection, and anemia. Hematology 2009; 1 87-93.

[31] Lamikanra, A. A., Brown, D., Potocnik, A., Casals-Pascual, C., Langhorne, J., Roberts, D. Malarial anemia: of mice and men. Blood 2007. DOI 10.1182/blood-2006-09-018069.

[32] Brinkman, H., de Pee, S., Sanogo, I., Subran, L., Bloem, M. W. High food prices and the global financial crisis have reduced access to nutritious food and worsened nutritional status and health. The Journal of Nutrition 2009; 140(1) 153S-161S.

[33] Berry, J., Mukherjee, P., Shastry, G. Taken with a grain of salt? Micronutrient fortification in South Asia. Economic Studies 2012; 58(2) 422-449.

[34] Das, J., Salam, R., Kumar, R., Bhutta, Z. Micronutrient fortification of food and its impact on woman and child health: a systematic review. Systematic Reviews 2013; 2(67)

[35] Gera, T., Sachdev, H., Boy, E. Effect of iron-fortified foods on hematologic and biological outcomes: systematic review of randomized controlled trials. The American Journal of Clinical Nutrition 2012; 96 309-24.

[36] Bhutta, Z., Das, J. K., Rizvi, A., Gaffey, M. F., Walker, N., Horton, S., Webb, P., Lartey, A., Black, R. E. Evidence-based interventions for improvement of maternal and child nutrition: what can be done and at what cost? The Lancet 2013; 382(9890) 452-477.

[37] The Micronutrient Initiative. Fortified Candies/Lozenges. The Micronutrient Initiative, Ottawa, Canada. Available from http://www.micronutrient.org/CMFiles/What%20we%20do/New%20Solutions%20-%20Emergencies/Lozenges.pdf (Accessed 22 July 2014).

[38] Bulusu, S., Joshi, T. P. Suck it and see: Fortified lozenges delivering multiple micro-nutrients to the community in India. Nutrition 2006; 3 16-17.

[39] Anand, K., Lakshmy, R., Janakarajan, V. N., Ritvik, A., Misra, P. Effect of consumption of micronutrient fortified candies on the iron and vitamin A status of children aged 3-6 years in rural Haryana. Indian Pediatrics 2007; 44 823-829.

[40] Sari, M., Bloem, M. W., de Pee, S., Schultink, W. J., Sastroamidjojo, S. Effect of iron-fortified candies on the iron status of children aged 4-6 y in East Jakarta, Indonesia. The American Journal of Clinical Nutrition 2001; 73 1034-1039.

[41] Canadian Food Inspection Agency. Dairy Vitamin Addition. http://www.inspection.gc.ca/food/dairy-products/manuals-inspection-procedures/dairy-vitamin-addition/eng/1378179097522/1378180040706 (accessed 15 July 2014).

[42] Institute of Medicine of the National Academies. Dietary reference intakes guiding principles for nutrition labeling and fortification. Washington, D.C.: National Academies Press; 2003.

[43] Hotz, C., Porcayo, M., Onofre, G., García-Guerra, A., Elliott, T., Jankowski, S., Greiner, T. Efficacy of iron-fortified ultra rice in improving the iron status of women in Mexico. Food & Nutrition Bulletin 2008; 29(2) 140-149.

[44] Stein, A. J., Meenakshi, J. V., Qaim, M., Nestel, P., Sachdev, H. P., Bhutta, Z. A. Potential impacts of iron biofortification in India. Social Science & Medicine 2008; 66(8) 1797-808. doi:10.1016/j.socscimed.2008.01.006

[45] Slamet-loedin, I. H. "Iron-clad" rice. Rice Today 2011; 10(3) 46.

[46] Mridula, D., Pooja, J. (2014). Preparation of iron-fortified rice using edible coating materials. International Journal of Food Science & Technology 2014; 49(1) 246-252. doi:10.1111/ijfs.12305

[47] Arcanjo, F. P., Santos, P. R., Arcanjo, C. P., Amancio, O. M., Braga, J. A. Use of iron-fortified rice reduces anemia in infants. Journal of Tropical Pediatrics 2012; 58(6) 475-80. doi:10.1093/tropej/fms021

[48] Angeles-Agdeppa, I., Saises, M., Capanzana, M., Juneja, L. R., Sakaguchi, N. Pilot-scale commercialization of iron-fortified rice: Effects on anemia status. Food & Nutrition Bulletin 2011; 32(1) 3-12.

[49] Beinner, M. A., Velasquez-Meléndez, G., Pessoa, M. C., Greiner, T. Iron-fortified rice is as efficacious as supplemental iron drops in infants and young children. The Journal of Nutrition 2009; 140(1) 49-53. doi:10.3945/jn.109.112623

[50] Grimm, K. A., Sullivan, K. M., Alasfoor, D., Parvanta, I., Suleiman, A. J. M., Kaur, M., Al-Hatima, F. O., Ruth, L. J. Iron-fortified wheat flour and iron deficiency among women. Food & Nutrition Bulletin 2012; 33(3) 180-186.

[51] World Health Organization. Recommendations on Wheat and Maize Flour Fortification. World Health Organization, Geneva, Switzerland 2009. Available from http://

www.who.int/nutrition/publications/micronutrients/wheat_maize_fort.pdf   (Accessed 21 July 2014).

[52]   Muthayya, S., Thankachan P., Hirve S., Amalrajan V., Thomas T., Lubree H., Agarwal D., Srinivasan K., Hurrell R. F., Yajnik C. S., Kurpad A. V. Iron fortification of whole wheat flour reduces iron deficiency and iron deficiency anemia and increases body iron stores in Indian school-aged children. Journal of Nutrition 2012; 142(11) 1997-2003.

[53]   Cercamondi, C. I., Egli, I. M., Mitchikpe, E., Tossou, F., Zeder, C., Hounhouigan, J. D., Hurrell, R. F. Total iron absorption by young women from iron-biofortified pearl millet composite meals is double that from regular millet meals but with less than that from post-harvest iron-fortified millet meals. Journal of Nutrition 2013; 143(9) 1376-1382.

[54]   Walczyk, T., Tuntipopipat, S., Zeder, C., Sirichakwal, P., Wasantwisut, E., Hurrell, R. Iron absorption by human subjects from different fortification compounds added to Thai fish sauce. European Journal of Clinical Nutrition 2005; 59 668-674.

[55]   Fidler, M., Davidson, L, Walczyk, T., Hurrell, R. Iron absorption from fish sauce and soy sauce fortified with sodium iron EDTA. The American Journal of Clinical Nutrition 2003; 78 274-278.

[56]   Theary, C., Panagides, D., Laillou, A., Vonthanak, S., Kanarath, C., Chhorvann, C., Sambath, P., Sowath, S., Moench-Pfanner, R. Fish sauce, soy sauce, and vegetable oil fortification in Cambodia: Where do we stand to date?. Food and Nutrition Bulletin 2013; 34(2) S62-72.

[57]   Thuy, P.V., Berger, J., Davidsson, L., Khan, N. C., Lam, N. T., Cook, J. D., Hurrell, R. F., Khoi, H. H. Regular consumption of NaFeEDTA-fortified fish sauce improves iron status and reduces the prevalence of anemia in anemic Vietnamese women. American Journal of Clinical Nutrition 2003; 78(2) 284-290.

[58]   Longfils, P., Monchy, D., Weinheimer, H., Chavasit, V., Nakanishi, Y., Schumann, K. A comparative intervention trial on fish sauce fortified with NaFe-EDTA and FeSO4+citrate in iron deficiency anemic school children in Kampot, Cambodia. Asia Pac J Clin Nutr 2008; 17(2) 250-257.

[59]   World Health Organization. Guideline: Sodium intake for adults and children. World Health Organization, Geneva, Switzerland 2012. Available from http://www.who.int/nutrition/publications/guidelines/sodium_intake_printversion.pdf (Accessed 10 July 2014).

[60]   World Health Organization. Salt reduction and iodine fortification strategies in public health. World Health Organization, Geneva, Switzerland 2013. Available from: http://www.who.int/nutrition/publications/publichealth_saltreduc_iodine_fortification/en/ (Accessed 10 July 2014).

[61] Zlotkin, S., Arthur, P., Antwi, K. Y., Yeung, G. Treatment of anemia with microencapsulated ferrous fumarate plus ascorbic acid supplied as sprinkles to complementary (weaning) foods. The American Journal of Clinical Nutrition 2001; 74(6) 791-795.

[62] Zlotkin, A., Shauer, C., Christofides, A., Sharieff, W., Tonderu, M. C., Zlauddin Hyder, S. M. Micronutrient Sprinkles to control childhood anaemia. Health in Action 2005; 2(1) 24-28

[63] Ip, H., Hyder, S., Haseen, F., Rahman, M., Zlotkin, S. Improved adherence and anemia cure rates with flexible administration of micronutrient Sprinkles: a new public health approach to anemia control. European Journal of Clinical Nutrition 2009; 63 165-172.

[64] Macharia-Mutie, C. W., Moretti, D., Van den Briel, N., Omusundi, A. M., Mwangi, A. M., Kok F. J., Zimmerman, M. B., Brouwer, I. D. Maize porridge enriched with a micronutrient powder containing low-dose iron as NaFeEDTA but not amaranth grain flour reduces anemia and iron deficiency in Kenyan preschool children. The Journal of Nutrition 2012; 142(9) 1756-63. doi:10.3945/jn.112.157578

[65] Troesch, B., van Stuijvenberg, M. E., van Stujivenberg, M. E., Smuts, C. M., Kruger, H. S., Biebinger, R., Hurrell, R. F., Baumgartner, J., Zimmermann, M. B. A micronutrient powder with low doses of highly absorbable iron and zinc reduces iron and zinc deficiency and improves weight-for-age z-scores in South African children. The Journal of Nutrition 2011; 141(2) 237-42. doi:10.3945/jn.110.129247

[66] Serdula, M. K., Lundeen, E., Nichols, E. K., Imanalieva, C., Minbaev, M., Mamyrbaeva, T., Timmer, A., Aburto, N. J. Effects of a large-scale micronutrient powder and young child feeding education program on the micronutrient status of children 6-24 months of age in the Kyrgyz Republic. European Journal of Clinical Nutrition 2013; 67(7) 703-7. doi:10.1038/ejcn.2013.67

[67] Giovannanini, M., Sala, D., Usuelli, M., Livio, L., Francescato, G., Braga, M., Radaelli, G., Riva, E. Double blind, placebo-controlled trial comparing effects of supplementation with two different combinations of micronutrients delivered as sprinkles on growth, anemia, and iron deficiency in Cambodian infants. Journal of Pediatric Gastroenterology and Nutrition 2006; 42 306-312.

[68] Jack, S., Ou, K., Chea, M., Chhin, L., Devenish, R., Dunbar, M., Eang, C., Hou, K., Ly, S., Khin, M., Prak, S., Reach, R., Talukder, A., Tokmoh, L., Leon de la Barra, S., Hill, P., Herbison, P., Gibson, R. Effect of micronutrient Sprinkles on reducing anemia. Arch Pediatri Adolesc Med 2012; 166(9) 842-850.

[69] Suchdev, P. S., Ruth, L. J., Woodruff, B. A., Mbakaya, C., Mandava, U., Flores-Ayala, R., Jefferds, M. E., Quick, R. Selling sprinkles micronutrient powder reduces anemia, iron deficiency, and vitamin A deficiency in young children in western kenya: A cluster-randomized controlled trial. The American Journal of Clinical Nutrition 2012; 95(5) 1223-30. doi:10.3945/ajcn.111.030072

[70] Varma J. L., Das S., Sankar R., Mannar M. G., Levinson FJ, Hamer D. H. Community-level micronutrient fortification of a food supplement in India: a controlled trial in preschool children aged 36-66 mo. American Journal of Clinical Nutrition 2007; 85(4) 1127-1133.

[71] Salam, R., MacPhail, C., Das, J., Bhutta, Z. Effectiveness of micronutrient powders (MNP) in women and children. BMC Public Health 2013; 13(3) S22-S32.

[72] Drover, D.P., Maddocks, I. Iron content of native foods. Papua New Guinea Med. J. 1975; 18 15-17.

[73] Kumari, M., Gupta, S., Lakshmi, A., Prakash, J. Iron bioavailability in green leafy vegetables cooked in different utensils. Food Chemistry 2004; 86(2) 217-222. doi: 10.1016/j.foodchem.2003.08.017

[74] Sharieff, W., Dofonsou, J., Zlotkin, S. Is cooking food in iron pots an appropriate solution for the control of anaemia in developing countries? A randomised clinical trial in Benin. Public Health Nutrition 2008; 11(9) 971-7. doi:10.1017/S1368980007001139

[75] Geerligs, P., Brabin, B., Mkumbwa, A., Broadhead, R., Cuevas, L. E. Acceptability of the use of iron cooking pots to reduce anaemia in developing countries. Public Health Nutrition 2002; 5(5) 619-24. doi:10.1079/PHN2002341

[76] Geerligs, P. P., Brabin, B., Mkumbwa, A., Broadhead, R., Cuevas, L. E. The effect on haemoglobin of the use of iron cooking pots in rural Malawian households in an area with high malaria prevalence: A randomized trial. Tropical Medicine & International Health 2003; 8(4) 310-315.

[77] Geerligs, P. D., Brabin, B. J., Omari, A. Food prepared in iron cooking pots as an intervention for reducing iron deficiency anaemia in developing countries: A systematic review. Journal of Human Nutrition and Dietetics 2003; 16(4) 275-281.

[78] Tripp, K., Mackeith, N., Woodruff, B. A., Talley, L., Mselle, L., Mirghani, Z., Abdalla, F., Bhatia, R., Seal, A. J. Acceptability and use of iron and iron-alloy cooking pots: Implications for anaemia control programmes. Public Health Nutrition 2010; 13(1) 123-30. doi:10.1017/S1368980009005928

[79] Kapur, D., Agarwal, K. N., Agarwal, D. K. Nutritional anemia and its control. The Indian Journal of Pediatrics 2002; 69(7) 607-616.

[80] Charles, C. V. Happy Fish: a novel supplementation technique to prevent iron deficiency anemia in women in rural Cambodia. PhD Thesis. University of Guelph; 2012

[81] Charles, C. V., Dewey, C. E., Daniell, W. E., Summerlee, A. J. Iron-deficiency anaemia in rural Cambodia: Community trial of a novel iron supplementation technique. European Journal of Public Health 2011; 21(1) 43-8. doi:10.1093/eurpub/ckp237

[82] Helen Keller International. Iron Deficiency in Cambodia: The Need for Iron Supplementation Among Preschool-aged Children. Phnom Penh, Cambodia 2001. Available

from http://www.hki.org/research/CmbNutrBul_vol2_iss6.pdf (Accessed 3 July 2014).

[83] Charles, C. V., Summerlee, A. J., Dewey, C. E. Anemia in Cambodia: Prevalence, etiology and research needs. Asia Pac J Clin Nutr 2012; 21(2) 171-181.

[84] Cambodia Ministry of Health. National guidelines for the use of iron folate supplementation to prevent and treat anemia in pregnant and post-partum women. Phnom Penh, Cambodia 2007. Available from http://www.a2zproject.org/pdf/National%20Guidelines%20for%20the%20Use%20of%20Iron%20Folate%20Supplementation%20to%20Prevent%20and%20Treat%20Anemia%20in%20Pregnant%20and%20Post-Partum%20Women.pdf (Accessed 3 July 2014).

[85] Kanal, K., Busch-Hallen, J., Cavalli-Sforza, T., Crape, B., Smitasiri, S. Weekly iron-folix acid supplements to prevent anemia among Cambodian women in three settings: process and outcomes of social marketing and community mobilization. Nutrition Reviews 2005; 63(12) 126-133.

[86] Allen, L.H. Iron supplements: scientific issues concerning efficacy and implications for research and programs. Journal of Nutrition 2002; 132(4) 4813S-4819S.

[87] Beard, J.L. Effectiveness and strategies of iron supplementation during pregnancy. American Journal of Clinical Nutrition 2000; 71(5) 288s-1294s.

[88] Ramsay, L. Use of health centres in rural Preah Vihear province, Cambodia. Unpublished manuscript 2014.

[89] Allen, L.H., Peerson, J.M., Olney, D.K. Provision of multiple rather than two or fewer micronutrients more effectively improves growth and other outcomes in micronutrient-deficient children and adults. Journal of Nutrition 2007; 139(5) 1022-1030.

[90] Aboud, F., Singla, D. Challenges to changing health behaviours in developing countries: a critical overview. Social Science & Medicine 2012; 75 589-594.

Chapter 9

A Review on the Assessment of the Potential Adverse Health Impacts of Carbamate Pesticides

Elsa Dias, Fernando Garcia e Costa,
Simone Morais and Maria de Lourdes Pereira

Additional information is available at the end of the chapter

http://dx.doi.org/10.5772/59613

1. Introduction

Carbamates are an important class of pesticides used worldwide in public health, among rural and urban settings. Indeed, due to their mode of action and effectiveness, the application of these compounds is one of the best options presently offered for pest control in modern agriculture. They are also used for gardening, and as therapeutic pharmaceuticals for veterinary medicine. Carbamates have been also used in medicine for myasthenia gravis, an autoimmune disease which affects the postsynaptic element of the neuromuscular junction, and as pre-exposure protection in military settings from chemical warfare nerve agents such as Sarin and Tabun. For example carbamates such as physostigmine, and pyridostigmine have been listed as human drugs. However, current environmental concerns of the deleterious health impacts of carbamate pesticides have been increasing. Humans and other non-target species are exposed to residues of these cholinesterase-inhibiting chemicals via nutritional sources (legumes, fruits, contaminated meat, and dairy products), water and/or through environmental/occupational settings due to inappropriate handling. As other pollutants, carbamates may induce deleterious effects on both biotic (micro and macro fauna and flora) and abiotic systems. The adverse effects of several carbamate pesticides include renal, hepatic, neurological, reproductive, immune, and metabolic functions in both humans and animals. Furthermore, some of them are classified as endocrine disrupting chemicals [1], and regarded as priority pollutants by the United States Environmental Protection Agency (US EPA) [2].

In this chapter a brief overview of the current knowledge on the carbamates' mode of action and toxicological aspects is presented. The role of *in vivo* studies (histological and hematological approaches), epidemiology and interdisciplinary research on assessment of the carbamates' environmental and potential public health effects is addressed and the major

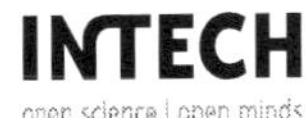

contributions are discussed. In addition, this chapter presents the results of some of our laboratory experiments that focus on the evaluation of aminocarb and thiodicarb renal and hepatic toxicity, lymphoid organ damage including the spleen and thymus, and adverse effects on male reproductive organs.

2. Mode of action and toxicology

Several key issues on carbamate pesticides such as mechanism of action, and toxicological aspects, including adverse human health effects were recently reported by our group [3]. Briefly, this paper also addresses other topics for a better understanding of toxicological effects, namely risk and exposure assessment, biomonitoring, and analytical methods for the detection of these chemicals on foodstuffs and biological fluids or tissues (e.g. blood, serum, urine, breast milk, hair). International legislation was also mentioned in this report.

Carbamates are esters of N-methyl carbamic acid, known as acetylcholinesterase-inhibiting agents (AChE). As with other pesticides like organophosphates, carbamates inhibit the acetylcholine esterase enzyme which catalyzes the hydrolysis of acetylcholine (Ach), a neuromediator agent, which results in ACh increase at a nerve synapse or neuromuscular junction, thereby increasing stimulation of those nerve endings [4]. Carbamates' cholinesterase-inhibiting effect is reversible compared to organophosphates which is irreversible.

The range of the toxicity of carbamates is variable [5]. Several carbamates have slight (LD_{50} > 200 mg/kg) to highly (LD_{50} <50 mg/kg) toxic activity in rodents (Table 1). For example thiodicarb (dimethyl N, N'-thiobis (methylimino) carbonyloxy bisethanimido thioate) is a conventional insecticide for controlling cotton bollworm [6]. It is categorized as class II, moderately toxic, by US EPA and World Health Organization (WHO). In addition, several factors including the route, duration, and frequency of exposure, contact with other pollutants, and compromised physiological condition (e.g. hepatic injury) may determine the degree of toxicity [7-8].

Among other pesticides, some carbamates were included in the list of endocrine-disrupting chemicals (EDCs) by WHO [1]. Due to the potential dangerous effects on both wildlife and human health, this issue has received considerable attention within the scope of public health. The potential of EDCs to interfere with the synthesis, secretion, transport, metabolism, and elimination of a wide range of hormones was already established. These hormonally active chemicals may induce a wide range of deleterious health effects such as developmental, behavioral and reproductive deficits. Agonistic and antagonist mechanism was described. Recently, De Coster and van Larebeke [9] presented an overview of relevant chemicals with endocrine disrupting features, including carbamate pesticides such as chlorpropham, carbaryl, benomyl, methiocarb, pirimicarb, and propamocarb. In this well designed review, authors provided different mechanisms such as the activation of the classical ERα and Erβ nuclear receptors, through estrogen associated receptors, and membrane-bound estrogen-receptors, among others.

3. Potential public health risks

A growing body of literature evidences the harmful effects of carbamates and other pesticides on human and environmental health. Carbamates have been analyzed in environmental analysis, food safety, toxicology, and occupational health. Due to the extensive use of carbamates for agricultural and non-agricultural purposes, their residues have been detected in soils, wastewater effluents, surface water and raw drinking water sources, as well as food products, around the world, and have received particular attention because of their toxicity. The control of the levels of the residues of these compounds in the environment and in crops has an outstanding importance. The presence of pesticide residues and/or their degradation products, which sometimes are more toxic than their precursors in the environment and in foodstuffs, calls for the use of very sensitive analytical methods, capable of determining these compounds at concentration levels equal to or lower than the maximum residue levels (MRLs) established by international organizations [10]. Except for occupational exposure or at home application, e.g. home gardens or the handling with domestic animals, people are exposed to pesticides mainly through diet. Human intake due to pesticide residues in food commodities is usually much higher than those related to water consumption and air inhalation. The evaluation of pesticide residues in food is nowadays a priority objective to ensure food quality and safety, as well as to protect consumers against potential health risks [3, 11]. Considering the chronic exposure through food, Jensen and co-workers [12] used the probabilistic approach to estimate the cumulative exposure to organophosphorus and carbamate pesticide residues from the consumption of fruit, vegetables and cereals in the population of Denmark. Despite the limitations and the uncertainties in the calculation of the dietary cumulative intake, the results showed that exposure for children aged up to 6 years were, on average, 2.4 times higher than the exposure for the general population. Tomatoes were the food source that provided about 67% of the total intake of acetylcholinesterase enzyme-inhibiting pesticides. An outbreak of food borne-illness was reported due to severe methomyl intoxication in Korea [8]. Six elderly people collapsed abruptly after eating 1-2 spoons of boiled rice mixed with bean sprouts and seasoned with soybean sauce. One patient died of cardiac arrest. Symptoms of toxicity presented quickly in the subjects and progressed rapidly, including chest tightness, an unusual sensation in the pit of the stomach, dizziness, ataxia, and finally, collapse. Three patients who drank ethanol with the meal experienced only mild toxic symptoms [8].

The relationships between possible exposure to pesticides and the implications for human health have been the matter of exhaustive and multiple reviews [9, 13-21]. The overall conclusions are that pesticides may induce chronic health complications leading to several diseases. For example neurodevelopmental or behavioral problems, birth defects, asthma, and cancer were documented in children [22].

Due to the relevance of hormones through the life cycle, EDCs may interfere with the developmental processes of humans and wildlife species. The extent of exposure to EDCs may severely affect the most vulnerable life stages including prenatal, early postnatal life, and children. Developmental exposures may induce alterations that, while not evident as birth defects, can promote permanent changes that lead to increased incidence of diseases throughout life [1].

Several recent reports indicate a correlation between EDCs and numerous chronic diseases such as cancer, diabetes, developmental deficits, obesity, and reproductive health disorders. For example, the potential influence of several endocrine disruptor pesticides on human health was reviewed by Mnif and colleagues [15]. Among other carbamates, aldicarb was demonstrated to inhibit the activity of 17 beta-estradiol and progesterone; carbendazim induced an increase of estrogen production and aromatase activity, although low estrogen effect was reported for carbaryl.

Deleterious health effects of some carbamates chronic exposure in occupational settings were already described, and environmental and public health impacts also considered [14]. Occupational pesticide exposure associated with cancer incidence is thoroughly discussed elsewhere. Alavanja and Bonner reviewed association between carbamates such as aldicarb and carbaryl with colon cancer and melanoma, respectively [23]. In this review and concerning the U.S. Agricultural Health Study (AHS), specific pesticide exposures ascertained by questionnaire prior to the onset of disease were found to be significantly associated with cutaneous melanoma (eg. for more than 56 days of exposure to carbaryl) [23]. Also positive relations between non-Hodgkin lymphoma and carbamate insecticides, among other pesticide exposures in occupational agricultural sceneries, were also lately reported [21]. The relationship between carbamate pesticides, namely carbaryl, and multiple myeloma occurrence was recently described [24].

The association between occupational exposure to organophosphate and carbamate pesticides and semen quality, as well as reproductive and thyroid hormone profiles of Venezuelan farm workers, was undertaken by Miranda-Contreras and colleagues [19]. These findings confirm the potential impact of occupational exposure to EDCs on male reproductive function. Features like sperm chromatin damage and reduction of semen were documented and adverse reproductive health outcomes were detected. The evidence available today shows that both men and women can experience adverse reproductive effects as a result of chronic exposure to carbamate pesticides.

Occupational pesticides non-intentional poisoning was also reviewed recently and carbamates were one of the main groups of pesticides-related mortalities in Brazil [25]. Multiple routes may be considered (inhalation, dermal, oral), with skin contact being one of most common routes of exposure. Protective measures for pesticides exposure related with dermal route of exposure were recently reviewed [26]. In fact, safe handling through personal protective equipment may reduce absorption of those chemicals. In the Republic of Korea, mortality studies due to organophosphate and carbamate poisoned patients (occupationally linked acute exposures or suicides) were recently reported in which 17 cases, under the age of 56.8 ± 19.2 years were found among a total of 146 [7]. Unlike other types of intoxication, there are definite antidotes for carbamates exposure. The mortality of these disease entities could be diminished with sufficient use of atropine, 2-pyridine aldoxime methyl chloride (2-PAM, known as pralidoxime) and vigorous airway management if used from the early stage of their occurrence [7].

4. *In vivo* studies

As for other hazardous chemicals, the contribution of laboratory experimental studies is relevant to understand the impact of carbamate pesticides on public health. Extensive research based on animal experiments, particularly mammals, has evidenced the toxicological effects of a wide range of carbamates. Table 1 displays some relevant contributions of predictive toxicology studies carried out in laboratory animals, based on several approaches. Results clearly show that a number of carbamates have led to a broad spectrum of adverse health effects on different tissues, organs, and systems (hepatic, renal, developmental, and repro-ductive) in a dose dependent manner with obvious implications on functions. In particular, exposure to carbamates during critical periods of life (eg. pregnancy, and fetal development) induces maternal health anomalies and developmental disability. Generally, apart from hepatic toxicity, harmful effects on reproductive health through altered spermatogenesis, and reduced semen quality have become a noticeable concern.

As shown on Table 1 the most characterized compounds are carbaryl and carbofuran. Alter-ations on brain, liver, and testis accompanied by testosterone level decay were reported after carbaryl exposure. In addition, nephrotoxic, hepatotoxic and intestinal disruption were documented after intoxication with carbofuran.

Recently, the toxicity of two new carbamates, ethyl-4-bromophenyl-carbamate and ethyl-4-chlorophenylcarbamate, was characterized [27, 28]. Authors reported low subchronic toxicity to rats as evidenced by low severity and reversibility of the majority of the observed alterations [28]. Still, degenerative changes in liver, binucleated hepatocytes, and focal coagulative necrosis were noted, and increased lesions were related to high dosage. Biochemical parame-ters, namely plasma enzymes such as gamma-glutamyltransferase, lactate dehydrogenase, and creatinine exhibited a slight increase.

Carbamate Pesticide	Animal	Exposure route & dosing	Tissue/Organ /system	Results	Reference
Aminocarb	Rat	Orally, 10, 20 and 40 mg/kg bw for 14 days	Blood, liver and kidney	Hemorrhagic focus on hepatic and renal parenchyma, toxic effects on lymphoid organs	[29]
Bendiocarb	Rabbit	Orally 5 mg/kg bw daily for 10 and 30 days	Testis	Decrease of testicular weight, degenerative changes on testicular parenchyma, and Leydig cells	[30]
		Per os daily at a dose of 5 mg/kg/bw, and after day 11 received the same dose every 48 h.	Liver	Affects the liver ultrastructure; regeneration of the damaged tissue	[31]

Carbamate Pesticide	Animal	Exposure route & dosing	Tissue/Organ /system	Results	Reference
Ethyl-4-bromphenyl-carbamate and ethyl-4-chlorphenyl-carbamate	Rat	Subchronic oral toxicities; drinking water (12.5, 25 and 50mg/kg/day) for 90 days 5, 50, 300 and 2000mg/kg single dose using an intragastric tube	Many organs Lung, brain, cerebellum, intestine, stomach, liver, kidney, heart, and muscle.	Low subchronic toxicity and reversibility on liver, and spleen. Both carbamates are low hazard; signs of toxicity at the higher dosages. The maximum dose of each carbamate did not cause clinical manifestations or liver and skin alterations	[28] [27]
Carbaryl	Rat	Orally Chlorpyrifos, carbaryl and a mixture for 90 consecutive days. per os	Liver, kidney, urine	No significant histopathological changes; mitochondrial enzymes were affected	[32]
	Rat	10, 30 mg/kg via intraperitoneal 35 days of exposure	Blood testis	Decline in the testosterone levels; increase in LH and FSH levels Decrease in number of germ cells	[33]
	Rat	oral gavage at 2 ml/kg preweaning age to senescence	Brain, plasma, liver	Dose-related increase at all ages, with differences across life span	[34]
Carbendazim	Rat	Orally at 0, 20, 100 and 200 mg/kg for 80 days prior to mating.	Testis	Adverse effects on spermatogenesis, resulting in reduced fertility	[35]
	Mouse	Mated mice 0, 150, 300, and 600 mg/kg/day by gavage.	Maternal Blood Fetuses	Dose of 150 mg/kg/day induced a very slight increase in postimplantation loss; maternal and developmental toxicity at 300 and 600 mg/kg/day	[36]
	Rat	Once daily p.o. at 10 ml/kg for a dose of 200 mg/kg/day.	Testis	Tubular dilation, tubular necrosis, and/or germ cell degeneration	[37]
Cartap, carbofuran	Rat	Each pesticide *per se* (50% LD50);	Serum	Alterations in the serum lipid profile; marked decrease in	[38]

Carbamate Pesticide	Animal	Exposure route & dosing	Tissue/Organ /system	Results	Reference
		combination of these two with 25% LD50 of each during 1 week Orally.		HDL; enhanced effect on levels of serum lipids in co-adiministration	
Carbofuran	Rat	4.0 mg/kg/bw for 7 days or 2.8 mg/kg/bw for 30 days daily by Ryle's tube.	Small Intestine	Intestinal distruption of the villi, and comet assay showed disintegration of DNA in enterocytes of animals exposed for 30 days; toxicity may modulate digestive functions in intestine	[39]
	Rat	Orally 1 mg/kg/bw dissolved in sunflower oil daily for 28 days	Kidneys blood	Nephrotoxic effects through augmented oxidative stress and attenuated antioxidant defense system	[40]
	Rat	P.o at 0–5 mg/kg/ bw for 5 weeks	Liver, bone marrow	Liver toxicity and clastogenic effects (micronucleated polychromatic erythrocytes)	[41]
Carbosulfan	Rat	Orally (0.5, 1, 2, and 4 mg/kg) during the embryonic period (1–15)	Brain	High developmental disability in pups (changes in sensorimotor functions, and high anxiety) in pups; growth rate changes in a dose dependent manner.	[42]
Methiocarb	Rat	Orally at doses 25, 10, and 2 mg/kg/ bw for 1, 5, and 28 days	Liver, kidney, brain, and testis	Possible lipid peroxidation, disturbances on the GSH levels in liver, kidney, testis, and brain	[43]
		25 mg/kg/ bw for 20 days, (i.g.)	Liver,and kidney	Oxidative damage on liver and kidney, which were partly, ameliorated by the pretreatment of vitamin E and taurine.	[44]
Methomyl	Mouse	Orally; 1 mg; 2 mg, 3 mg and 4 mg/kg/bw for 30 days and effective dose of 4 mg/kg/bw for 5, 10, and 20 days	Liver and serum	Harmful effects on cell metabolism, cell membrane permeability, and hepatic detoxification system	[45]

Carbamate Pesticide	Animal	Exposure route & dosing	Tissue/Organ /system	Results	Reference
	Rat	Orally daily for 65 days at 2 doses (0.5 and 1.0 mg kg$^{(-1)}$ bw)	Testis, epididymis, and serum	Decreased the fertility index, testicular damage, sperm quality affected	[46]
Pirimicarb	Mouse	Oral gavage 2.14, and 10.7 mg/kg/day pirimicarb, and dichlorvos plus pirimicarb daily for 30 consecutive days	Liver and serum	Prominent changes in liver oxidative markers, as endogenous metabolites in serum and liver; PI, either alone or in combination lead to changes on liver glucose, fat and protein metabolism, energy metabolism and oxidative balance	[47]
		Orally daily at 10, 20, or 40 mg/kg/bw during 30 days	Liver, kidneys, spleen, testis and thymus	Organ toxicity to high doses	[48]
Thiodicarb	Rat	Intraperitoneal, 2.9 and 5.8 mg/kg daily for 28 days	Vital organs, particularly liver and heart	Significant increase in AST on 7th day. No much changes on the various biochemical profiles except inhibiting AChE. No adverse specific damage to vital organs, mainly liver and heart	[49]

Table 1. Laboratory animal findings on main carbamate pesticides effects. Abbreviations: bw-body weight; i.g.-intragastrically.

4.1. Case studies: Effects of thiodicarb and aminocarb on male reproductive system

As presented in Table 1, the effects of thiodicarb on various biochemical parameters and blood enzymes were investigated in adult male wistar rats following its daily intraperitoneal administration at rates of 2.9 and 5.8 mg/kg for 28 days [49]. The findings of this research indicated that thiodicarb did not significantly affect or alter the various biochemical profiles except inhibiting AChE following intraperitoneal administration up to 28 days.

The systemic toxic effects of thiodicarb on rats have been well described by our group [48]. Several approaches such as hematological, biochemical, histopathological, and flow cytometry were used in this paper to characterize the subacute effects. Marked systemic organ toxicity was reported including renal and testis degeneration, appreciated cellular loss on thymus, hemorrhagic focus on liver, and disruption within the spleen. T lymphocytes displayed high values. This paper also evidenced some hemorrhage on interstitial tissue of testis.

To complement the above mentioned work, and in order to fully characterize the effects of thiodicarb on the male reproductive system of rats, experiments were conducted under the guidelines for ethics on animal experimentation using a similar protocol for epididymis (another reproductive organ). Briefly, three months old rats purchased from Harlan Iberica (Spain) were divided into two groups, and kept under appropriate conditions. Thiodicarb was dissolved in water and was given every day (40 mg/kg body weight) for a period of 30 days. For comparison, animals given water only were used. After one month, animals were anesthetized, and sacrificed for epididymis sampling and further histological analyses. No apparent macroscopic changes were noted in organs of thiodicarb-exposed rats. However the observations at light microcope level evidenced a reduction of sperm mass within the lumen (Figure 1). However no changes were noted on the epithelium lining the ducts.

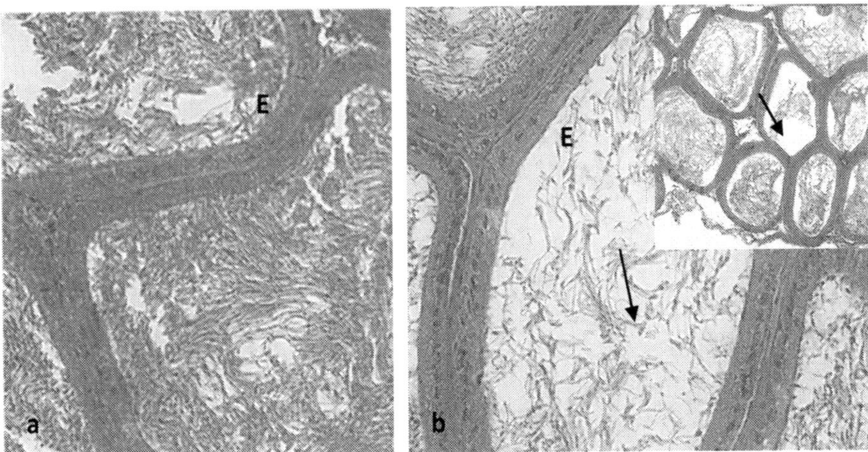

Figure 1. Histological sections of rat epididymis (E) from (a) control; and thiodicarb (40 mg/kg body weight) exposed animals during one month period (b). A considerable decrease on sperm is noted in the lumen (arrow); Inset – a general view displaying a reduction on sperm (arrow); haematoxylin and eosin stain. Original magnification: (a) x200; (b) x200; inset x40.

Aminocarb (4-dimethylamino-3-methy-N-carbamate) is a phenylsubstituted methylcarbamate pesticide broadly used to control the growth of insect pests such as Lepidoptera and Coleoptera species affecting agriculture and storage of legumes, fruits, and grains. The toxicity of this carbamate on rats was thoroughly characterized through histological, hematological, and biochemical approaches as shown on Table 1. The results of this study evidenced multi-organ damage and the extension of lesions were dose-dependent. Studies on progress using a similar experimental dosing procedure (30, and 40 mg/kg body weight, respectively) were conducted in male rats aiming to evaluate the effects of aminocarb on testis and epididymis using histological assays. The results clearly show harmfull effects on both testis and epididymis (Figures 2 and 3). Epidydimis revealed a reduction of sperm compared to control. The testis presented some degenerative changes such as vacuolation, germ cell loss with obvious decrease of seminiferous epithelium, and release of immature germ cells into the lumen.

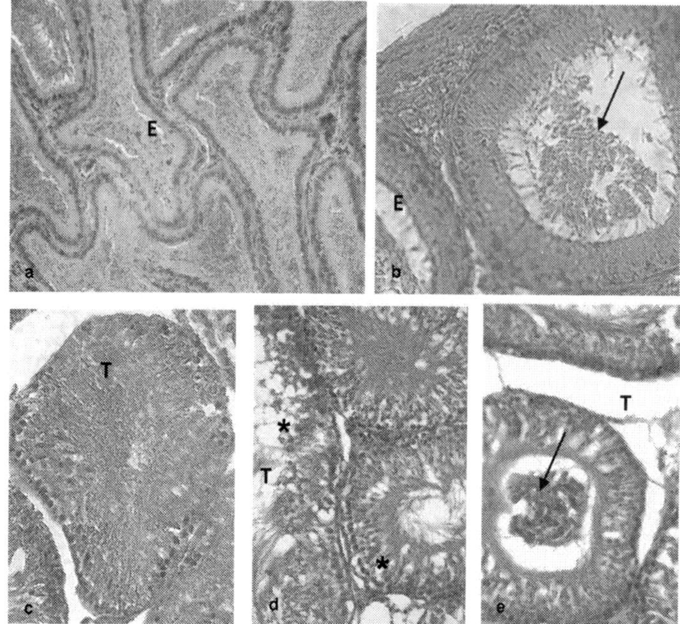

Figure 2. Epididymis (E) of (a) control and aminocarb-dosed rats (20mg/kg) for 14 days (b) displaying a decrease on sperm (arrow); testis (T) from control (c) and pesticide exposed rat (d-e) evidencing strong vacuolation (*), and immature germ cells (arrow); haematoxylin and eosin stain. Original magnification: (a,) x100; (b) x200; (c-e) x200.

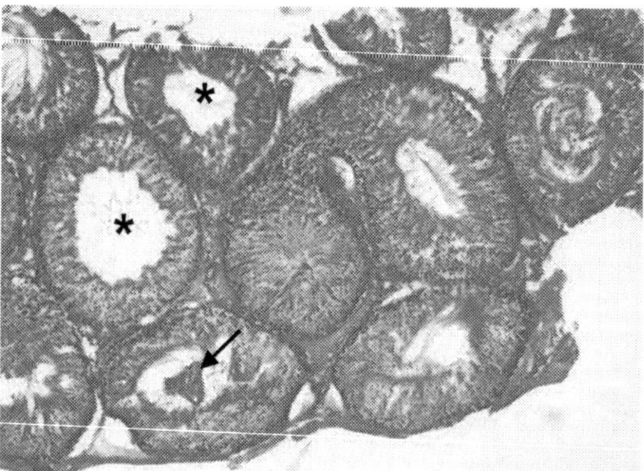

Figure 3. Representative histological section of testis from aminocarb-exposed rat (40 mg/kg/body weight) during 14 days. Immature germ cells (arrow) within the lumen of seminiferous tubules; some tubules (*) denoted a decrease on germ cell layers; haematoxylin-eosin stain. Original magnification: x100.

Overall taken together, the results mentioned above clearly evidence the deleterious effects of both carbamates (thiodicarb and aminocarb) on male organs namely testis and epididymis. In fact disrupted spermatogenesis, and subsequent changes in epididymis ducts may compromise the reproductive potential. These findings are consistent with the results from studies on other carbamates reported on Table 1.

5. Conclusion

Although efforts have been made globally and a significant progress was accomplished, the impact of carbamates (mainly of those that exhibit endocrine disruptor behavior) on human and environmental health still remains a public health problem and a challenge.

Insights from endocrine disruptor research in animals have a huge impact on current practice in toxicological evaluation. The effects of exposures should be studied in adulthood but also, and particularly, in fetal development, perinatal life, childhood and puberty.

Continuous efforts to undertake multidisciplinary research based on *in vitro* technologies and *in vivo* toxicological studies, coupled to the epidemiological studies of exposure in humans are mandatory in order to improve our knowledge on the underlying mechanisms and health consequences. Also, protection programs, including educational ones, on the appropriate use of pesticides to minimize population exposures as well as preventive health monitoring are needed principally in developing countries.

Acknowledgements

The present work was financed by FEDER Funds through the Programa Operacional Factores de Competitividade – COMPETE, and National Funds through FCT – Fundação para a Ciência e Tecnologia, under the projetc CICECO-FCOMP-01-0124-FEDER-037271 (Ref. FCT PEst-C/CTM/LA0011/2013). Authors are greatly indebted to the Serviço de Patologia Clínica, Centro Hospitalar Baixo Vouga, EPE, Aveiro, Portugal (Director: Dr. Elmano Ramalheira). HoribaABX, SAS, (Portugal), and Siemens Healthcare Diagnostics (Portugal) are also acknowledged. Authors are grateful to Tânia Fernandes.

Author details

Elsa Dias[1,2], Fernando Garcia e Costa[3], Simone Morais[4] and Maria de Lourdes Pereira[1*]

*Address all correspondence to: mlourdespereira@ua.pt

1 Departamento de Biologia & CICECO, Universidade de Aveiro, Aveiro, Portugal

2 Serviço de Patologia Clínica, Centro Hospitalar Baixo Vouga, EPE, Aveiro, Portugal

3 Departamento de Morfologia e Função, CIISA, Faculdade de Medicina Veterinária, Universidade de Lisboa, Lisboa, Portugal

4 REQUIMTE, Instituto Superior de Engenharia do Porto, Porto, Portugal

References

[1] World Health Organization (WHO). State of the Science of Endocrine Disrupting Chemicals 2012. United Nations Environment Programme and the World Health Organization, 2013 Geneva.

[2] United States Environmental Protection Agency (US EPA). Water Quality Standards; Establishment of numeric criteria for priority toxic pollutants; States'compliances. Federal Register 1992; 57(246): 60848 (57FR 60848).

[3] Morais S, Dias E and Pereira ML. Carbamates: human exposure and health effects. In: Jokanović M. and Cheyenne WY. (eds.) The Impact of Pesticides. Academy Press 2012. p21-38.

[4] Jokanovic M. Medical treatment of acute poisoning with organophosphorus and carbamate pesticides, Toxicology Letters 2009; 190: 107-115.

[5] International Programme on Chemical Safety (IPCS, 1986), Environmental Health Criteria 64, Carbamate Pesticides: a General Introduction, World Health Organization, Geneva, http://www.inchem.org/documents/ehc/ehc/ehc64.htm#subsection-number:1.1.7.

[6] Saber M, Parsaeyan E, Vojoudi S, Bagheri M, Mehrvar A and Kamita SG. Acute toxicity and sublethal effects of methoxyfenozide and thiodicarb on survival, development and reproduction of Helicoverpa armigera (Lepidoptera: Noctuidae). Crop Protection 2013; 43: 14-17.

[7] Kim KH, Kwon IH, Lee JY, Yeo WH, Park HY, Park KH, Cho J, Kim H, Kim GB, Park DH, Yoon YS and Kim YW. Clinical significance of national patients sample analysis: factors affecting mortality and length of stay of organophosphate and carbamate poisoned patients. Healthcare Informatics Research 2013; 19(4): 278-285.

[8] Gil HW, Jeong MH, Park JS, Choi HW, Kim SY and Hong SY. An Outbreak of Food Borne Illness Due to Methomyl Pesticide Intoxication in Korea. Journal Korean of Medical Science 2013; 28: 1677-1681.

[9] De Coster S and Larebeke N. Endocrine-disrupting chemicals: associated disorders and mechanisms of action. Journal of Environmental and Public Health 2012, doi: 10.1155/2012/713696 52 pages.

[10] Crespo-Corral E, Santos-Delgado MJ, Polo-Diez LM and Soria AC. Determination of carbamate, phenylurea and phenoxy acid herbicide residues by gas chromatography after potassium ter-butoxide/dimethyl sulphoxide/ethyl iodide derivatization reaction. Journal of Chromatography A 2008; 1209: 22-28.

[11] Sagratini G, Mañes J, Giardiná D, Damiani P and Picó Y. Analysis of carbamate and phenylurea pesticide residues in fruit juices by solid-phase microextraction and liquid chromatography–mass spectrometry. Journal of Chromatography A 2007; 1147: 135-143.

[12] Jensen BH, Petersen A and Christensen T. Probabilistic assessment of the cumulative dietary acute exposure of the population of Denmark to organophosphorus and carbamate pesticides. Food Additives and Contaminants 2009; 26(7): 1038-1048.

[13] George J and Shukla Y. Pesticides and cancer: insights into toxicoproteomic-based findings. Journal of Proteomics 2011; 74(12): 2713-2722.

[14] Imran H. and Dilshad KA. Adverse Health Effects of Pesticide Exposure in Agricultural and Industrial Workers of Developing Country. In: Stoytcheva M (ed.), Pesticides-The Impacts of Pesticides Exposure, InTech; 2011. p155-178.

[15] Mnif W, Hassine AIH, Bouaziz A, Bartegi A, Thomas O and Roig B. Effect of endocrine disruptor pesticides: a review. International Journal of Environmental Research and Public Health 2011; 8: 2265-2303.

[16] Watts M. Human health impacts of exposure to pesticides. 2012 http://awsassets.wwf.org.au/downloads/pr_attachment_human_health_impacts_of_exposure_to_pesticides_20mar13.pdf (assessed on 25 july 2014).

[17] Corsini E, Sokooti M, Galli CL, Moretto A and Colosio C. Pesticide induced immunotoxicity in humans: a comprehensive review of the existing evidence. Toxicology 2013; 307: 123– 135.

[18] Hernández AF, Parrón T, Tsatsakis AM, Requena M, Alarcón R and López-Guarnido O. Toxic effects of pesticide mixtures at a molecular level: their relevance to human health. Toxicology 2013; 307: 136-145.

[19] Miranda-Contreras L, Gómez-Pérez R, Rojas G, Cruz I, Berrueta L, Salmen S, Colmenares M, Barreto S, Balza A, Zavala L, Morales Y, Molina Y, Valeri L, Contreras CA and Osuna JA. Occupational exposure to organophosphate and carbamate pesticides affects sperm chromatin integrity and reproductive hormone levels among venezuelan farm workers. Journal of Occupational Health 2013; 55: 195–203.

[20] Sugeng AJ, Beamer PI, Lutz EA and Rosales CB. Hazard-ranking of agricultural pesticides for chronic health effects in Yuma County, Arizona. Science of the Total Environment 2013; 463–464: 35–41.

[21] Schinasi L and Leon ME. Non-Hodgkin lymphoma and occupational exposure to agricultural pesticide chemical groups and active ingredients: a systematic review and

meta-analysis. International Journal of Environmental Research and Public Health 2014; 11: 4449-4527.

[22] Roberts JR, Karr CJ and Council on Environmental Health. Pesticide exposure in children. Pediatrics 2012; 130(6): e1765-e1788.

[23] Alavanja MC and Bonner MR. Occupational Pesticide Exposures and cancer risk: a review. Journal of Toxicology and Environmental Health Part B 2012; 15(4): 238-263.

[24] Kachuri L, Demers PA, Blair A, Spinelli JJ, Pahwa M, McLaughlin JR, Pahwa P, A Dosman JA and Harris SA. Multiple pesticide exposures and the risk of multiple myeloma in Canadian men. International Journal of Cancer 2013; 133: 1846-1858.

[25] Santana VS, Moura MCP, Ferreira e Nogueira F. Occupational pesticide poisoning, 2000-2009, Brazil. Revista de Saúde Pública 2013; 47(3): 1-8.

[26] MacFarlane E, Carey R, Keegel T, El-Zaemay S and Fritschi L. Dermal Exposure Associated with Occupational End Use of Pesticides and the Role of Protective Measures. Safety and Health at Work 2013; 4(3): 136-141.

[27] Prado-Ochoa MG, Gutiérrez-Amezquita RA, Abrego-Reyes VH, Velázquez-Sánchez A, Muñoz-Guzmán MA, Ramírez-Noguera P, Angeles E. and Alba-Hurtado F. Assessment of Acute Oral and Dermal Toxicity of 2 Ethyl-Carbamates with Activity against *Rhipicephalus microplus* in Rats. BioMedical Research International 2014a, *in press*. doi: 10.1155/2014/956456.

[28] Prado-Ochoa MG, Abrego-Reyes VH, Velázquez-Sánchez AM, Muñoz-Guzmán MA, Ramírez-Noguera P, Angeles E and Alba-Hurtado F. Subchronic toxicity study in rats of two new ethyl-carbamates with ixodicidal activity. BioMedical Research International 2014b, *in press*. doi: 10.1155/2014/467105.

[29] Dias E, Morais S, Ramalheira E and Pereira ML. Characterization of the toxicological effects of aminocarb on rats: hematological, biochemical and histological analyses. Journal of Toxicology and Environmental Health A. 2014; 77: 849-855.

[30] Almasiova V, Holovska K, Tarabova L, Cigankova V, Lukacinova A and Nistiar F. Structural and ultrastructural study of rabbit testes exposed to carbamate insecticide. Journal of Environmental Science Health 2012; 47: 1319–1328.

[31] Holovska K. Almasiova V and Cigankova V. Ultrastructural changes in the rabbit liver induced by carbamate insecticide bendiocarb. Journal of Environmental Science and Health 2014; 49: 616–623.

[32] Wang HP, Liang YJ, Zhang Q, Long DX, Li W, Li L, Yang L,Yan XZ and Wu YJ. Changes in metabolic profiles of urine from rats following chronic exposure to anticholinesterase pesticides. Pesticide Biochemistry and Physiology 2011; 101: 232–239.

[33] Fattahi E, Jorsaraei SGA and Gardane M. The effect of carbaryl on the pituitary-gonad axis in male rats. Iranian Journal of Reproductive Medecine 2012; 10(5): 419-424.

[34] Moser VS, Katherine LM, Phillips PM and Lowit AB. Time-course, dose-response, and age comparative sensitivity of N-Methyl carbamates in rats. Toxicological Science 2010; 114: 113–123.

[35] Yu G, Guo Q, Xie L, Liu Y and Wang X. Effects of subchronic exposure to carbendazim on spermatogenesis and fertility in male rats. Toxicology and Industrial Health 2009; 25: 41–47.

[36] Farag A, Ebrahim H, ElMazoudy R, and Kadous E. Developmental toxicity of fungicide carbendazim in female mice. Birth Defects Research 2011; 92:122–130.

[37] Moffit JS, Her LS, Mineo AM, Knight BL, and Phillips JA, and Thibodeau MS. Assessment of inhibin B as a biomarker of testicular injury following administration of carbendazim, cetrorelix, or 1,2-dibromo-3-chloropropane in wistar han rats. Birth Defects Research Part B 2013; 98:17–28.

[38] Rai DK, Rai PK, Gupta A, Watal G, and Sharma B. Cartap and carbofuran induced alterations in serum lipid profile of wistar rats. Indian Journal of Clinical Biochemistry 2009: 24(2): 198-201.

[39] Gera N and Kiran R, Mahmood A. Subacute effects of carbofuran on enzyme functions in rat small intestine. Toxicology Mechanisms and Methods 2009; 19:141-147.

[40] Kaur B, Khera A, and Sandhir R. Attenuation of cellular antioxidant defense mechanisms in kidney of rats intoxicated with carbofuran. Journal of Biochemistry and Molecular Toxicology 2012; 26(10): 393-398.

[41] Gbadegesin MA, Owumi SE, Akinseye V and Odunola OA. Evaluation of hepatotoxicity and clastogenicity of carbofuran in male Wistar rats. Food and Chemical Toxicology 2014; 65:115–119.

[42] Banji D, Banji OJ, Ragini M and Annamalai AR. Carbosulfan exposure during embryonic period can cause developmental disability in rats. Environmental Toxicology and Pharmacology 2014; 38: 230–238.

[43] Ozden S. and Alpertunga B. Effects of methiocarb on lipid peroxidation and glutathione level in rat tissues. Drug and Chemical Toxicology 2010; 33: 50-54.

[44] Ozden S, Catalgol B, Gezginci-Oktayoglu S, Karatug A, Bolkent S and Alpertunga B. Acute effects of methiocarb on oxidative damage and the protective effects of vitamin E and taurine in the liver and kidney of Wistar rats. Toxicology and Industrial Health 2012; 29(1): 60–71.

[45] Manawadi S and Kaliwal BB. Methomyl induced alteration in mice hepatic-oxidative Status. International Journal of Biotechnology Applications 2010; 2(2): 11-19.

[46] Shalaby MA, El Zorba HY and Ziada RM. Reproductive toxicity of methomyl insecticide in male rats and protective effect of folic acid. Food and Chemical Toxicology 2010; 48: 3221–3226.

[47] Wang P, Wang HP, Xu MY, Liang YJ, Sun YJ, Yang L, Li L, Li W and Wu YJ. Combined subchronic toxicity of dichlorvos with malathion or pirimicarb in mice liver and serum: A metabonomic study. Food and Chemical Toxicology 2014; 70: 222-230.

[48] Dias E, Gomes M, Domingues C, Ramalheira E, Morais S, and Pereira ML. Subacute effect of the thiodicarb pesticide on target organs of male wistar rats: biochemical, histological, and flow cytometry studies. Journal of Toxicology and Environmental Health A. 2013; 76(9): 533–539.

[49] Satpal, Jain SK and Punia JS. Studies on Biochemical Changes in subacute thiodicarb toxicity in rats. Toxicology International 2010; 17: 30-32.

Chapter 10

Use of Natural Latex as a Biomaterial for the Treatment of Diabetic Foot — A New Approach to Treating Symptoms of Diabetes Mellitus

Suélia de Siqueira Rodrigues Fleury Rosa, Maria do Carmo Reis,
Mário Fabricio Fleury Rosa, Diego Cólon, Célia Aparecida dos Reis and
José Manoel Balthazar

Additional information is available at the end of the chapter

http://dx.doi.org/10.5772/59135

1. Introduction

Diabetes mellitus (DM) is one of the most investigated health issues today, and it is becoming a major concern for academicians and decision makers in Public Health, mainly due to its complications, which are associated with high rates of morbidity and mortality. This disease interferes with various aspects of the daily lives of the individuals affected and imposes various lifestyle restrictions. Some of its chronic complications are the most common causes of non-traumatic lower-limb amputations. In most cases, amputation is initially preceded by an ulcer on the foot. The diabetic foot, as defined by the World Health Organization (WHO), is a foot with an infection, ulceration, and/or destruction of deep tissue associated with neurological abnormalities and various degrees of peripheral vascular disease in the lower limbs. The various socioeconomic impacts of this disease in its more advanced stages, which result from prolonged hospitalization, rehabilitation, and the great needs for home care and social assistance, provide motivation for public health policies and research for new ways to prevent and treat the diabetic foot from a multidisciplinary perspective [1, 4]. In this chapter, we present the results of a study on factors that contribute to the prevention and treatment of diabetic foot ulcers using natural latex biomaterials made from *Hevea brasiliensis*, in the form of biomaterials applied to humans (in this case, in direct contact with the human skin). The chapter is organized in the following way: in section 2, it is defined what a diabetic foot is, to provide the context for addressing the problem. The use of natural latex biomaterials made from *Hevea brasilien-sis* is discussed in the context of biotechnology, wherein *Hevea brasiliensis* is used as a raw

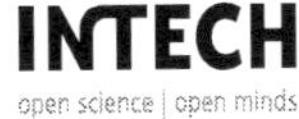

material in the prevention and treatment of diabetic foot. In section 3, the diabetic foot is described by a mathematical model and it is presented how the use of biomaterial latex acts as modifier of the dynamics of the system to believe this application as a minor theory and/or auxiliary hypothesis in the biotechnological process as it applies to humans. In section 4 and 5 the chapter closes with a presentation of a "natural latex insole" prototype capable of preventing and treating diabetic foot ulcers.

2. International consensus on the diabetic foot

Among the consequences of DM are the increased incidences of amputation of the lower limbs and mortality. Many scientific studies have been conducted to increase understanding of diabetes and established a general framework for its treatment, prevention, and assistance. In light of these and other needs, the Brazilian Federal Government launched on December 17, 2011 a major public health policy, which is the National Plan on the Rights of the Disabled Person, or as it is more commonly known, the *VIVER SEM LIMITES (living without limits)*. The main objective of this initiative was to establish new fronts and intensify actions that were already being developed by the Government and/or the private sector for the benefit of persons with disabilities. This initiative established a set of public policies that were articulated along four axes: (1) access to education, (2) social inclusion, (3) health care, and (4) accessibility. These public policies were established by means of a plan of action that articulated and organized innovative initiatives in multiple subject areas designed to make it possible to achieve improvements in the quality of life, dignity, and rights of persons with disabilities. The research presented in this chapter fits into the context of this policy, as it is being conducted within the Center for Research, Development, and Innovation in Assistive Technology and Accessibility at the University of Brasilia (UnB), in partnership with the Engineering and Biomaterials Laboratory—BioEngLab®, Faculdade Gama (FGA), University of Brasília (UnB), which gives priority to the multidisciplinary asymmetry upon which this study is based. Diabetes mellitus is classified among the chronic diseases that are mostly asymptomatic or almost asymptomatic. These are diseases that do not endanger the life of a person in the short term. Shown by many researchers to be very costly, not only to the affected individuals and their families but also to national governments, it is the sixth most common cause of primary diagnosis in hospitalizations [1-6]. In Brazil, the prevalence of DM is approximately 15% in the age group above 35 years, according to [5]. In a perspective analyses, some studies [7-11] have reported that approximately 50% of patients are unaware of the diagnostics and that 24% of patients known to be diabetic make use of no treatment. This causes a variety of complications, among which the diabetic foot is notable, as it is considered a serious problem with often devastating consequences (the related ulceration, which can involve amputation of the toes, feet, or legs). Diabetes has been associated with several structural and functional alterations of the feet that can result in higher plantar pressures, anatomical deformities (claw toes, charcot neuro-osteoarthropathy), limited joint mobility, and skin changes (callus formation) [12]. The diabetic foot exhibits morphological alterations, and its distribution of the various tissues influences its functioning, resulting in a set of changes in the patient. This study focuses on biomechanical changes, with emphasis on the vertical ground reaction force involved. In [13], that is a major study of the biomechanics of gait analysis, the vertical ground reaction force was measured and the movement of the ankle joint was filmed in patients with diabetic neuropathy. That study showed that the values of the 1st and 2nd vertical ground reaction force peaks are greater in patients with diabetic peripheral neuropathy. The vertical ground reaction force was found to have different characteristics among the different groups studied; thus, methods to reduce the vertical ground reaction force are required to decrease the likelihood of developing plantar ulcers. In Brazil, because of the tropical climate and cultural norms, walking barefoot and using inappropriate or insufficient diabetic foot care (lack of good hygienic habits, hydration, transport type, etc.) are common [14]. According to the literature [15-17], the causes of foot injuries are strongly related to increased pressure in certain areas and deformities of the feet and toes. This is because of diabetic neuropathy (DN), which is considered to be the main permissive factor for developing foot ulcerations in diabetic patients. Lesions are generally caused by unanticipated and undesirable events that are complicated by possible gangrene and infection, because of deficiencies in the healing process, which can lead, in extreme cases, to amputation. It is known that ulcerations may lead to a decrease in the quality of life, prolonged hospitalization, consequent absenteeism, early retirement, and high economic costs associated with treatment and reduced working capacity of individuals of productive age. Recent studies provide information pertaining, in greater quantity and accuracy, to dramatic changes. In elderly patients affected by the disease, foot abnormalities can result in loss of stability that can lead to falls and consequently to death. Previous studies have used various tests, such as capturing a controlled gait, foot anthropomorphic measurements, and clinical examinations, to understand these changes. The results of previous studies have shown that pressure and shear stress variables are applied at distinct points and affect the frontal regions of the foot (the forefoot) more than the heel regions [18-22]. Among the changes that occur are reduced sensitivity to pain, vibration, and temperature; hypotrophy of small muscles; distention of the dorsal veins in the feet; and decreased postural sensitivity, which results in changes in gait and contributes to the formation of calluses [23, 24]. As some studies [4,5, 16, 17-21] have reported, these changes indicate that the feet of diabetic persons must be well cared for, protected, and accommodated accordingly, because of the risk of ulcers developing as result of repetitive trauma or, for instance, the presence of foreign objects inside footwear and/or inadequate accommodations. Another important factor involving the diabetic foot is that motor neuropathy also leads to muscle weakness and subsequently to intrinsic muscle atrophy of the feet. These changes result in deformities, such as claw and hammer toes (dominance of the flexors over the extensors), foot cavus (pronounced curvature of the foot), and pressure points in some areas of the feet (mainly in the metatarsal head, plantar, and dorsal regions of the feet), which change the normal gait pattern when walking [25]. Autonomic neuropathy leads to the reduction or total absence of sweat secretion, making the foot dry and the skin more susceptible to breakage than normal. Skin dryness favors the formation of fissures and cracks that, if not treated properly, can develop into ulcers with or without infection. Natural protection and skin integrity become less efficient, exposing the foot to the risk of mechanical lesions [26, 27]. It is evident that intrinsic and extrinsic factors contribute to abnormal pressure on the foot and the possible stress of accommodation. This chapter presents a new contribution to DM treatment and more specifically the diabetic foot problem. This contribution was developed by examining some of the extrinsic factors that contribute to the emergence of injuries that affect the diabetic foot and asking: how can these extrinsic factors be changed. This is the question that guided this research, which mobilizes a multidisciplinary group of researchers (in the areas of engineering, health, and human sciences) who believes that this study will contribute to customized biomechanical and behavioral changes. The following changes can be made with the proposed approach: decreasing the ground reaction force, increasing foot moisture, protecting against foreign objects, and modifying the DM gait performance index. Studies conducted in [28-34] to assess high-risk diabetic individuals have reported lower recurrence of ulcerations in groups given specially made shoes. These studies have also reported that special footwear can be beneficial to patients without expert foot care assistance and to those with severe foot deformities [28-34]. For this reason, to devise a treatment for ulcerated diabetic feet, it is vital to identify the worst-affected areas of the foot before pressure ulcers develop, using pressure gauges to establish the likelihood of preventing foot injuries through the use of customized insoles that redistribute pressure in high-pressure plantar regions during patient gait. The use of latex biomaterials in customized shock-absorbing insoles that are intended to prevent the emergence of diabetic foot ulcers constitutes a potential new contribution to diabetic foot treatment, as described in this chapter. The authors have questioned the usefulness of high foot plantar pressure in identifying neuropathy and consequent ulceration, because of the high coefficient of variation of plantar pressure. However, several other studies [35-33] have confirmed the role of mechanical stress on the development of ulceration, as well as the importance of relief of mechanical stress in the treatment of the neuropathic diabetic foot. Once patients are affected by DM, the ulcers and subsequent infection are its main complications [36]. Unless diabetic foot ulcers are properly diagnosed and treated, amputation is a frequent outcome. Other predisposing factors that have been identified as being related to increased plantar pressure include body mass, sensory deficit, and the presence of foot deformities [37]. Although diabetic patients are usually obese, body mass is a factor that can be related to the appearance of high plantar pressures and ulcers even if not combined with other factors (neuropathy, deformity). Diabetic foot treatment depends on the degree of commitment of the limbs, taking into consideration the presence and/or severity of ischemia and/or infection. Currently, there are a few options for the treatment of lesions, such as wound dressings (for which various types of bandages are available on the market), debridement of devitalized tissue, revascularization, local application of growth factors, oxygen therapy, human dermis (Dermagraft®), and amputation of extremities, the last of these being the option most frequently adopted [38-42]. Considering that diabetic foot patients are affected by serious shortcomings in scar healing, this process has been widely investigated [43-45]. Optimization of the tissue regeneration process has been studied and discussed in various lines of research, covering aspects such as pathophysiology, risk factors, anti-inflammatory drugs, and chemical substances that may influence the healing process [46-50]. Among the resources that have been proposed, low-intensity light-emitting diode (LED) therapy and the use of natural latex derived from the *Hevea brasiliensis* [50] rubber tree are noteworthy. The authors believe that this biotechnology association offers the potential for a new treatment approach, involving the use of a latex insole with LED light emission, through which healing can be induced. This treatment approach was developed by making use of the results obtained in the construction phase of the first shock-absorbing insole.

3. Participants, experimental set-up, and definitions

To ensure the suitability of the assumptions and methodological procedures pursued by the developers of the aforementioned treatment approach, the approval of the Research Ethics Committee of the State Secretariat for Health of the Federal District – Brazil (SES/DF/BR) was requested. This request was approved under Protocol 428/11. To carry out the data collection for testing and treatment in humans, two DM patients were selected, one of whom presented foot ulcerations and the other of whom did not. Both signed an Informed Consent Form (ICF), supported by a correlational descriptive and qualitative study of the relationship between the systematic collection of data and the immersion of the researcher in the context being studied [51]. The two individuals were personally contacted and invited to participate in the research. The instrument for obtaining data was a structured questionnaire with closed-ended questions and history taking (date of birth, sex, date of diagnosis, type of medicine, DM type, among other items) and application of the Michigan Neuropathy Screening Instrument questionnaire (a tool to assess symptoms related to diabetic neuropathy). The research group enrolled a patient without ulcers (who had never exhibited any ulceration) but who had pressure peaks, to test the first proposed method for correcting the performance indexes through the use of a shock-absorbing insole. We also enrolled a patient with an established ulcer who had not received prior treatment, to test for wound healing (scarring) through the use of a healing insole with red LED light.

3.1. Patient in need of plantar pressure correction

The first stage of the research was performed with the patient without any diabetic foot ulceration in the lower limbs. The focus of this stage of the research was on evaluating the effectiveness of the insole padding material in reducing plantar pressure. The patient was a 33-year-old female with Type 1 diabetes who had been diagnosed 24 years ago. She was married, had no children, had completed higher education and was a graduate student. She was a resident of the central region of the Federal District – Brazil, had a Class B license, was able to communicate and get around, and was an insulin pump user. Initially, an interview was conducted for data collection to characterize her gait condition, taking into consideration any gait change the patient exhibited while walking. Measurements were taken of the patient's height, body weight, glycemic index (using an Accu-Chek active lancing device, with meas-uring strips and lancets), basal temporal dose, heartbeat, percentage of oxygen and anthropo-morphic foot dimensions (via calipers). Subsequently, a questionnaire was administered to assess the patient's quality of life, the patient's mechanical activities (such as walking, climbing stairs, driving, and performing household chores), items related to financial considerations, side effects of medications, and lifestyle (overall dimensions). This patient was advised not to consume alcohol or any sort of medication for 24 h prior to the beginning of the experiment. The subject was informed about the experiment, and a trial run was conducted before the readings were taken. To determine where the latex shock absorbers should be placed in the insole that would be made for her, a pedographic test analysis was conducted. The equipment used was the emed®-n50 Novel platform (4 sensors/cm² resolution, frame rate of 50 Hz, dimensions of 700 x 403 x 15.5 mm, 6080 sensors, sensor resolution (sensors/cm²) of 1 or 4/4/4, frequency of 50 Hz, pressure range of 10–1270 kPa, accuracy of ± 5% ZAS, temperature range of 10–40°C, maximum total force of 193,000 N) (emed® HMFT-novel-projects v23.3.44, © 2013 by Novel GmbH), which collects plantar pressure distribution data using sensors, data collection circuits, and appropriated software. The initial phase of the orthostatic recording was a "break-in" phase that began with the patient adopting a stable standing position in bare feet. The individual responsible for data collection then instructed the patient to remain in a standing position for 30 seconds with her eyes open for each dual-foot acquisition. She was asked to maintain the standing position and balance her body weight evenly on the right foot and left foot. This protocol was repeated three times to check whether the blood glucose checked at the time of testing (acute assessment) interfered with the results. Just before the plantar pressure assessment portion of each test, the patient's capillary glycemia was measured using a digital pulp puncture glucose meter (Accu-Chek System Active Glucose Meter, lancing device, measuring strips, lancet, and cotton). Figure 1 shows the equipment and system for the testing carried out to identify the highest pressure peak locations.

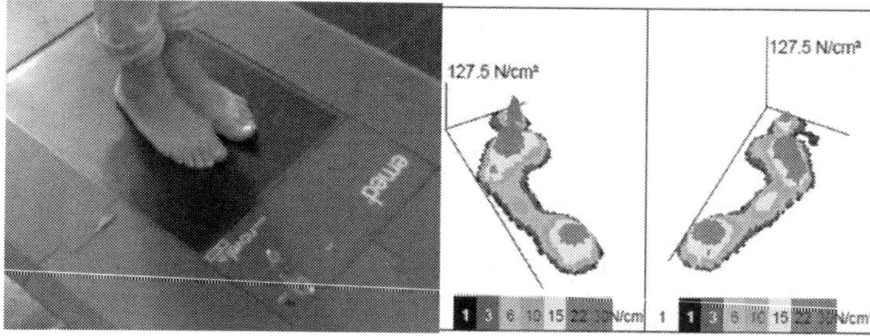

Figure 1. Photo image of the test carried out to measure foot pressure, taken by the authors with the patient's consent. The plantar pressure distribution image was produced by the emed®-n50 Novel software. The photo image highlights the frontal region of the foot as exhibiting the highest concentration of pressure. Image provided for data sample of plantar pressure: metatarsal head=MTH, hallux=toes, midfoot, and heel.

The second type of test was a static postural balance test conducted using kinetic data obtained with the AccuSway Plus force platform manufactured by AMTI. The sampling frequency was 100 Hz, and each data collection cycle lasted 30 seconds. For each cycle, four attempts were made with the patient's eyes open. The patient was asked to keep her eyes fixed on a point that was highlighted on the wall at the patient's eye level at a distance of 2.0 meters. The patient was also asked to extend her arms parallel to her body. Adhesive tape was used to mark the position where the patient should step on the platform for the four attempts. It should be noted that previous attempts were made and eliminated because of errors, such as variation of support, imbalance, arm movement, and noise in the room. To correct these errors, testing and data collection were conducted during hours with less activity/noise in the lab (saturday nights). The variables of interest that were measured were the magnitudes of the anterior–posterior (shift in y (cm)) and medial–lateral (shift in x (cm)) force centers and the average velocity of the shift from the force center (Vm in cm/s). These measurements were obtained for use in a comparative analysis with and without the patient foot insole. It should be noted that the insole selected was the one that promoted the largest plantar pressure reduction. Eight different latex insole models were made with different shock-absorbing formats, different associations, and protocols. These eight models were tested to identify the one that provided the patient with acceptable comfort, usability, and reduced pressure. The repeatability criterion was applied in the research, and the same insole model was made several times so that one from the lot that yielded the highest scores in the patient evaluation could be identified. For each insole, she completed a questionnaire, video was captured, and an evaluation was conducted by the authors. Figure 2 shows details of the test.

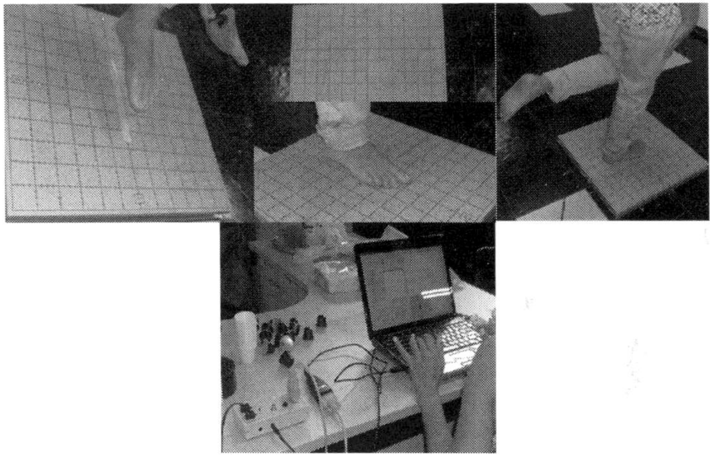

Figure 2. Pictures taken by the authors with details of the test conducted on the AccuSway Plus force platform manufactured by AMTI, with a sampling rate of 100 Hz and each collection cycle lasting 30 seconds. This platform was used to record static pressure and postural balance data, in compliance with the Nyquist criterion, with a postural static frequency value of 5 Hz.

Light Emitting Diodes (or LEDs) are semiconductor diodes that emit light when there is electrical current across them. They are manufactured in several wavelength bands (from 405 nm blue till 940 nm infrared) and in different emission patterns, that is, normal or LASER (Light Amplification by Stimulated Emission of Radiation). The LASER LED emit coherent light with a very narrow wavelength band (single color) while the ordinary LED emits in a wider band (several wavelengths). Both types of LEDs have different therapeutic purposes [49]. The blue light has renewing and anti-bacteria effects in the skin, and the red light has anti-inflammatory and scarring effect. The light intensity (emitted by the LEDs) necessary to obtain the desired therapeutic effects are lesser than LASER diodes, due to good interaction between the human skin and incoherent light (Rigau, 1996). Specifically, the blue light LED (470nm) has anti-bacteria action against *propionibacterium acnes*, by a process known as photo-inactivation (that is, the remotion of electrons from the bacteria's external citoplasmatical membrane by oxygen molecules) and the 660 nm red light also has anti-inflammatory effect and stimulate cellular multiplication. The LASER LED light has a directional effect while the ordinary LED is more spread in the area. The equipment consists of LED arrays (or cells) mounted outside and below the latex insole and they are placed only in the ulcerative regions in the feet, after a clinical examination. The light intensity is 25 J/cm² and the scarring effect is then expected. An electronic circuit controlling the LED array has a timer that terminates the process after a programmed time interval and a buzz to indicate the end.

3.2. Patient in need of established ulceration correction

In this chapter, it is presented two cases, but reference in [52], a study conducted previously have been all reported cases. The second stage of the research was conducted with the participation of the patient that had diabetic foot ulcers. This stage focused on correcting the established ulcer through the use of a healing insole associated with a red LED light. After the initial assessment, the subjects were divided into two study groups: control group (CG) and experimental group (GE). In GC: Treatment with foam dressing with silver and GE: treatment with the inducer tissue formation system.

The GC was made up of four patients and a total of five diabetic foot ulcers. These patients underwent conventional treatment for a minimum of 30 days and monitored weekly by the responsible team. A few of these patients were followed until complete healing of the ulcer. Before applying the foam dressing with silver, a nurse performed the wound debridement of devitalized tissue and hygiene with 0.9% saline and gauze. After cleaning, the ulcer had its bed dry with gauze and was found ready to receive the healing. After placing the foam with silver on the wound, gauze was placed over it and the closing was done by bandages. The exchange of this dressing was performed every 5 days at home by the patient or by its own family (except in the clinical evaluation days, where the curative was made by ambulatory nurse). Is worth mentioning that even when the dressing change was performed at home, it was necessary for the patient to carry out cleaning of the wound with 0.9% saline and gauze. The silver foam is foam made of antibacterial wound dressing impregnated with silver ions that are released continuously, to the extent that the exudate (fluid) is absorbed. The foam half silvered promotes moist environment for healing important factor.

The GE was made up of six patients and a total of nine diabetic foot ulcers. These patients underwent treatment with the healing inducer system for varying periods of tissue neoformation, and monitored weekly by the responsible team. Some of these patients used the system inducing tissue formation until complete ulcer healing. It is noteworthy that the inducing tissue formation system consists of a healing insole and an electronic circuit for tissue regeneration. After clinical evaluation to characterize the sample, it was taken the mold of the patient's foot for making the healing insole, since it is customized to each individual patient. Individuals from GE group were also monitored weekly by the responsible staff. At each time, the nurse performed the procedure debridement of devitalized tissue and cleaning the ulcer with 0.9% saline and gauze. The clinical and demographic characteristics such as age, sex, occupation, height, weight and the associated diseases in six patients belonging to the study, illnesses are listed in Table 1:

Patients and Group	age (years)	sex	height (m)	weight (kg)	occupation	Associated diseases
Patients 1 - GC e GE	46	F	1.59	98	homemaker	hypertension
Patients 2 – GE	53	M	1.75	72	Brazil server	hypertension
Patients 3 - GC e GE	57	F	1.72	87	homemaker	Nothing
Patients 4 – GE	64	M	1.78	82	businessman	hypertension
Patients 5- GC e GE	68	M	1.60	68	retired	hypertension
Patients 6 - GC e GE	62	F	1.57	60	homemaker	hypertension

Table 1. Clinical and demographic characterization of patients with diabetic foot ulcer.

Patients Group	Typeof DM	Time of Diagnosis DM	Number of ulcers already presented from the diagnosis	Number of ulcers treated in the study	Amputation (quantity and area)
Patients 1 - GC e GE	2	17	5	2	Off
Patients 2 - GE	2	12 anos	2	1	Off
Patients 3 - GC e GE	2	24 anos	6	4	two - 2nd toe (right foot) and 5th toe (left foot)
Patients 4 - GE	2	18 anos	4	1	Off
Patients 5- GC e GE	2	29 anos	3	1	two - 1st toe (hallux) and the 2nd to 5th toes (left foot)
Patients 6 - GC e GE	2	8 anos	3	2	two - the 2nd to the 5th toe, hallux and part of the foot (right foot)

Table 2. Data from patients relating to DM and diabetic foot ulcers.

Exploring the data in Table 1, it appears that patients in both groups have an average age of 58.3 years, with a minimum age of 46 years and maximum of 68 years; 50% of patients are female and 50% male; the average height of patients is 1,66m; 50% of patients have weight above average weight (77.8 kg). Regarding occupation, it was predominant householding, comprising two patients (33.3%). And 83.3% of patients, in addition to DM, also have hypertension. Is worth mentioning that, according to Table 1, among the 6 patients included in the study, 4 patients were part of both groups: experimental and control; only 2 patients were part only in the experimental group and no patients were part only in the GC. Below is the division of the total number of ulcers (11) by group: i) GC: 5 ulcers and ii) GE: 9 ulcers. In GE, among 9 ulcers, 3 were part of both groups: GC and GE. Such an occurrence is because after these 3 ulcers were accompanied by a month in the GC, they were transferred to GE, in an attempt to accelerate the healing process through the use of the inductor system tissue formation. In Table 2 it is shows the other data collected from patients regarding DM and diabetic foot ulcers.

In accordance with the Table 2, 100% of the patients show type 2 DM (the most common form of the disease); 3 patients (50%) have had a minimum of 4 ulcers since diagnosis of diabetes mellitus. The highest number of ulcers was recorded by the patient 3, who during all the time of diagnosis of DM, has recorded six ulcers. The most alarming observed data in this table is the number of amputations, as 50% of patients have two amputations caused by diabetic foot ulcers. The patient was 46 years of age, had been diagnosed with DM 15 years previously, and was a homemaker. The ulcer, which was present since two months ago, was located in region 2 (1st metatarsal head) of the right foot. This injury arose through a callus caused by mechanical stress due to the use of inadequate footwear. This patient was also more susceptible than the first patient to cracks, dry skin, fissures, and calluses, which influence the appearance of ulcers. This patient has presented five ulcers since the DM diagnosis. She is 1.59 m in height and weighs 98 kg, with illnesses associated with hypertension. This stage of the research was conducted on the premises of the Regional Hospital of Taguatinga (HRT), located in Taguatinga – Federal District-Brazil. This hospital was chosen to conduct all the steps in this stage of the study, because the medical staff included a diabetes physician who was a representative member in Brazil of the International Working Group on the Diabetic Foot, which provided support for this research and saw the potential that this study had to provide benefits to human health. Dr. Hermelinda Cordeiro Pedrosa participated in this experimental study as the main medical contributor. After the clinical evaluation conducted to characterize the patient's ulcer, the patient's diabetic foot was prepared so that a cast mold could be taken for the production of the healing insole, which is customized and personalized for each patient. The process of taking and making the mold is explained in the sections that follow. It should be noted that the patient's foot was cleaned and sanitized prior to being wrapped in plastic to obtain a copy of the mold. A home-use-only procedure was conducted to treat the ulcer using the tissue-healing insole. The patient first cleaned the ulcer with a 0.9% saline solution and gauze. After the cleaning procedure, the diabetic foot was ready for the insole. The patient then wore the latex insole, which was sterilized and sealed in its own packaging, and put it on by securing it with Velcro at the top. The next step was to secure the LED cell on the outside of the insole in the region of the wound, so that the light would reach the insole and the wound. In addition, the patient was advised to put a piece of plastic wrap on the LED cell to avoid contamination. The patient turned on the tissue regeneration electronic circuit using its on/off switch button and started the LED light emission in the direction of the wound, aided by the natural latex insole. During the treatment, the patient was required to stay at rest and not move the LED cell. The circuit emitted light for approximately 35 minutes. At the end of this time interval, the circuit automatically triggered an alarm. When the alarm went off, the patient had to turn off the circuit with the on/off button and remove the LED cell. After the patient removed the LED cell, gauze was placed on the outside of the insole at the wound site, using a bandage to hold the gauze in place. The gauze and bandage absorbed the discharge from the wound. The patient was advised to wear the healing insole all day or at least for a period of approximately 10 hours. The patient was also advised to make use of resting footwear along with the healing insole. Once a day, the patient repeated the entire process of cleaning the wound, replacing the insole and using the tissue regeneration electronic circuit. It should be noted that the insole was disposable and had to be replaced every day. Three times a week, the patient charged the tissue regeneration electronic circuit for a period of eight hours. It was tested for a period of two months. The patient performed the treatment with the insole and was monitored weekly by the research team. The clinical evaluation conducted by the medical team complied with the standard used in traditional methods. Figure 3 illustrates part of the procedure described above.

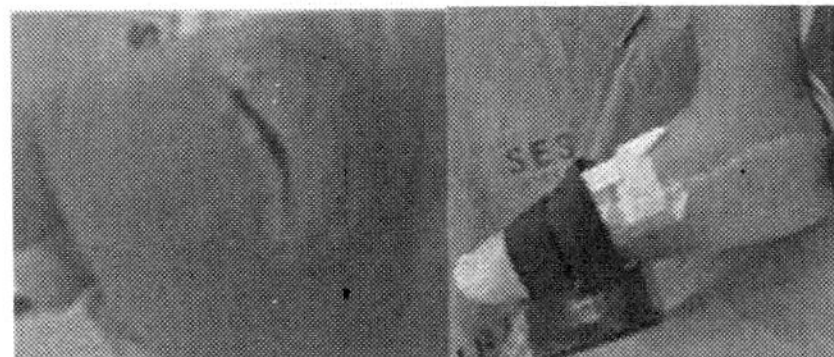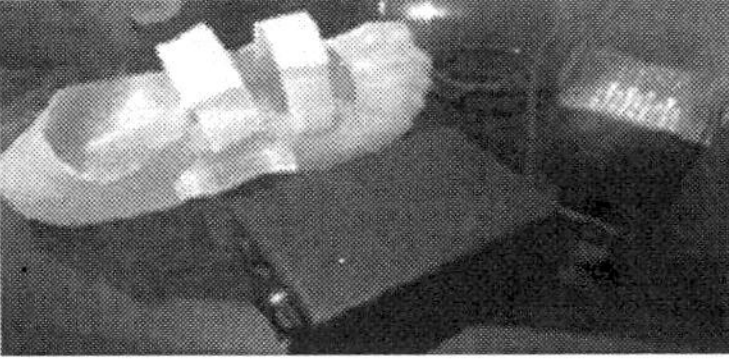

Figure 3. Photo images made by the authors of the established untreated ulcer on the patient, the system applied to the patient's foot as described for home care, and the complete system, with emphasis on the tissue regeneration electronic circuit.

3.3. Mathematical model

With the realization that injuries that occur in the diabetic foot have a mechanical etiology, many efforts have been made to achieve the stabilization and correction of these physical phenomena and correlate them to the occurrence of ulceration and the plantar pressure distribution. The pressure and shear stress variables in people with diabetes are applied at different points and produce effects in the frontal regions of the foot (forefoot) that are more pronounced than in the heel regions. The results show that the peak pressures do not all occur at the same shear stress point, a fact that underscores the need for a thorough analysis of the diabetic foot using a simple mechanical approach. To obtain a mathematical model for the system presented, we used the Bond Graph (BG) tool, which is an alternative to traditional modeling practices. The central idea of the behavioral study of the diabetic foot stance was to implement a custom-made insole derived from natural latex biomaterials to perform plantar pressure control. To accomplish this objective, the variables associated with the insole (or controller) customized design needed to be represented by the model. The use of the mathematical modeling as a biological system function representation and the use of its essential aspects to understand how it functions, based on some variables and conditions, is consistent with the production and standardization process for the technologies applied to these systems in actuality. The scenario involving biological variables and modern control systems, such as the manufacturing of latex-based shock-absorbing insoles for the prevention and cure of diabetic foot ulcers, naturally leads us to reflect upon control systems application in the area of biotechnology, in particular its use directly to control biological variables, like the plantar pressure. In this study, we suggest a control systems approach hypothesis, in which Latex materials should be used as the modifier factor of feet's system dynamics. The biotechnology revolution is based on massive scientific advances that have been made over the last sixty years. These advances have given scientists an extremely detailed understanding of life processes, have allowed life forms to be deliberately manipulated at the genetic level, and have enabled the creation of novel organisms containing genes from other species. To understand the history of the biotechnology revolution, it is useful to look at the development of the science that helped to create it. There was a significant merging of chemistry and biology (still seen by many as two distinct fields of science) in the early 1950s, as connections were made between the molecular structure of deoxyribonucleic acid (DNA) and its role in inheritance. The revolutionary techniques of genetic engineering and genome sequencing stem from this convergence [53]. Nevertheless, in the context of biotechnology, i.e., applications of science and engineering principles, materials processing, biological agents, biomaterials, mathematics, and obtaining supplies of goods and services, this study seeks to initiate discussions about derived biomaterial devices used as controllers or actuators (in the electrical engineering point of view) in the dynamics of biological systems, aiming to forge a system that best suits the linkage among engineering, biomaterials, and biological systems. For the research in question, taking into consideration that control engineering addresses the analysis and design for goal-oriented systems, in which modern control theory addresses systems that possess the qualities of self-organization, adaptability, robustness, learning, and optimality [55], use of biomaterials as a controller and / or actuator dynamics in the system presents itself as a minor theory and/ or auxiliary hypothesis possibility within the context of the paradigm [54]. From this perspective, the basic principle of mathematical modeling a physiological system is to simulate its action and thus be able to assess the parameters that may affect the system. Because of the natural aspects of the human body, which consist of many complex interactions, mathematically modeling a physiological systems allows for the development of diagnostic procedures that may be more effective in terms of the techniques applied, thus creating safer results, according to [52]. Simple mathematical models can generate complex patterns, and nature's complicated phenomena can be modeled using simple rules for generating a model for the system to assess, in this case, the insole's influence on the system parameters [56]. The challenges inherent to our proposal led us to develop various mathematical models to represent the foot dynamics. We employed the BG tool, which is an alternative to traditional modeling techniques and provides state space mathematical representations of nonlinear systems. By providing a graphical representation of a dynamic physical system, the BG tool facilitates the understanding of the influence of each element and visualization of the energy flow (gain and loss) throughout the system under study. In this respect, the BG tool differs from traditional modeling techniques. The concept on which the BG tool is based is unified representation of a dynamic system in which the elements interact with one another through ports within the system at which exchanges of energy occurs [57-58].

3.4. Static model

The first modeling procedure performed by the authors was to propose a mechanical model analogous to the diabetic foot that is capable of representing its behavior in terms of pressure variables. In formulating this analogous model, viscous and elastic elements were used in an attempt to express the structural characteristics of the pressure variables in physiomechanical terms. There are two basic component arrangements for physiological representations that are described in the literature: the Maxwell model and the Kelvin or Voight model [59]. These are viscoelastic models that represent approximations of actual material's behavior and that are sometimes combined to roughly and qualitatively represent the behavior of complex materials. The Kelvin or Voight model consists of a spring with elasticity k placed parallel to a viscous shock absorber (or damper) B. If a stress is applied at time t=0, the elongation of the spring may not be instantaneous because it may be slowed down by the shock absorber. The stress is distributed between the two components, the deformation occurs at a variable rate, and after a certain amount of time that depends on the shock absorber's viscosity, the spring approaches its maximum elongation. When the cause of the deformation is removed, the reverse process occurs: the deformation decreases over time, and the initial length tends to be restored. The Maxwell model consists of a spring and a shock absorber (damper) in series. According to this model, the material continues to deform as a constant stress is applied. The objective of the modeling is to represent important aspects of the system so that a design for a shock-absorbing insole can be developed that can govern or change the foot system response by reducing peak pressure. If we make an analogy with mathematical models, a classic example in the literature is the motorcycle and the rider; we follow the same strategy to propose a suspension derived from biomaterials, with a load distribution based on the construction of shock absorbers, i.e., generating energy loss (pressure) applied to the ground by the diabetic foot to decrease energy transfer. The representation of the diabetic foot is presented in Figure 4.

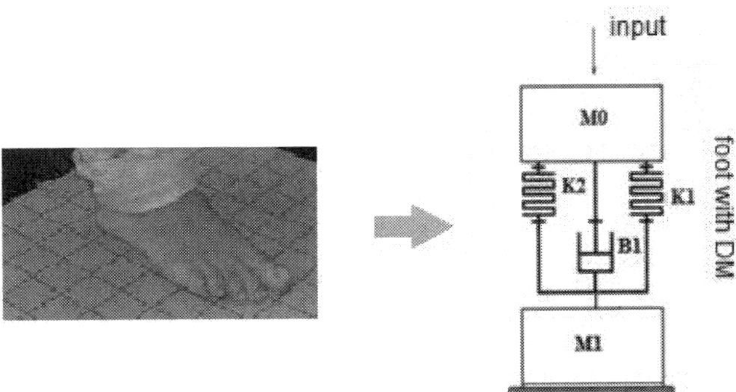

Figure 4. Photo of the foot in static position and proposal for a simple translational mechanical model.

The masses (M_0 and M_1) are the foot masses. The M_1 mass, which represents the forefoot, is connected in series with a spring (K_1) and a shock absorber (B_1). This representation shows that the force applied in passive diabetic walking has a greater impact in this region. The use of the shock absorber (B_1), which is responsible for reduced angulation and the low torque that this promotes in the system dynamics, is justified to represent the delay in activating the muscles that directly influence the pressure center (PC). Finally, for the heel region, which is responsible for driving the movement, a spring (K_2) was used. During both the compression of the spring and the movement back to equilibrium length, the force is always in the opposite direction of the displacement. Figure 5 illustrates the shock-absorbing insole system made from latex and a new model with a greater number of degrees of freedom (three in this case) and energy-damping shock absorbers that generate heat. This heat increases moisture and consequently hydration, as visually verified by the authors.

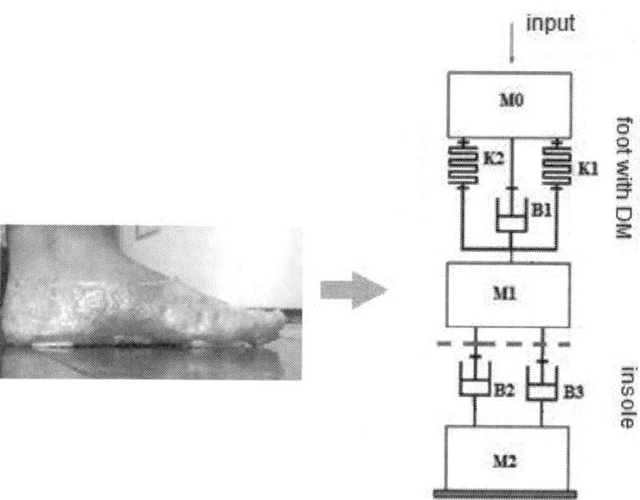

Figure 5. Photo of the foot in the static position with the insole and a proposed simple translational mechanical model with the insole element incorporated into its structure.

As explained by [60], the methodology for obtaining a model using the BG tool consists of three steps: i) specifying the analogous system based on the actual physiological model, ii) determining the energy areas, and iii) defining the simplification of the hypotheses and the input and output system variables. Following these steps to transform the analogous system into a graph of links, the following procedures were followed: 1) identification of the physical domain represented by the system and identification of the capacitive (C), resistive (R), inertial (I), sources of flow (SF) and effort (SE) elements present in the system; 2) identification of other energy variables, such as mass element velocities, and naming and assigning them type 1 junctions; 3) identification of the differences in efforts — in this case, differences in velocity, and assignment of type 0 junctions to these differences in velocity; and 4) connection of the elements identified in step 1 with their respective efforts or differences in effort, as represented by the type 1 junctions. Assignment of the causalities, automatically performed by the 20-Sim simulation software (a modeling and simulation program for mechatronic systems developed by Controllab Products). The motion equations for the systems presented in Figure 4, which represent the diabetic foot, are given by the following equations:

$$M_0\ddot{x}_1 + B_1\dot{x}_1 - B_1\dot{x}_2 + K_1x_1 - K_2x_2 + K_2x_1 - K_2x_2 = P(t)$$
$$M_1\ddot{x}_2 - B_1\dot{x}_1 + B_1\dot{x}_2 - K_1x_1 + K_1x_2 - K_2x_1 + K_2x_2 = 0 \tag{1}$$

The parameters of the system are M_0, the foot mass; M_1, the forefoot mass; K_1, human skin elasticity in the frontal region; and K_2, human skin elasticity in the heel region. The displacements are represented by the variables x_1 and x_2. The system input is the force $P(t)$, that is equal to the person's weight when the foot touches the ground. The motion equations for the system presented in Figure 5, which represents the diabetic foot in interaction with the insole, are the following:

$$M_0\ddot{x}_1 + B_1(\dot{x}_1 - \dot{x}_2) + K_1(x_1 - x_2) + K_2(x_1 - x_2) = P(t)$$
$$M_1\ddot{x}_2 - B_1(\dot{x}_1 - \dot{x}_2) - K_1(x_1 - x_2) - K_2(x_1 - x_2) = B_2(\dot{x}_2 - \dot{x}_3) + B_3(\dot{x}_2 - \dot{x}_3)$$
$$M_2\ddot{x}_3 + B_2(\dot{x}_3 - \dot{x}_2) + B_3(\dot{x}_3 - \dot{x}_2) = 0 \tag{2}$$

The parameters of the above system are M_2, the insole mass; and B_2 and B_3, the viscous shock absorbers made of latex. The displacements are x_1, x_2, and x_3. The system input is again the force $P(t)$. In analyzing this system, the eigenvalues of the characteristic equation were determined. Based on the consideration that a system is stable if all eigenvalues have a negative real part, the systems are asymptotically stable if and only if all eigenvalues have negative real parts, or equivalently, if all the Δ (characteristic polynomial) roots have negative real parts. Note that for systems without the insole, there is a null coefficient, and the system is critically stable, that is, may present undamped oscilattions. For systems with the insole inserted, according to the Hurwitz criterion, $M_0 > M_1$, which produces equation [3]:

$$\Delta_{foot}(s) = \left(s^4 + \left(\frac{B_1}{M_0} + \frac{B_1}{M_1}\right)s^3 + \left(\frac{B_1^2}{M_0M_1} + \frac{K_1}{M_0}\right)s^2 + \frac{B_1K_1}{M_0M_1}s - \frac{K_1K_2}{M_0^2}\right) = 0 \tag{3}$$

The terms K_1 and K_2 are spring constants that have positive values and units of N/m. The inclusion of an insole element with two shock absorbers for the proposed system changes the characteristic equation and renders the system marginally stable, a condition that is necessary and sufficient for ensuring stability in theory, according to equation [4]:

$$\Delta_{foot+insole}(s) = \left(s^5 + \left(\frac{B_1}{M_0} + \frac{B_2}{M_1} + \frac{B_2B_3}{(B_2+B_3)M_2} + \frac{B_2B_3}{(B_2+B_3)M_3}\right)s^4 + \right.$$
$$+\left(\frac{B_1}{M_0}\left(\frac{B_2}{M_1} + \frac{B_2B_3}{(B_2+B_3)M_2}\right) + \frac{B_1}{M_0}\left(\frac{B_2B_3}{(B_2+B_3)M_3}\right) + \left(\frac{B_2B_3}{(B_2+B_3)M_3}\right)\bullet\left(\frac{B_2}{M_1} + \frac{B_2B_3}{(B_2+B_3)M_2}\right)\right)s^3 +$$
$$\left. +\left(\frac{B_1}{M_0}\left(\frac{B_2B_3}{(B_2+B_3)M_3}\right)\bullet\left(\frac{B_2}{M_1} + \frac{B_2B_3}{(B_2+B_3)M_2}\right)\right)s^2 + \frac{K_2(B_2B_3)^2}{((B_2+B_3)^2M_0M_1M_2)}s\right) = 0 \tag{4}$$

Making use of the mathematical and static models presented, this study seeks to evaluate whether the use of latex insole shock absorbers is able to act in the areas of major diabetic foot plantar pressure to avoid the eruption of ulcers.

3.5. Hevea brasiliensis latex biomaterials

In the process of developing the insole, only materials found in the market were considered. The most commonly used materials are silicone, polyurethane, ethylene vinyl acetate (EVA), and viscoelastic foam. Based on this review, the raw material chosen for use in this study was latex biomaterial. This biomaterial is made from the natural latex of the *Hevea brasiliensis* rubber tree, which is low cost, high in quality, highly durable, and has biocompatible physical and chemical characteristics of antigenicity, hypoallergenicity, resistance, elasticity, softness, flexibility, and strength. Recent scientific studies have shown that the materials used in insoles must have these characteristics to ensure the patient's comfort, control foot temperature, and minimize the risk of developing allergies. It is noteworthy that latex has been used to make esophageal prostheses, biomembranes, and esophageal flow controller modules. The use of latex to make insoles is extremely advantageous for the foot because it is a material that is easily moldable and has beneficial properties for the healing of wounds. The material properties of latex, which is a milky sap and a living organism prior to vulcanization, vary with temperature and so will be altered by the temperature of the foot when used in a shock-absorbing insole. At the same time, the shock absorbers are responsible for reducing pressure, which is the basis of the bioinspired system. Because the insole is a biomaterial and because of the properties of latex, it is possible to obtain a variable density through the manufacturing process, the handling, and the sourcing of the latex. Another important fact is that the viscous damping coefficient is closely related to the viscosity of the fluid, which implies that it is influenced by temperature: a temperature increase results in a decrease in the viscous damping coefficient. For this reason, we find that the higher the temperature, the "softer" the latex. In addition, the diabetic foot displays temperature and moisture changes (most often, the feet are warm and the skin is rather dry). An advantage of latex in this regard is that when vulcanized at temperatures of 35 to 45°C, it retains moisture and hydrates the patient's skin. Furthermore, latex is a non-Newtonian biomaterial, which implies that its viscosity can be controlled by factors such as geometry and temperature. Latex, which is a whitish secretion extracted from the rubber tree (*Hevea brasiliensis*), is used as biomaterial in medical devices [51]. In addition to its biocompatibility, its tensile characteristics, maximum traction force, ductility, and toughness influence the ease with which the material can be molded into complicated shapes. Latex is also being tested in humans as tissue neoformation induction material, and has been used for patients with chronic ulcers of the lower limbs and myringoplasty. Insoles are another application of latex for the treatment of diabetic foot, with or without ulceration. Research has begun into its healing effects and its suitability for use in the treatment of burns and other types of wounds.

There are several products made from biomaterials on the market for the treatment of pressure ulcers. Typically, these products come in the form of films, foams, gels, or membranes. Their fundamental characteristics are light weight, odorless application and removal, sealing against microorganisms, oxygen and water vapor permeability, ease of manufacturing, biodegradability, and biocompatibility. Among these products are the following: i) Latex biomembrane: this latex component, obtained from the polymerization of polyisoprene, induces angiogenic formation and scarring and accelerates the regenerative process of chronic wounds via chemical debridement action; ii) Aloe vera biomembrane: this product induces the formation of new blood vessels and tissue repair; iii) Hyaluronic acid: this is obtained from fermentation of gram-negative bacteria or by isolation of animal structures, such as synovial fluid, skin, and cockscomb and is used for soft tissue filling and healing functions; iv) Collagen and alginate membrane: this product, which is 90% type I and III collagen, is obtained from bovine skin or tendon and 10% alginate. From these products, a gel can be produced that provides moisture and slow dispersion of collagen in injured tissue, thereby inducing chemotaxis for granulocytes, macrophages, and fibroblasts. The raw material used in this study in the preparation of latex devices was natural latex extracted from the *Hevea brasiliensis* rubber tree, purchased on the domestic market. Some standard features, such as a low sulfur content and high viscosity, were needed for this material. A high concentration of sulfur gives latex a sticky consistency and low viscosity after vulcanization, which turns the production process into a time-consuming manufacturing process. A raw material that could met these criteria was identified: a latex extracted from rubber plantations in Florianópolis, Santa Catarina, Brazil. This latex was bi-centrifuged at 8000 xg in an α-Laval A-4.100 centrifuge with a water-cooled continuous passage. From the natural latex, the final product was prepared by mixing and resting it for two hours to produce prototypes with essential features such as elasticity, softness, strength, good texture, impermeability, absence of bubbles, and hypoallergenicity.

4. Devices developeded for diabetic foot treatment

4.1. Compound preparation— Mold-making

The development process for the insole padding material consisted of two steps: i) mold-making and ii) product preparation. The mold-making process consisted of the following steps. The mold of one foot (of average size) required 800 g of alginate and 1200 ml of water. The alginate and water were mixed well with a spoon for approximately 60 seconds until a homogeneous and creamy mixture was obtained. The mixture had to be stirred quickly to avoid consolidation (clotting) or hardening of the mixture. As soon as the mixture was ready, a foot was dipped into the container holding the material, and a setting time of approximately 3 minutes was allowed to pass. The mixture changes color when it set. After setting, the foot was removed from the container slowly and carefully. A plaster cast of the foot was then made by pouring a mixture of special plaster and water into the void where the foot had been located. This plaster mixture had to be moderately consistent. The plaster took approximately 2 to 3 hours to harden. After the plaster hardened, the mold was removed, and wet sandpaper was used to make the mold surface smoother. In the case of a patient with foot ulcers, the foot had to be wrapped with plastic wrap. This mold-making process for the insole for the diabetic foot is completely individualized and customized: the shape and proportions of the insole are dictated by the characteristics of the patient's feet. This makes it possible to provide customized comfort, softness, and well-being. It should be noted that it is a simple and quick procedure that does no harm and does not cause discomfort to the patient. This mold-making process permits molding of the entire foot or the plantar region only.

4.2. Insole preparation process

This stage of the insole preparation process consists of two main steps: preparation and characterization of the product. In this stage of the process, indispensable product requirements, such as softness, comfort, hygiene, and shock absorption, were taken into account. The mold was washed with soapy water, dried with hot air, sterilized through autoclaving, removed, and dipped into the latex and remained in the compound for 1 minute. This point represents the beginning of the polymerization that determines the final preparation of the product. The mold was then slowly and gradually removed and placed in an oven and was heated at a temperature of 70ºC (for vulcanization) at intervals of 10 minutes. The mold then cooled outside the oven for at least 20 minutes. It is noteworthy that the dipping and heating steps were repeated until the healing insole was approximately 1.5 mm thick. After the vulcanization period, the insole was kept at room temperature for 24 hours to complete the preparation process. At the end of the process, the mold was removed under running water. The function of the insole is to redistribute pressure uniformly across the plantar surface of the foot by reducing excess pressure in regions that are at risk of injury and transferring this excess pressure to no-risk areas. This is recommended to prevent the onset of foot injuries and also to help in the treatment of wounds in the final stages of healing. Other features are related to the support surface elevation up to the sole of the feet and the ability of the insole to provide custom comfort, as it is formed according to the anatomical shape of the foot to provide a sensation of softness and well-being. Taking into consideration the correct distribution of plantar support between the feet, the insole is designed to improve the support base and improve stability between the feet. The fully individualized and customized preparation of this insole based on the anatomy and characteristics of the patient's feet permits the shock absorbers to be positioned at the exact and ideal points, which is necessary for deep absorption of shock impacts while walking and an exact plantar pressure distribution. In addition, this customized preparation process perfectly accommodates any foot deformities present (feet cavus or flat foot, bunions, claw toes, and hammer toes, among others). In contrast, in the fabrication of insoles with cushioning systems that are not made in a personalized and individualized manner with respect to size, shape, and proportions, with only the standard model of the shoe-size system considered, it is impossible to accommodate any foot deformities that may be present. In this preliminary study, in addition to the above specifications, the degree of plantar pressure and its distribution, which consequently influences its amount, location, and size, were considered in the customization and individualization of the shock absorbers. For other insoles described in the technical and market literature, only one standard model is considered in the preparation of the shock absorbers and in their positioning. The dimensions of this standard model are practically the same, regardless of the location on the insole. This is an important fact: if shock absorbers must be made according to the size, shape, and proportions of the wearer's foot, mainly in relation to the pressure exerted on that position, the required dimensions of the shock absorbers determined during the preparation process may vary widely from one wearer to another. When you have a custom-designed and individualized insole, the control over the degree of pressure and specifically the position and size of the shock absorbers are highly controllable, which was among the aims of this preliminary study. Lack of customization and individualization in insole and shock absorber development does not allow for such control in quantity, position, and size. Other insoles with cushioning systems that do not present such differentiation as a way to compensate for such control are made with numerous shock absorbers (which increases the cost) or have shock absorbers only in the calcaneus and forefoot regions. In the first case, the shock absorbers cover all or nearly all of the top surface of the insole, which may bring have disadvantages for wearers, such as pain and discomfort, until they become accustomed to the insole, which might take a long time. In the second case, the cushioning of impact typically occurs in the heel and sometimes also in the forefoot, first and foremost, leaving other regions exposed to impact. Doctors and specialists claim that the area's most prone to plantar pressure peaks and future plantar ulcers are the hallux, toes, metatarsal heads, middle of the foot, and heel. With a simple examination using adequate equipment, plantar pressure peaks, which occur at locations that are highly susceptible to the formation of plantar ulcers, can be identified on the foot. Each of these peaks should then receive treatment with shock absorbers. The shock-absorbing insole proposed in this preliminary study may be an essential addition to therapies to fight diabetes if applied in a preventative manner before the appearance of wounds or if applied after resolution of the case with the objective of assisting in specific treatment and avoiding the recurrence of the wound. Figure 6 shows the prototype of this shock-absorbing insole.

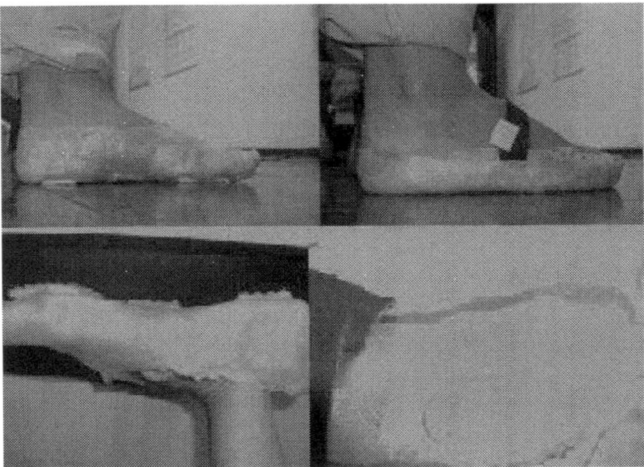

Figure 6. Photo of the shock-absorbing insole prototype with the shock-absorbers highlighted.

Figure 7 shows the pressure capture results, including the locations of pressure peaks, for patient 1 while wearing the insole shown in the previous figure. This new pressure distribution was captured under the same capturing conditions described previously.

Based on the results of previous studies, the authors adopted the strategy in this study of seeking to provide support through qualitative and quantitative changes in the forces applied to the foot by the ground, by means of an interaction passively controlled by the insole in the

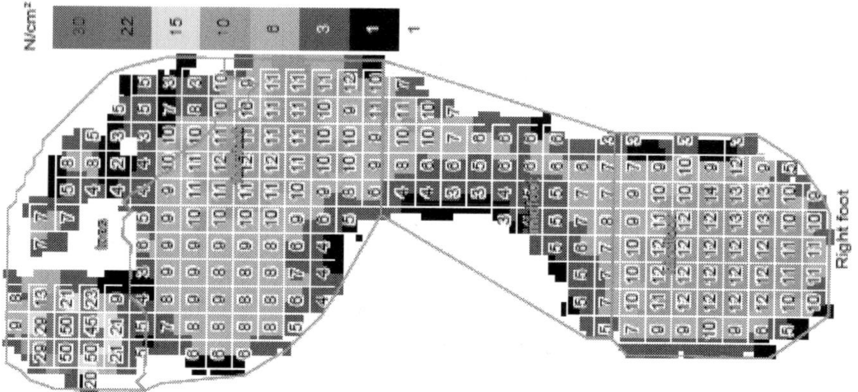

Figure 7. Results of using the insole to reduce plantar pressure.

foot-to-floor interface. This strategy has two main aspects: "control" which in essence is simply the regulation of a given element, and "organic," which pertains fundamentally to the organism controlled. The insole is intended to support the patient's walking and have the potential to change plantar pressure by controlling the parameters that affect it, as shown in this study. The regions with greater force concentrations can thereby be enhanced, leaving those with lesser force concentrations with greater loads than they usually bear. Removing the load or its redistribution is an attempt at a method that directly interacts with the system response to minimize overload and turn it into offload. Body balance was evaluated using stabilometry, which is a method of analyzing balance through the quantification of body oscillations. For this purpose, we used the AccuSway Plus® force platform, connected to a computer that recorded the movements of the pressure center (PC) on the platform plane (X, Y) in the anteroposterior (Y) and lateral (X) directions, by means of the force exerted on the platform by the soles of the feet, captured by the software. Assessing how the shock-absorbing insole can interfere with the control of a diabetic patient's semi-static posture can open up possibilities for developing a passive insole system with biofeedback, to compensate for neuromuscular deficits in DM patients. These muscular responses delimit an area within a base to indicate body stability. Associated with this support base concept is a stability limit that has been shown in many studies to be considerably reduced in cases of some diseases, such as Parkinson's disease and diabetes. In this context, based on the stability evaluation results, one question was asked: is it possible to maintain stability limits with the introduction of the shock-absorbing insole? That is, can performance indexes be changed to demonstrate a response that promotes better balance than without the insole? The results of qualitative assessments by observation show that the introduction of the insole helps to reduce passive stiffness of the muscle-to-tendon structure. This fact was verified in tests of time remaining in balance showing that the tendency of the body to fall forward was reduced, i.e., the momentum magnitude of the gravitational force was reduced. With the introduction of two shock absorbers and a mass, the conservation principle of mechanical equilibrium, as presented in equations [1] and [2], is verified, focusing only on external forces more common while maintaining an upright posture. In future studies, we intend to include the analysis and direct assessment of internal forces, such as disturbances generated by the delayed activation of the muscles, which can be evaluated as hysteresis or looseness, by analogy to translational/ rotational mechanics. In addition, the insole can be classified as an anticipatory postural adjustment element that causes an underestimation of the magnitude of the ground reaction force in maintaining a postural orientation. The data collected from the force platform tests with and without the insole were captured 5 times for 30 seconds apiece. The following stabilometric parameters, suggested by [51] were also analyzed: i) average displacement and standard deviation (SD) of the pressure center in the anteroposterior (YAvg) and latero-lateral (XAvg) directions, with XAvg (cm) and YAvg (cm); ii) displacement average velocity (VAvg, cm/s); iii) the circular area (Area) that corresponds to the area that best fits the trajectory of the pressure center. As an initial hypothesis, for a single-foot analysis, it was believed that without the insole, a DM patient would present greater imbalance than with the insole, because of the motor deficit developed. It is known that there is a relationship between the static balance deficit and the number of falls. Thus, the lower the patient's ability is to maintain his balance, the greater the probability is of the patient having a fall. In a state of dynamic equilibrium, both the center of mass and the support base move, and the center of mass will never align with the support base during the movement's single-foot stance phase. Ankle mobility influences balance in that the more the ankle moves, the greater the capacity of the individual to maintain balance. In Figure 8, the change in amplitude as defined by item i) above is plotted to illustrate the amplitude variation attributable to the introduction of the insole.

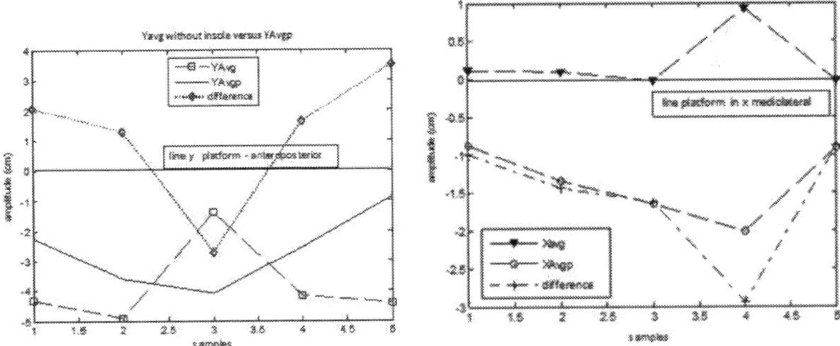

Figure 8. Comparisons between the displacement variations in X and Y with and without the insole.

In related studies, the authors confirmed that the introduction of the insole to the feet of DM patients using appropriately made (customized) shock-absorbers has shown that the effectiveness of the postural control insole is directly related to the pressure center displacement amplitude. Large amplitude variations in movement indicate poor-quality balance control, whereas acceptable control is indicated by small amplitudes of displacement in the Y and X directions. Increases in oscillation in the single-foot static upright posture were also verified.

These oscillation increases can occur because of a decrease in the corrective torque generated by the insole to control the oscillations and body velocity and because of an increase in the time required to feel the presence of the insole, transmit and process a response, and activate the muscles. Figure 9 illustrates the velocity amplitude changes caused.

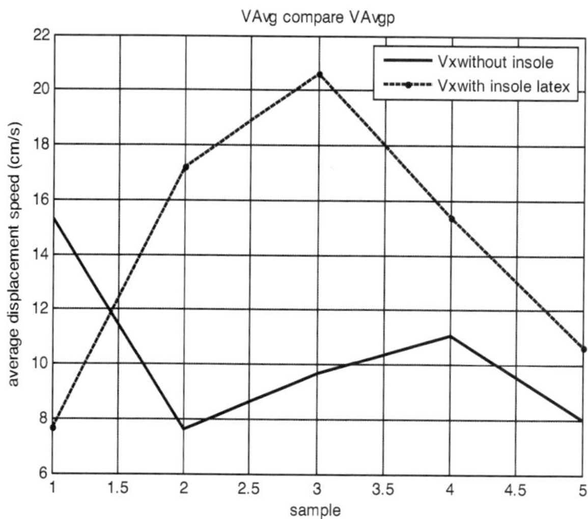

Figure 9. Comparison of average single-foot velocity with and without the insole.

A correlation exists between the displacement average velocity values VAvg (cm/s): an increased displacement velocity — that is, a higher speed in perceiving imbalance and attempting to stabilize the pressure center — decreases the imbalance. This may be because wearing the insole: i) reduces the ground reaction force; ii) reduces the resulting vector amplitude, and iii) generates greater body stability through greater velocity to control these oscillations. Figure 10 shows the velocity variation for each collection captured.

The circular area that corresponds to the area that best fits the trajectory of the pressure center is shown in Figure 11.

When we analyze the response variation data in the time domain, we obtain useful information, but to supplement the analysis. For a system without shock absorbers, the antiresonance corresponds to the absence of movement in all coordinates where the response is considered. Peaks in this frequency response occur in the time part of the diagram where the maximum response was observed because of entry excitation represented by the ground reaction force on the foot. We note that the vibration amplitude changes when we modify the oscillation frequency of the applied force. This result also shows that by varying the oscillation frequency of the force, both increases and decreases in vibration amplitude occur at different points on

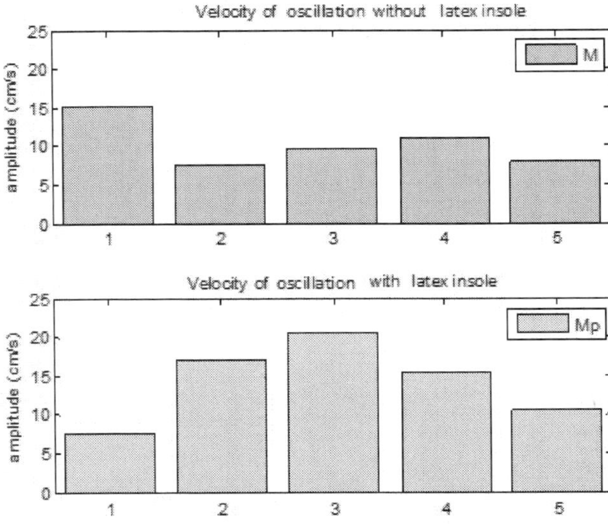

Figure 10. Comparison of the variation in velocity with and without the insole.

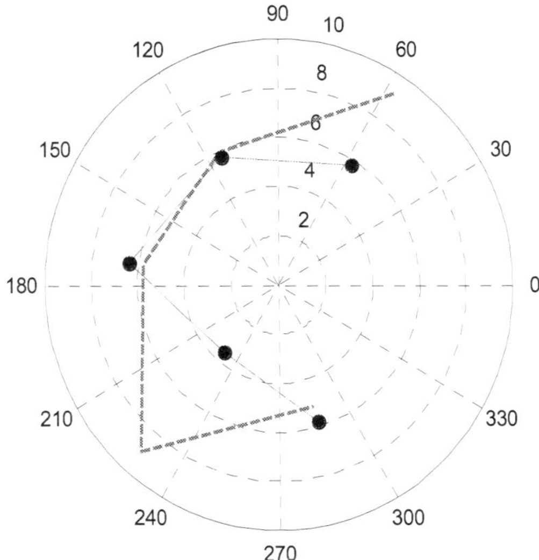

Figure 11. A graph generated in radar format to show that the stability region with the insole was increased by increasing the limits. The red line indicates the area with the insole, and the blue line indicates the area without the insole.

the time scale. In the time domain, there are natural frequencies and respective modal forms associated with these frequencies, which are inherent in each insole structure designed. These are basically characteristics that depend on inertia and rigidity. The introduction of shock absorbers with viscosity and mass characteristics and softness and flexibility features affect the response of the foot structure when it is excited by a force of some type.

5. Healing insole

The healing insole is disposable and sterile. The same preparation process used for the latex biomaterial centrifuged to 60% was used for the insole. In the process of preparing the insole, latex was placed in acrylic molds that were previously cleaned and dried. The latex biomaterial was spread out until it formed a thin layer covering the surface. Rather than resting the latex in the oven horizontally, it was rested completely upright so that all excess latex drained. This contributed to the insole becoming clearer. An oven was not used for the insole polymerization; it was polymerized at room temperature, which also promoted transparency. This process was repeated 6 times to reach a final insole thickness of 0.5 mm. The latex insoles were sterilized in ethylene oxide. Some small holes, approximately 2 mm in diameter, were made in the insoles so that during use, exudation (secretion) could be eliminated from the wound. This research examined an innovative method of tissue regeneration for diabetic ulcers consisting of the combined and simultaneous action of the latex biomaterial and low-intensity red LED light. The tissue regeneration electronic circuit is formed by a signal-emitting cell that is based on the tissue neoformation principle involving the use of LEDs. The LED cells are placed only on ulcerated regions of the foot. The cells are placed outside the insole and are covered with a sheet of latex. They emit radiation with a fluency of 25 J/cm². Figures 12 and 13 refer to patient 6. This patient is 62 years old and 8 years of diagnosis of DM, her profession is housework. The ulcer 1 (Figure 12) is situated in the region 7 (instep) the existence of time to approximately 7 months already told before amputation. The ulcer appeared through a bruised evolving dramatically with infection coming to osteomyelitis, not to provide answers to antibiotic treatment was necessary amputation of the second to the fifth toe. Then his picture of infection and osteomyelitis have not healed completely and reached the 1st toe (hallux), which was necessary to perform a further amputation. Thus, the present research, to heal these surgeries amputations, applied the treatment with silver foam during the patient's stay in the GC and then the inductor system tissue formation while in the GE.

The ulcer 2 (Figure 13) due to complications arose from the first, and also by mechanical trauma, caused by lack of rest. The wound is situated in area 3, the existence of time to approximately 5 months. As already mentioned, ulcers 1 and 2 (Figures 12 and 13) were followed for 1 month in the GC. Then, in an attempt to accelerate the healing process, the wounds were also accompanied in GE using the inductor system tissue formation. Figures 14 and 15 show the results. This patient already had three ulcers from diagnosis of DM and two amputations.

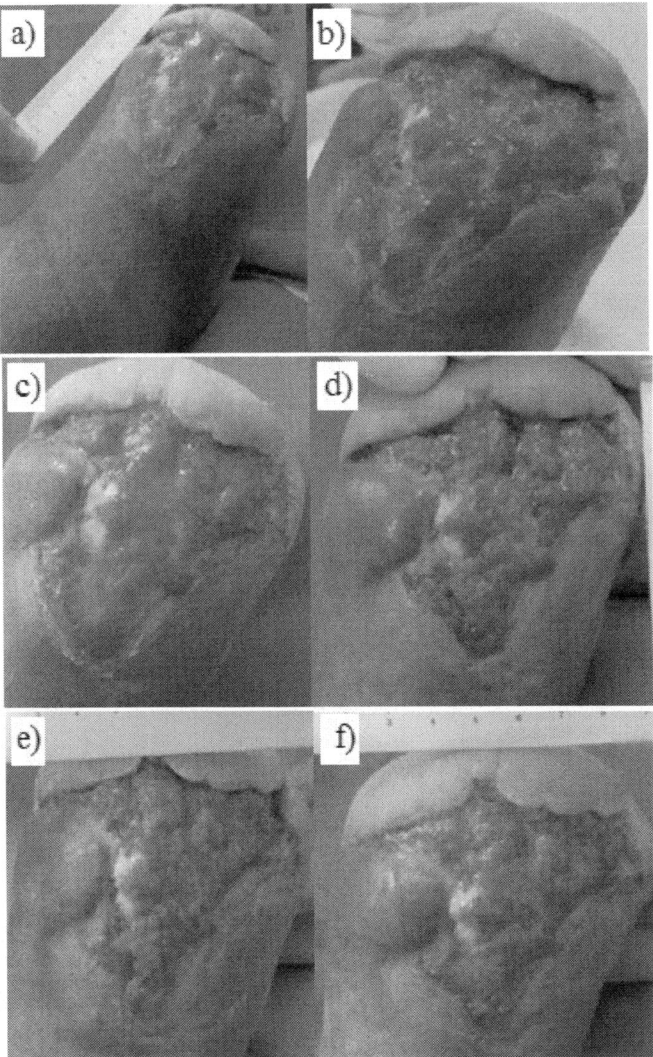

Figure 12. Clinical photo follow-up Patient 6 (1 ulcer)-GC: a) the ulcerated foot region; b) pre-treatment (initial); c) post-treatment (1 week); d) two weeks; and) 3 weeks; f) 4 weeks.

The two figures (Figure 14 and Figure 15) pertain to the patient 6, pictured in the preceding Figure 12 and Figure 13. In each ulcer in this patient, it was evaluated the behavior of two different methods of healing: foam with silver (GC) and system inducing tissue formation (GE). Because of the location of the ulcer 1 this patient, ulcers on both 1 and 2 were applied only to

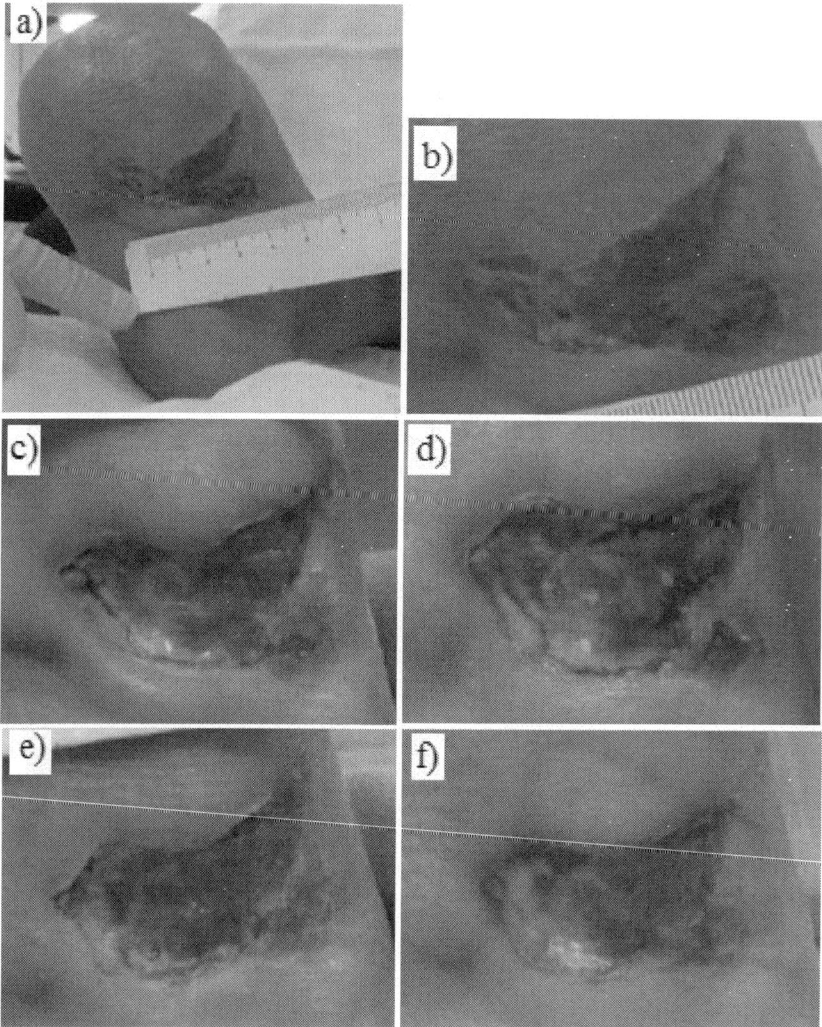

Figure 13. Clinical photo follow-up. Patient 6 (2 ulcer)-GC: a) region of the ulcerated foot; b) pre-treatment (initial); c) post-treatment (1 week); d) two weeks; and) 3 weeks; f) 4 weeks.

slide latex and electronic circuitry for tissue regeneration. Again being demonstrated that within the inductor tissue formation system can be used only blade latex and LED light to induce healing. Comparing the images in Figure 12 (GC) and Figure 14 (GE), one observes a faster ulcer healing 1 while in the GE. It is also noticed that the GE ulcer 1 showed better color, higher and more debridement of granulation tissue and reepithelialization. The same assess-

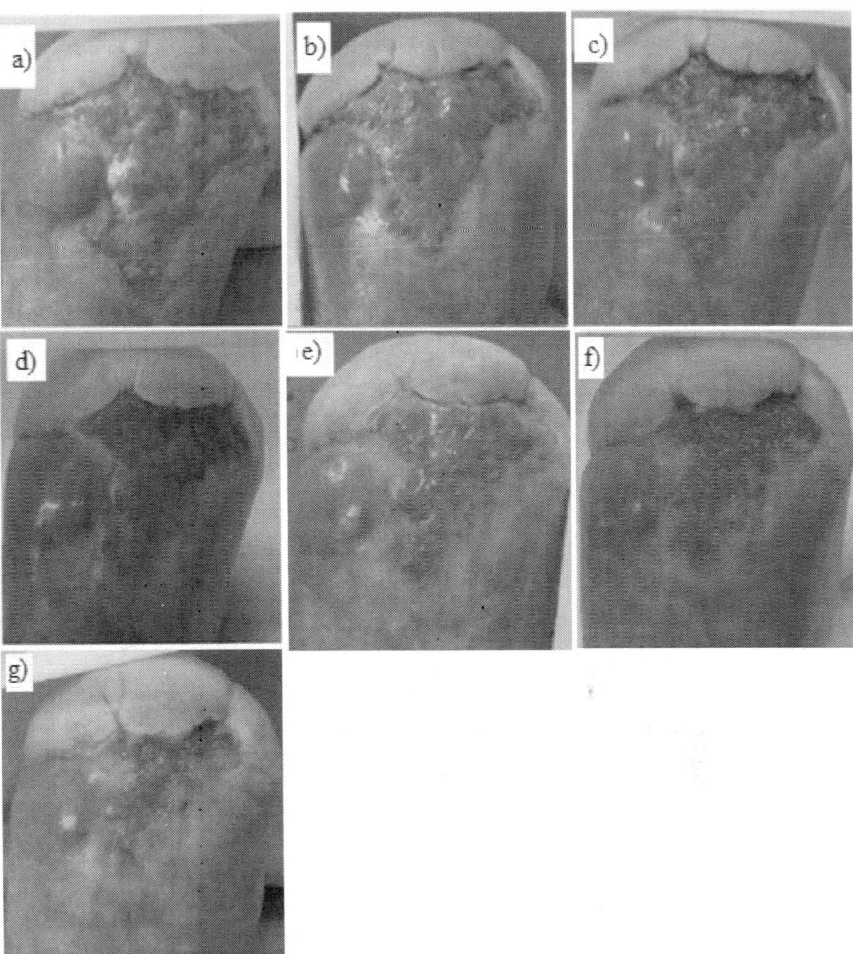

Figure 14. Clinical photo follow-up. Patient 6 (1 ulcer)-Experimental Group: a) early (before the inductor system tissue formation); b) post-treatment (after using the inductor system tissue formation)-1 week; c) two weeks; d) 3 weeks; e) 4 weeks f) 6 weeks g) 8 weeks.

ment can be made between Figures 13 and 14, which displays the ulcer healing was also second fastest while in the GE. Both this patient's ulcers were followed up at 6 GE for 8 weeks. Figures 14 and 15, it was observed that after 8 weeks of treatment with the inducer system for tissue formation, both ulcer decreased significantly in size.

An analysis of the progression of healing of ulcers, conducted by the patient's medical staff, showed full reepithelialization in eight weeks, as illustrated in Figure 16.

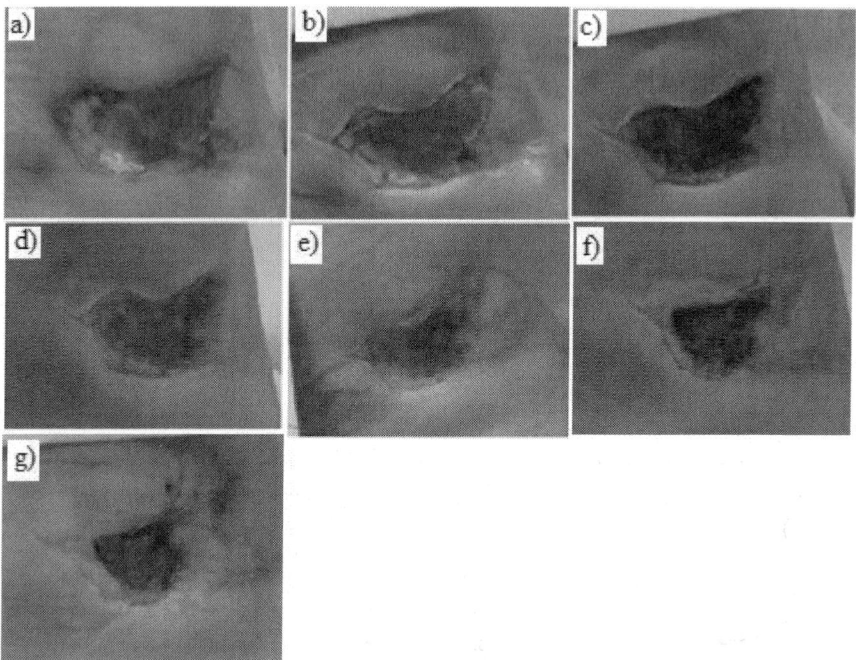

Figure 15. Clinical photo follow-up. Patient 6 (2 ulcer)-Experimental Group: a) early (before the inductor system tissue formation); b) post-treatment (after using the inductor system tissue formation)-1 week; c) two weeks; d) 3 weeks; e) 4 weeks f) 6 weeks g) 8 weeks.

The wounds were photographed on a weekly basis using a digital Sony DSC-H70 camera with 16.1-megapixel resolution. The images were taken with the patient positioned lying down in a chair, with the camera mounted on a tripod parallel to the wounds, and with a focal length of 15 centimeters. A metric ruler was placed alongside the wound for subsequent computational analysis. The digital images obtained were analyzed using the ImageJ® software to quantify the total area of the ulcers. The latex and LED light action gradually favored contraction around the edge of the wound. The coloring of the wound also improved considerably over the course of the 9 weeks. After a week of treatment, the wound appeared more reddish in color. Furthermore, there was a significant increase in granulation tissue. At the beginning of treatment, the wound had a slight depth, and over the course of the 9 weeks of treatment, new tissue gradually formed, making the lesion appear to be filling and healing. In order for low-intensity LED therapy to have positive effects, a protocol of application is essential. The biological effects of this type of therapy depend on the irradiation parameters, such as the wavelength, fluence, irradiation time, and emission mode. A rating of this study was to compare the behavior of two different methods of healing in the same patient. This fact refers to the patient 1, in which the silver foam

(GC) of the right foot ulcer (metatarsal area) and tissue formation-inducing system (GE) to the ulcer of the left foot (the heel area) was applied. Comparing the ICU in both cases in the 2nd, 4th, 6th and 8th week, patient 1 showed better results in GE. This means that the system inducing tissue formation favoring the evolution of healing better than the foam with silver.

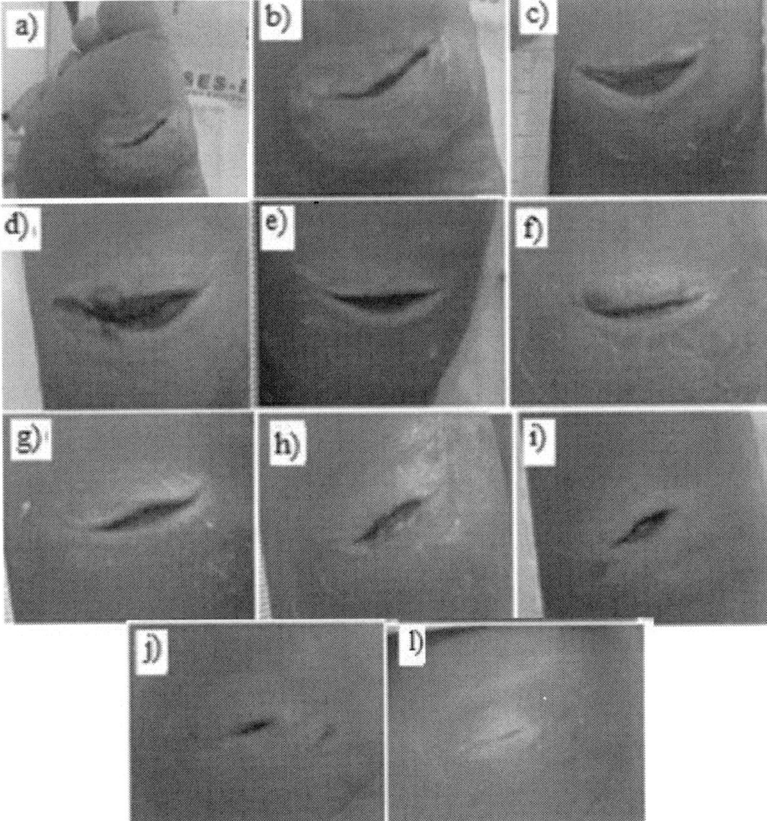

Figure 16. Clinical photo follow-up. Patient 1 – a) ulcerated foot region, b) pre-treatment (initial treatment), c) post-treatment (1 week), d) 2 weeks, e) 3 weeks, f) 4 weeks, g) 5 weeks, h) 6 weeks, i) 7 weeks, j) 8 weeks, l) 9 weeks.

6. Conclusions and contributions

Diabetes mellitus is a chronic disease and is characterized by a variety of complications, including diabetic foot stands, considered a serious and often devastating consequences on the results of ulcerations problem. The formation of sores that become infected and poorly healing can lead to gangrene and even amputation of toes, feet or legs. The essence of this study is intended, under the etiological-mechanical approach, to the intersection of an external element (latex-derived insole – the passive control) with diabetic passive stride. There is impact on the variation of some key variables such as change in mass and contact with soil. Then, we also analyze the parameter sensibility/robustness of the dynamical model obtained, and the effect of the addition of the insole controller in this sensibility. This study showed that the modeling of the diabetic gait is a challenging task, having previous researches already presented contributions which must be added to those brought up by this study. This parametric study's results provide the first steps towards the discovery of tendencies, aiming to obtain new perspectives with regard to this complex disease. Thus this research considers the disease's main etiology and parameters related to the patient's gait, anthropometry and social reality, for he/she might perform certain roles that require their feet to bear different loads – for instance, hairdressers and teachers. This must influence the design process of future insoles, which will function as controllers derived biomaterials acting directly on the dynamics of the gait. The center of pressure of the human foot is displaced in carriers of diabetes, which attests the necessity of a study of the patient's gait prior to the manufacturing of the insole. Second, presented in this study will be an intellectual preparation for the emergence of a new concept, proposed with the idea of controllers derived biomaterials. This methodology will be critical to the creation of a "bioinspired" theory in the field of Biomedical Engineering, which will further assist in the construction of the concept (which says what the thing is) called controlling derived biomaterial (this study insole latex). Based on the literature, it was observed that the introduction of assistive devices is common for changing the stride. But this study presented, that element was characterized and analyzed as a controller that, through qualitative and quantitative changes in the charges applied to the foot, proved possible to correct the diabetic stride. Finally, a search for a new possibility for the treatment of diabetic foot. Accordingly, an inductor system for new tissue formation novel diabetic foot with light emitting circuit LEDs and use of natural latex has been developed. This system consists of a healing insole and an electronic circuit for tissue regeneration. Cicatrizing insole is derived from the rubber tree latex brasiliensis and made a personalized and individualized. This innovative method of healing diabetic foot ulcers consists of the joint and simultaneous action of biomaterial latex and light irradiation of low intensity LEDs. The clinical findings were analyzed qualitatively and quantitatively, which showed that the results obtained by the experimental test suggests that the inducing tissue neoformation system is characterizing.

Author details

Suélia de Siqueira Rodrigues Fleury Rosa[1*], Maria do Carmo Reis[1], Mário Fabricio Fleury Rosa[2], Diego Cólon[3], Célia Aparecida dos Reis[4] and José Manoel Balthazar[5]

*Address all correspondence to: suelia@unb.br

1 Engineering and Biomaterials Laboratory – BioEngLab®, Biomedical Engineering, University of Brasilia, Brasil

2 University of Brasilia-Post-Graduate Program of Sciences and Technology in Health, Brasil

3 University of São Paulo-Polytechnic School, Automation and Control Laboratory, Brasil

4 Estadual Paulista Júlio de Mesquita Filho, School of Sciences, Mathematics Department of Bauru, Brasil

5 Paulista State University Júlio de Mesquita Filho, Institute of Geosciences and Exact Sciences of Rio Claro, Brasil

References

[1] Centers for Disease Control and Prevention. National Diabetes Fact Sheet: National Estimates and General Information on Diabetes and Prediabetes in the United States, 2011. U.S. Department of Health and Human Services, Centers for Disease Control and Prevention 1–12; 2011.

[2] Shavelson D. The Biomechanics of the Diabetic Foot, Global Perspective on Diabetic Foot Ulcerations, Dr. Thanh Dinh (Ed.), ISBN: 978-953-307-727-7; 2011.

[3] Fabrikant J. Plantar Faciitis (Fasciosis Treatment Outcome Study: Plantar Fascia Thickness Measured by Ultrasound and Correlated with Patient Improvement; Foot, vol 21 no 2, Mar 12, 2011, p79-83.

[4] Pedrosa HC. Introdução. In: Fábio Batista. (Org.). Uma abordagem multidisciplinar sobre pé diabético. São Paulo: Andreoli, v. p. 2010, p27-28.

[5] Goske S, Erdemir A, Petre M, Budhabhatti S, Cavanagh PR. "Reduction of plantar heel pressures: insole design using finite element analysis," Journal of Biomechanics,Vol. 39 (13), 2006, p2363-70.

[6] Boulton AJM. (1988). The Diabetic Foot. Medical Clinics North America. v. 72(6): 1513-30, 1988.

[7]   Zequera ML, Solomonidis S. Performance of insole in reducing plantar pressure on diabetic patients in the early stages of the disease. In: 32nd annual international conference of the IEEE EMBS. 2010.

[8]   Nteleki B, Houreld NN. Review Article: The use of phototherapy in the treatment of diabetic ulcers. JEMDSA; 17(3), 2012, p128-132.

[9]   Pai S, Ledoux WR. The shear mechanical properties of diabetic and non-diabetic plantar soft tissue. Journal of Biomechanics. 45(2), January 10, 2012, p364–370.

[10]   Bowker JH, Pfeifer MA. "Levin and O'Neal's the Diabetic Foot", seventh edition, Mosby, Philadelphia, 2008.

[11]   El-Hilaly R, Elshazly O, Amer A. "The role of a total contact insole in diminishing foot pressures following partial first ray amputation in diabetic patients," Foot (Edinburgh, Scotland), vol. 23, issue 1, 2013, p6-10 (DOI: 10.1016/j.foot.2012.10.002).

[12]   Savelberg HH, Ilgin D, Angin S, Willems PJ, Schaper NC, Meijer K. Prolonged activity of knee extensors and dorsal flexors is associated with adaptations in gait in diabetes and diabetic polyneuropathy. Clinical Biomechanics (Bristol, Avon), 25, 2010, p468-475.

[13]   Cardoso VS. Estudo da marcha e de alterações biomecânicas no pé de pacientes com diabetes [dissertation]. São Paulo: Universidade de São Paulo, Faculdade de Medicina; 2009 (accessed 2014-07-09). http://www.teses.usp.br/teses/disponiveis/5/5135/tde-02062009-100404/.

[14]   Sociedade Brasileira de Diabetes. Consenso brasileiro de tratamento e acompanhamento do diabete mellitus. Rio de Janeiro: Diagrafic; 2007.

[15]   Formosa C, Gatt A, Chockalingam N. "The importance of clinical biomechanical assessment of foot deformity and joint mobility in people living with type-2 diabetes within a primary care setting", Primary Care Diabetes, Vol. 7, Issue 1, 2013, p45-50, ISSN 1751-9918, DOI: 10.1016/j.pcd.2012.12.003.

[16]   Zequera ML, Solomonidis S. Performance of insole in reducing plantar pressure on diabetic patients in the early stages of the disease. In: 32nd annual international conference of the IEEE EMBS. 2010.

[17]   Melai T, Ijzerman TH, Schaper NC, de Lange TL, Willems PJ, Meijer K. et al. Calculation of plantar pressure time integral, an alternative approach. Gait & Posture, 34, 2011, p379–383.

[18]   Cavanagh PR. Plantar soft tissue thickness during ground contact in walking. J Biomech, Vol. 32, June 1999, p623-628.

[19]   Rao S, Saltzman CL, Yack HJ. Relationships between segmental foot mobility and plantar loading in individuals with and without diabetes and neuropathy. 2, s.l.: Elsevier Gait & Posture, Vol. 31, 2010, p251-255.

[20] Sicco AB, Maas M, Michels RPJ and Levi M. Role of intrinsic muscle atrophy in the etiology of claw toe deformity in diabetic neuropathy may not be as straightforward as widely believed. Diabetes Care. Jun 2009; 32(6): 1063–1067. Doi: 10.2337/dc08-2174.

[21] Richardson JK, Thies SB, DeMott TK, Ashton-Miller JA. Gait analysis in a challenging environment differentiates between fallers and nonfallers among older patients with peripheral neuropathy. Elsevier, Archives of physical medicine and rehabilitation, Vol. 86, 2005, p1539-1544.

[22] Sacco IC1, Bacarin TA, Canettieri MG, Hennig EM. Plantar pressures during shod gait in diabetic neuropathic patients with and without a history of plantar ulceration. J. Am. Podiat. Med. Assoc., Vol. 99, 2009, p285-294.

[23] Martinelli AR, Mantovani AM, Nozabieli AJL, Ferreira DMA, Barela JA, de Camargo MR, Fregonesi CEPT. Muscle strength and ankle mobility for the gait parameters in diabetic neuropathies, The Foot, Volume 23, Issue 1, 2013, p17-21.

[24] Melai T, Schaper NC, IJzerman TH, de Lange TLH, Willems PJB, Meijer K, Lieverse AG, Savelberg HHCM, Increased forefoot loading is associated with an increased plantar flexion moment, Human Movement Science, Volume 32, Issue 4, August 2013, p785-793, ISSN 0167-9457, http://dx.doi.org/10.1016/j.humov.2013.05.001

[25] Fregonesi CEPT, Camargo MR. Gait parameters in patients with diabetes mellitus. Revista Brasileira de Cineantropometria & Desempenho Humano 2010, 12(2),p155-163.

[26] Lavery LA, Armstrong DG, Wunderlich RP, Mohler MJ, Wendel CS, Lipsky BA. Risk factors for foot infection in individuals with diabetes. Diabetes Care, 29: 2006, p1288-1293.

[27] Kwon, OY, Tuttle, LJ, Johnson, JE, Mueller, MJ. "Muscle imbalance and reduced ankle joint motion in people with hammer toe deformity." Clin. Biomech. 24, 2009, p670-675.

[28] El-Hilalyemail R, Elshazly O, Amer A. The role of a total contact insole in diminishing foot pressures following partial first ray amputation in diabetic patients Received: April 30, 2012; Received in revised form: June 26, 2012; Accepted: October 18, 2012; DOI: http://dx.doi.org/10.1016/j.foot.2012.10.002 The Foot, Volume 23, Issue 1, p6-10.

[29] IJzerman, TH, Schaper NC, Melai T, Blijham P, Meijer K, Willems PJ et al. Motor nerve decline does not underlie muscle weakness in type 2 diabetic neuropathy. Muscle Nerve, 44, 2011, p241–245.

[30] Keijsers NLW, Stolwijk NM, Louwerens JWK, Duysens J. Classification of forefoot pain based on plantar pressure measurements, Clinical Biomechanics, Volume 28, Issue 3, March 2013, p350-356, ISSN 0268-0033, http://dx.doi.org/10.1016/j.clinbiomech.2013.01.012.

[31] Cheuy VA et al. Intrinsic foot muscle deterioration is associated with metatarsophalangeal joint angle in people with diabetes and neuropathy, Clin. Biomech. 2013, http://dx.doi.org/10.1016/j.clinbiomech.2013.10.006

[32] Stucke S, McFarland D, Goss L, Fonov S, McMillan GR, Tucker A, Berme N, Guler HC, Bigelow C, Davis BL, Spatial relationships between shearing stresses and pressure on the plantar skin surface during gait. Journal of Biomechanics 2 February 2012; 45(3): p619-622. doi:10.1016/j.jbiomech.2011.11.004.

[33] Melai T, Schaper NC, Ijzerman TH, de Lange TLH, Willems PJB, Meijer K, Lieverse AG, Savelberg HHCM. Increased forefoot loading is associated with an increased plantar flexion moment, Human Movement Science, Volume 32, Issue 4, August 2013, p785-793, ISSN 0167-9457, http://dx.doi.org/10.1016/j.humov.2013.05.001.

[34] Keijsers NLW, Stolwijk NM, Louwerens JWK, Duysens J. Classification of forefoot pain based on plantar pressure measurements, Clinical Biomechanics, Volume 28, Issue 3, March 2013, p350-356, ISSN 0268-0033, http://dx.doi.org/10.1016/j.clinbiomech.2013.01.012

[35] Melai T, Ijzerman TH, Schaper NC, de Lange TL, Willems PJ, Meijer K et al. Calculation of plantar pressure time integral, an alternative approach. Gait & Posture, 34, 2011, p379-383.

[36] Sawacha Z, Guarneri G, Cristoferi G, Guiotto A, Avogaro A, Cobelli C. Integrated kinematics–kinetics–plantar pressure data analysis: A useful tool for characterizing diabetic foot biomechanics, Gait & Posture, Volume 36, Issue 1, May 2012, p20-26, ISSN 0966-6362, http://dx.doi.org/10.1016/j.gaitpost.2011.12.007.

[37] Phethean J, Nester C. The influence of body weight, body mass index and gender on plantar pressures: Results of a cross-sectional study of healthy children's feet, Gait & Posture, Volume 36, Issue 2, June 2012, p287-290, ISSN 0966-6362, http://dx.doi.org/10.1016/j.gaitpost.2012.03.012

[38] Cheuy VA, Commean PK, Hastings MK, Mueller MJ. Reliability and validity of a MR-based volumetric analysis of the intrinsic foot muscles. J. Magn. Reson. Imaging, 2013. http://dx.doi.org/10.1002/jmri.24069

[39] Cheuy VA, Hastings MK, Commean PK, Ward SR, Mueller MJ. Intrinsic foot muscle deterioration is associated with metatarsophalangeal joint angle in people with diabetes and neuropathy. Clinical Biomechanics, Volume 28, Issue 9, p1055-1060. Received: May 21, 2013; Accepted: October 8, 2013; Published Online: October 30, 2013. DOI: http://dx.doi.org/10.1016/j.clinbiomech.2013.10.006

[40] Tong JW, Ng EY. Preliminary investigation on the reduction of plantar loading pressure with different insole materials (SRP — Slow Recovery Poron®, P — Poron®, PPF — Poron®+Plastazote, firm and PPS — Poron®+Plastazote, soft). Foot 20 (1), 2010 p1-6.

[41] Andrade TAM, Leite SN, Frade MAC. "Neoformação tecidual em camundongos in‐ duzida pela biomembrana de látex da seringueira Hevea Brasiliensis". 21º Congresso Brasileiro de Engenharia Biomédica, Salvador, BA, 2008, p152-155.

[42] Cunha ALCP. Desenvolvimento de adesivos biológicos degradáveis. Dissertação de Mestrado Faculdade de Ciências e Tecnologia, Universidade de Coimbra, Coimbra, 2008.

[43] Frade MAC, Assis RVC, Coutinho Netto J, Andrade TAM, Tiraboschi Foss N. The vegetal biomembrane in the healing of chronic venous ulcers. Anais Brasileiros de Dermatologia.87(1):2012, p45-51.

[44] Bastos JLN. Estudo comparativo de sistemas a base de LASERs, LEDs e ultra-som (US) de baixa intensidade no reparo tecidual em tendão calcâneo. Dissertação de Mestrado, Universidade de São Paulo, São Carlos, SP, 2008.

[45] Bagnato VS, Corazza AV, Corazza LFG, Jorge J. Fotobioestimulação comparativa do LASER e LEDs de baixa intensidade na angiogênese de feridas cutâneas de ratos. In: X Congresso Brasileiro de Física Médica, 2005, Salvador.

[46] Caetano KS, Frade MA, Minatel DG, Santana LA, Enwemeka CS. Phototherapy im‐ proves healing of chronic venous ulcers. Photomed. Laser Surg., v.27, n.1, 2009, p111-118.

[47] Nteleki B, Houreld NN. Review Article: The use of phototherapy in the treatment of diabetic ulcers. JEMDSA; 17(3): 2012, p128-132.

[48] Reis, MDCD. "Sistema indutor de neoformação tecidual para pé diabético com circui‐ to emissor de luz de LEDs e utilização do látex natural." (2014). Tese Doutorado p. 163, Universidade de Brasilia.

[49] Reis MC, Soares F, da Rocha, Adson F, Carvalho JL, Rodrigues, SSFR. Insole with Pressure Control and Tissue Neoformation Induction Systems for Diabetic Foot. In: 32nd Annual International Conference of the IEEE Engineering in Medicine and Biol‐ ogy Society, 2010, Argentina. Proceedings of the 32nd Annual International Confer‐ ence of the IEEE Engineering in Medicine and Biology Society. Danvers, MA, EUA: PubMed, 2010. v. 1. p5748-5751.

[50] Reis MC, Rocha AF, Rodrigues, SSFR. Desenvolvimento de uma Palmilha Derivada do Látex Natural para Pé Diabético. In: The 6th Latin American Congress of Artificial Organs and Biomaterials-COLAOB, 2010, Gramado-RS. The 6th Latin American Con‐ gress of Artificial Organs and Biomaterials-COLAOB, 2010. v. 1. p356-366.

[51] Alves-Mazzotti, AJ, Gewandsznajder, F. O método nas ciências naturais e sociais: pesquisa quantitativa e qualitativa. Second edition. São Paulo: Pioneira, 2001.

[52] Rodrigues SS. Desenvolvimento de um sistema para controle de fluxo esofagiano para tratamento da obesidade. Tese (Doutorado em Tecnologia)-Departamento de Engenharia Elétrica da Universidade de Brasília, Brasília, DF, 2008.

[53] Rhodes C. International Governance of Biotechnology: Needs, Problems and Potential (Science Ethics and Society). London: Bloomsbury Academic, 2010. Retrieved July 15, 2014, from http://dx.doi.org/10.5040/9781849661812

[54] Kuhn, TS. The Structure of Scientific Revolutions. Chicago and London: The University of Chicago Press, 2012.

[55] Dorf, RC, Bishop, RH. Sistemas de controle modernos. Rio de Janeiro: LTC, 2009.

[56] Karnopp D, Margolis DL, Rosenberg RC. System Dynamics: Modeling and Simulation of Mechatronic Systems, third edition. New York: Horizon, 2000.

[57] Gawthrop P. Metamodelling: *Bond Graphs* and dynamic systems. Prentice Hall, 1996.

[58] Paynter H. An epistemic prehistory of *Bond Graphs*. In P. Breedveld and G. Dauphin-Tanguy, Eds., *Bond Graphs* for Engineers. Amsterdam: North-Holland, 1992, p3–17.

[59] Rosenberg RC. Reflections on Engineering systems and *Bond Graphs*, Journal of Dynamic Systems, Measurement, and Control, 115(1): 1993 p242-251.

[60] Rosa SSRF, Souza ÊKF, Urbizagástegui PAA, Peixoto LRT, Rocha AF, Modeling of the human tibia bone using Bond Graph Rev. Bras. Eng. Bioméd., v. 29, n. 4, p329-342, dez. 2013. DOI: http://dx.doi.org/10.4322/rbeb.2013.042

The Changing Face of Threats to the Public

The Public Health perspective on Migratory Health – Displaced Populations in Global Disease Epidemics

Charles Fokunang, Estella Tembe-Fokunang,
Zacharia Sando, Marceline Ngounoue Djuidje,
Barbara Atogho Tiedeu, Frederick Kechia,
Jerome Ateudjieu, Valentin Ndikum,
Raymond Langsi, Dobgima Fomnboh,
Joseph Fokam, Luc Gwum, Obama Abena,
Tazoacha Asongani, Vincent Pryde Titanji and
Lazare Kaptue

Additional information is available at the end of the chapter

http://dx.doi.org/10.5772/59069

1. Introduction

The interest of migratory health displaced population and the impact on global disease epidemics has generated a lot of public health interest within the framework of movement in search for *greener pastures*. Many studies conducted to show a link between disease, travel and migration show some indications of historical connections that continue to have an impact on current medical programmes and daily activities [1]. The perspective of traditional medical services that concerns migrant health considers the recognition, identification and management of specific diseases, and health issues in displaced populations at the time and location of their destination [2]. In this paper we consider migrants population to be a group of people moving from one geographical location or environment to another for many reasons such as political instability, outbreak natural disaster, war, epidemic outbreak, for better life, search for fertile grazing field for livestock, asylum seeking and religious intolerance [2], The various sovereign states are making more effort to put in place measures that protects immigrants population. The process of restricting migratory population in isolation for some period before liberation for health control is still adopted in developed countries. This quarantine operation

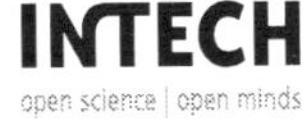

is intended to screen immigrants for potential diseases of public health concern and possible free transmission within the community. [3] The adoption of border control and restriction migrants into host countries has significantly reduced some those potential indicators that public health concerns and the constraints of increasing disease burden that in most cases are difficult to implement a developed health management system, due to inadequate health personnel and service providers.

The study of the disease epidemics, disease mapping and monitoring, and the platform of health information system reporting and analysis of researched report of diseases in the migratory community is always considered in several ways in those countries where pro-grammes and planning are developed to handle the cohort of migratory or mass displaced population. One of the main concern of the mass movement of immigrants is the screening process to profile their state of health before the population are received in the host countries. There is also the problem to develop a programme or platform to monitor the evolution of diseases and the quality of life of the displaced population at any given time, and building a health record data base [4].

1.1. Quarantine strategies associated to migratory health

The quarantine-strategies in migration health practices has ensured that much of the interest in health and migration is directed towards communicable diseases [5]. Generally, migrant medical screening is focused on conditions that prevails in different magnitudes between the migrant and host population, such as tuberculosis, and other poverty related diseases in the case of low income economies [6 Incidence of the Hansen diseases [7], and those suffering from syphilis infection [8]. In cases where medical screening are adopted and has been applied to evaluate and report public health and disease situation in the migrant population, in some cases to give an insight into the national and global health statistics. At the moment disease evaluation studies has shown some known health problems in the short and long run within the displaced migrant populations. The increasing interest in study on international migration has shown new areas and information on the migration health particularly studies in the Central African sub regions where, political instability has increased migration of displaced population within and the concentration in border countries.[9]. In addition to communicable diseases, attention is now focused on pre-existing non-infectious diseases [9] and other health domains, including behaviour [1, 10], morality [3, 11] and genetic diversity or ethnic profiles [4, 12]. Studies on displaced population concerning their behavioural pattern and psycho-social analysis has shown a public health concern especially in the sub-sahran African regions where regulation on drug and substance of abuse are difficult to put into action and the population are not under any restriction to possess and consume substances of abuse alcohol and other narcotics. Studies on genetic diversity and ethnicity within the mapped populations has indicated that genotype by environment interactions is correlated to linkage factors to non-infectious and other common diseases among the communities. This study has led to the strong consideration of implementing a health counselling programmes to manage the migrant population ethnicity and health issues [8, 12].

Epidemiological studies is currently inclusive of chronic diseases [13] like cancer malignancies [14], kidney renal failure [15] and severe cardiovascular diseases [8, 16], mental and psycho-social health [17] maternal and child health [12, 18]. Lifestyle diseases and associated health issues (metabolic diseases), frequent tobacco use, alcohol use and substance of abuse, are critically being studied and considered in relation to the process of migration in some migrant receiving countries [19]. Due to variations in migrant demographics between receiving nations, international comparisons involving the pooled analysis of several host nations can be very challenging for interpretation and unreliable for use.

The global and national popularity in research towards thepotential epidemics in migrant population has been on the increased [20]. The strategies to provide and develop health information systems on migrant population is also on the increase although the outcome of study is limited by other constraints such as ethnic diversity that is reported in most current displaced migrant communities. The displaced populations usually are made up of mixed cohorts that unevenly distributed within the displaced population receiving nations. The displaced population usually in most cases are asylum applicants, refugees, and temporary migrants like the potential students, economic migrants, and other more complex to define categories of migrants, [20]. Migratory population becomes difficult to manage in increased volume and pressure and in some situation the receiving countries have limited logistical facilities in place to cope with the influx of the uncontrolled population, especially cases with health concerns. To reduce the population pressure measures are put in place to develop strategies that uses health population principles in studying migration process which involves observations geared towards immigration health policy management programme potentially developed for the developing economies [21].

1.2. Population based approach

In migratory population the health-based approach in migratory health gives consideration into the factor of migration and health as a closely linked process that can be affected by short term and other local factors. [7, 20]. It has been shown by many indications that the population based approach are possibly less associated with the administrative principles of population displacement [22] and very closely linked to those important factors or characteristics that drives or motivate migration at national and global level. The population based consideration makes it possible for for the study of the long term effect that migration have between the different health communities and the effect on the different cohorts under consideration. This approach can enhance the consideration of many factors at a more global view point and many countries are making efforts to integrate the population based approach in the national and global health programmes and also address some poverty related diseases like TB, HIV/AIDS and malaria. [5, 23].

Following the information in table 1 below, the major problem of the different health milieu and the evolution of the migration of displaced population considers problems of disease associated with migratory related diseases within the framework of population-based risk that could add more value to the disease control programs during the period-of-entry screening for individual conditions [3, 11, and 24]. The study on migration and history of displaced populations supports the quantitative and analytic investigation on health variables important for study of disease burden in migratory population [24, 25].

General Trends	Outcome indicators
Point of exit and extend of medical need identified and the state of detected disease	State of disease progression - Care provision facilities - Access to basic health care
Migrant population in host community needing health attention and service:	Disease severity and epidemic survey assessment •Sensitization of health care services and providers • Disease diagnosis facilities, treatment and monitoring
Potential health problems among migratory population	Potential health factors-depression - trauma, stress - vulnerable exposure - tribal and religious conflicts, disease stigmatization
Migratory population exposure and predisposition to ill-health cause by change in environment.	Migration cohorts of war victims, civil unrest, asylum claimant Child trafficking
Health problems acquired in host communities by socio cultural interaction	Health factors linked to poverty, starvation, famine and hunger - linguistic and cultural problems - Unemployment constraints
Sensitization on access and health care facilities and service providers in the displace community	Groups of migrant services include farm and factory jobs • Prostitution • Housemaids • Drug trafficking and abuse

Table 1. The influence of immigrant health environments evolution of migratory community [25]

1.3. Population health approach

The population health approach to migration health is focused on the issue on standardized examination of two key factors that are: (1) sustained stable and disparate health environments and (2) the movement of mixed populations between regions or environment of varied prevalence of key health indicators and potential outcomes [2, 14,24].

1.3.1. The main trends in migratory health variability

It is important to note that a number of migratory related diseases results from some genotype by environmental interactions [25], The variation in health problems in migratory population identified in most cases, and some the determinants of health impacts can be attributed to frequent population socio-cultural cross fertilization [26], also economic and social, genotypic variations, and psycho social behaviours.

These variables greatly affects the population and evaluation of the evolution of disease within the cohort population. Some examples of endemic disease are in most cases caused by in hygienic conditions, water borne and vector transmitted diseases. With no frontier control some vector transmitted diseases like malaria, yellow fever can rapidly spread across countries [9]. Environmentally-related non-communicable disease epidemiological variations are caused by some deficiencies micronutrients [27] and geographically-defined exposure risks, such as health outcomes related to extreme weather or altitude, climate change [28].

. Social and economic influences can be important contributing factors in the development and maintenance of disparity in health and disease outbreaks between populations. Problems related to poverty, low education, housing and nutrition are shown to be closely associated to disease or illness prevalence and illness outcomes in low income countries [29]. The capacities and technical knowhow of medical and health sectors can influence health through the availability, accessibility of health facilities and state of the art medical equipment [30] and accessibility and ability to afford health promotion, disease prevention and treatment services [31,32]. Some of the major hindrance to manage disease burden in migratory population and slow response health delivery system include the problem of language barrier [33], socio-cultural cross fertilization and integration [34, 35], drug abuse, food tolerance and adoption of new menu and conformity to the norms and practice of host community, social interaction [36]. The displace populations in the case of massive displacement can have a great influence on the host countries and can drastically cause a hospitality problem by indigenes as a result of the pressure to deal with their new inhabitants who are considered as of great threats [37, 38]. Most displaced population are under the influence of micro environmental factors that are linked to disease burden.

These micro factors could be caused by the process of migration, during the travel period between origin and destination. These factors are usually observed within the refugees' communities, displaced populations and disadvantaged migrant communities such as the trafficked or smuggled groups of the migrant population, groups with psycho-social behaviours like depression, trauma and torture victims [39-41]. Other migration-specific health issues have been recorded in the groups of migrant worker [44, 45], the population of migrants' children [46] and some groups of returning migrant returning from family visits and or attending major ceremonies outside the immigration zones [47].

1.3.2. The impact of genetic diversity and biological interaction

The impact of genetic diversity and biological interactions of health and disease may be a contributing factor to migrant adaptation and sustainability. However, in non-endemic regions these influences, and their association to mobility of population, can be poorly appreciated during the early stages of migration mainly due to inadequate of awareness, sensitization, knowledge or experience in the healthcare delivery sector [47]. The changes in disease progression and disease burden are dynamic and in most cases evolving at a steady rate in developing countries. This disease dynamism pattern expression is an indication of the complex nature of data base record analysis and management [24]. Socio -economic environments can rapidly change in our current global world especially if those changes have influence on health determinants, consequential changes in health outcomes observed over relatively short periods of time [2, 15], In case where there are basic health improvement facilities such as putting in place modern facilities for the provision of good source of portable drinking water, proper housing conditions, food and basic clothing facilities in more ways can have a great impact on reducing disease burden and greatly address public health problems resulting from disease epidemics. [20]. Conflict, environmental change, natural disasters and population growth are known to result in new risk exposures and acquisition of adverse health outcomes over a short period of time [5]. Investigation at the global and national level of genotype by environment interactions on disease progression, psycho social behavioural patterns of the migratory population that may have a negative influence on the health of the population. [11, 17]. The aspect of climatic oscillation has the potential to influence disease epidemic as the migrant population are predisposed to diseases resulting from the climate changes and the slow process of human adaptation [28, 40]. The future of the health situation of displaced communities usually differs from the population of the host countries in many ways within the same community due to the genotypic variation of these two cohort coexisting in same environment.

The changes in the health indicators of displaced population are linked to complex individual health status at the time of migration which makes the health management programmes at the host countries difficult to implement [33, 44],.

2. Modern migration and population mobility

Migration phenomenon has generally been considered as a fluid process that is constantly undergoing changes, that needs to be assessed in terms of rate of change and global magnitude of population movement. In the last decades, the process of migration and movement of other mobile populations has been greatly influenced by the following factors:

1.   The decolonialization of many nations and post-independence adaptation in Africa, the Middle East, Asia, Latin America and the Caribbean [3, 8, 41];

2.   Large refugee displacement following conflicts and civil disturbances in Africa, South East Asia, the Balkans, Central America and Central Africa; *and*

3.   The fall of the former Soviet Union has caused some socio-political, and economic problems to the extent that the institution for the legal and administrative restrictions on the ability of migrants to travel, work and move internationally have undergone a significant change at the global and national. One of the contributing factors has been linked to a complete shift in the demography of migrant population [17, 21]. In most traditional migrant-receiving regions such as Australia and North America where huge influx of migration has been recorded in the past, there has been a shift in the patterns of migration from Central Europe to new exploratory countries in Asia, South Africa, Central and South America and the Middle East countries [20, 33]

2.1. The Grazer displaced population and Trans-humans

In the sub Saharan African countries facing a long period of dry season, the grazer population are faced with problem of extreme shortage of vegetation for their animals and therefore have to travel for long distances and away from home for months in search of greener pastures and water for their herds [25, 46], in an activity termed trans-humans. During the trans-humans period the grazer population generally from the Fulanis and Masai population are vulnerable to many forms of disease attack[8, 47], There is poor medical care, poor nutritional intake leading to mineral deficiencies and disease epidemic outbreak. This period of trans-humans has led to significant loss of grazer herds, and human life [45].The grazer population are general nomads and are constantly involved in gazer land disputes with the local indigenous population [45].

2.2. Concern to expanding immigrant foreign born population

There is a global and national concern with the expanding immigrant population due to the fact that these group of people have been shown to reproduce at a rate that is difficult for host countries to managed. The long term implication response to growing immigrant born population has been summarized in table 2.

Critical Issues	Implications
Increased demands for health service and access	Increased in Health Budget spending of host countries Provide adequate diagnostic and treatment services
Implementation of training programs for health providers and personnels	Adequate translation and interpretation services Set up information and communication systems (health information)
Increased in the migration of health professionals from migrant source regions	Address Issues of unemployment and job competition with indigenes, Social issues of labour exploitation of immigrants.
Training/certification of professional migrants who have linguistic skills	Sensitization in cultural awareness and sensitivity programs and training expensive to be introduced

Table 2. Long Term implication Response to Growing Immigrant -Foreign Born Population Component

2.3. Health environments and displaced population

In low income economies the health environments are limiting to manage the immigrant population mobility. In the Central African regions for example the lack of health environmental settings has been a health concerns in conflict areas to cope with the increasing displaced population. This problem has not been limited to regulated, traditional immigration and emigration. It also involves refugee and humanitarian movements and an increase in irregular arrivals (refugee claimants, asylum seeking, smuggling and trafficking in humans).

The different support structures at global and national level involved in supporting and addressing the problems of displaced population work with a common vision of reducing environmental crisis, prevent or control disease outbreaks and maintaining peace and mutual coexistence of the interacting population. Great efforts have been made at the international and national levels enhance international mass displacement of migrant population during period of crisis, civil riot, natural disaster or political instability in a region. The role of international bodies involved in conflict management has been very important in managing massive population influx. These organizations directly implicated in peace and conflict management and health intervention include medicine without borders (*medicine sans frontier*) the United Nations High Commission for Refugees (UNHR), UNICEF, and the AU in the African sub regions [26]. Other bodies like the International Organization for Migration has played an important role in managing the problems of global displaced population [37]. New approach put in place globally through the improvement of health facilities and capacity building of health personnel and delivery systems can enhance the management of displaced population at point of entry [15]. With worldwide fluctuations in socio-political landscape, terrorist attacks dynamics, civil societal change, the nature, speed and access to international travel has also undergone marked changes in regulation and evolution of travel trends. The global travel patterns have been affected by changes in information and communication technology, transportation technology, accessibility, and affordability [5, 24]. Growth in air travel has functionally reduced previous limits on the rapid international movement of large numbers of individuals. The high volume of international travel supports greater population exchange and return flows between migrant origin and destination locations. Increased international travel has also been an integral component to support the growing process of globalization [2, 9, and 41], the progressive integration of global economic and communications sectors has been achieved by, a corresponding growth in the international demand and flow of labour and manpower. Recent report by the International Labour Organization (ILO) show an increasing global trend in foreign-born migrant labour market [22]. The trend of occupational mobility among migrant population from one location to another is on the increase leading to the slogan too many skilled migrants chasing few. In most cases occupational mobility is well structured managed by job agencies and outsourcing contract houses in most cases targeting illegal migrants workforce for exploitation [14, 39].

2.4. Geopolitical changes

One of the major factor affecting population mobility and migration is geo-political changes such as the collapse of the former Soviet Union, the fall of the Berlin wall, independence of smaller countries like Southern Sudan, Eritrea etc [41]. The implication of socio-economic and political factors of migration have other consequences on the population trends and dynamics of displaced mass population globally. [19].

2.5. The epidemiological implications of mobility across differentials in disease prevalence

Contrary to the developed countries, where infections that were historically considered as major causes of illness and death are decreasing in incidence and prevalence or have been eliminated, sub-Saharan Africa is still suffers from poverty related diseases and new diseases emerging like Ebola, konzo, buruli ulcer especially in west and central Africa.[38. 40]. Well-developed health facilities and sensitization programmes for healthy living and clean environmental, the adoption of environmental protection agency programmes on a global basis has significantly reduced disease burden in most developed nations. In the last decade diseases of global economic importance has attained a level that can be managed within the different sub regions [3.11] and large improvement of immunization programmes and vaccine development initiatives has significantly reduced infectious diseases under a manageable scale [32, 35], and some of these diseases like polio, measles, mumps etc. are in the process of complete eradication.

The level of public health sensitization programs towards disease eradication also varies from regions to region and this disparity has led to problems in understanding the disease burden in the different migrant communities. Where there is mass movement of displaced population across borders the outbreak of disease can become a national or international public health concern. [17].The disparity in epidemic outbreaks of diseases that are not usually predictable is not restricted to communicable disease pressure but also cut across non communicable diseases. The issue of developed framework geared towards the control of non-infectious diseases in migrant communities has been properly developed in advance countries than in the poor resource nation, due to the priorities given to strategic health development process This developed health structures enhance the process and potential to diagnose, treat and control non infection diseases in well developed countries when compared with the cases shown in sub Saharan Africa. Availability and services for complex and expensive medical interventions like heart bypass, chemotheraphy, organ transplant etc and other health delivery services varies based on the health priorities and logistics implementation between one country to another [1, 6, 23].

The variation in public health spending are linked to social and economic attributions, health service delivery facilities and access of the displaced population to health care and medical insurance [27]. In areas where there is limited international migration and national massive population occupational mobility the variation in disease epidemics is less significance and disease survey data base is easy to develop. On a global scale there is a concerted effort in the different regions to improve on health programmes, policies and infrastructures and delivery systems that can enhance the reduction of disease burden in the displaced population. In the last two decades there has been a general global increase in disease epidemics with potential health implication on disease burden of some poverty related disease like tuberculosis (TB), sexually transmitted infection (STIs), HIV/AIDs, Ebola Konzo, buruli ulcer and Chagas' disease. Within the migrant communities problems of disease co-infections are common and mostly observed from displaced population where the diseases are endemic [21, 33, and 42]. The trends in disease epidemic progression in developed countries has been shown for long un sustainable infections such as HIV/AIDS, hepatitis B and C. This trends are significantly different for developing countries of the Middle East, Asia and Africa where the diseases are very common and mostly recorded in foreign born migrant population [11, 44]. Disease epidemics linked to mass displaced population can influence local and community disease trends for the host migrant countries for both communicable and non-communicable diseases [20]. Displaced migrant population from resource poor countries have limited access to health facilities, disease diagnostics, health insurance, health promotion programmes, and therapeutic interventions for disease. The migrants have the potential of disease predisposition in an advanced stage than is normally seen by health personnel and service providers in the migrants host countries [16, 20]. An overview of health problems within the migratory population gives an indication that all epidemic situation linked to migration is correlated with the situation where the migrant population are less privileged than the migrant host population. Many migrants population base on life style related non communicable and non-infectious disease tend to show health indicators that are far superior than those of host population [21, 25, 41].A number of factor such as nutrition, psycho social behavior changes with time tends to change within the migrant population. In some cases the displaced migrants may show some adverse health effects closely related to those of host population. [1, 6]. In most cases some of the benefits and privileges derived from immigrant communities may be short lived and may be lost with time when the host country can no longer cope with the massive influx of population.

2.6. Short term impact of migration on health and disease epidemic

Migration has been closely linked to the influences on the potential disease epidemics with some short and long term implications on host country and there are significant disparity in disease health indicators. The disparity in disease indicators has led to the obligation of the international and national communities to develop health policies and programmes to address international population mobility as shown in table 3 below.

Critical Issues	Implications
Main entry point of monitoring and checks	Practice of immigrant health screens for defined diseases at entry points very difficult and time consuming
Migratory health intervention integrated programmes in migrant nations	Programmes are likely to be user friendly and more adopted than the nationwide intervention programmese
General movement of displaced population	May become a more important determination factor influencing many health outcomes, with age, sex, genetic diversity factor, behavior, educational, ethno-religious issues, and wealth attainment
Mobile population health policy frameworks (Mobile health, e-health)	may significantly need integration and harmonization at all jurisdictional levels with international economic, trade and security strategies.

Table 3. Health policy issues resulting from international population mobility

Where diseases of rare occurrence, has been reduced to very low levels, the occurrence of a few cases may have significant health impact at local and international scale [3]. This health impact can lead to a public health concern at the local necessitating an increase health response.

There are cases of global public health control strategies developed from the 2003 SARS events [22, 30, and 42], the case of zoonotic avian-to-human influenza transmission [4], and the records on spontaneous outbreaks of viral haemorrhagic fevers [1. 20. 43] and the health impact of HIV/AIDS incidences recorded in developed countries [27, 35] transmitted by overseas visitors or migrant population. Regular mass displacement of new migrants from high disease endemic zones contribute significantly to the existing diseases due to low incidence of migrant host population. There is a need for long term health care programme to put in place policies and strategic plan to manage disease burden in host migrant communities for a more effective international and global integration. Countries that rely on historical, and local disease epidemics data for health policy, legislation and implementation may have less impact in the case where the disease burden develops above a manageable dimension at national and global level within the different control programmes [4, 21, and 27]. Concerning non-infectious diseases, migration-associated pressures result from the need to provide service delivery in culturally or linguistically sensitive programmes for the prevention or treatment of illness in migrant communities. There has been increase public health concern cause by introduction of new diseases through mass displaced populations into areas where there has been no known incidence of the disease. This situation can be worsen by the rapid growth of the new migrant populations with a gap in linguistic, socio- cultural cross fertilization, psycho social behaviours that may potentially cause problems in disease recognition, diagnosis and possible therapy [2, 31].In some recorded cases of the delay in diagnosis and possible treatment can lead to important health implications affecting the population [8.34], difficulties in the management of health programmes. With the increasing growth and freedom of migration coupled with increased number of occupational mobility there is a potential danger of increasing global and national health disease burden in situations of mass displacement of migrant population [11].

2.7. The public health problems associated with complex emergencies and refugee situations in developing countries

In many displaced migrant populations caused by war, natural disasters, civil disobedience and other macro environmental problems, there are always public health problems caused by disease burden that are either communicable or non-communicable in nature in the affected area. Other consequences of massive displaced population include food insecurity, famine, lack of basic access to health care, and the difficulties in developing a standard health programme, policies for a good standard of care [5, 13, 31].The impact of mass displacement of population on public health disease management programmes has had a significant impact in low income economies The other drawback caused by mass displaced population includes increasing death and morbidity ratios. In most low resource countries like in sub-Saharan Africa, there is high mortality rates due to significant increase in disease burden, extreme poverty, unemployment and the most common causes of death within the displaced population are associated with water borne diseases like diarrheal and dysentery, measles, acute respiratory infections, malaria and most recent in sub Saharan Africa, ebola virus disease [9, 14, 37]. High prevalence of acute malnutrition have contributed to high case fatality rates. In conflict-affected African countries, such as Sudan, the Central African Republic, Mali, Chad etc., war-related injuries have been the most common cause of death among civilian populations; however, increased incidence of communicable diseases, neonatal health problems, and nutritional deficiencies (especially among the elderly) have been reported [35, 39, 45]. Studies have shown that in massive displaced communities some of the standard procedures put in place to manage and control high mortality and morbidity includes a sustainable food security, improvement in hygiene and sanitation, portable good source of drinking water supply, shelter and clothing,; reduction in water borne related diseases, well developed immunization programmes; good mother and child health care, neonatal health monitoring systems, and strategic management and control of communicable and non-communicable endemic diseases; and the implementation of enhanced special feeding programs where migrants of special dietary needs are put under selected or special diet and follow up for the improvement of their nutritional status.

2.8. Migration of displaced population from farmers' grazier conflicts in sub-Saharan Africa

The movement of population of grazers from one locally to another over a wide area in search of greener pastures has led to tribal conflicts and problem of human coexistence. Studies have been conducted on the conflict problems arising from grazer activities and in an attempt to appreciate some of the main causes of conflict and also to give an insight into the implication on local and national migration, and how they can be managed within the framework of effective and sustainable community development [46, 47]. In a global scale conflict results from a serious misunderstanding, communication problems, dispute, difference of opinions among individual and groups of people in a community. In most cases conflicts leads to threats that can be directed to an individual or groups restriction to some privileged, or access to some properties or resources [46]. Within the grazer population conflicts are usually linked to land disputes between crop farmers and grazers in areas where both parties compete for a limited space of land for their main activities of farming and grazing (Normadic herds' men and farmers' population). The conflict has caused in some cases the grazier population to adapt a persistent nomadic lifestyle which predispose them to disease attack and little access to medical care. The long period of trans humans requires that grazer population travel long distance in search for green vegetation or pastures and water for their livestock. During the long period of transhumans there is less access to medical protection and the livestock suffer severe disease infection due to little veterinary visits [45]. Access to proper food is limited and the herders go for long period of poor feeding, under feeding, lack of balance diet. The health consequences are tissue wasting, diarrheal, cholera attack from poor water source [23].

3. Future impact of population mobility on global health

Some of the drawbacks resulting from increased migration and population mobility is the constant increased pressure in developing in the migrant receiving countries a structured health planning programmes Population migration is an essential part of the current process of globalization. Studies have shown that migration trends, forecast on the movement or the migration of workforce may stay stable or take a steady rise with time. The variation in health indicators at the global and regional scale are likely to expand despite the mobilization effort at the international level to develop control strategies for population displacement.International efforts and prgrammes have been developed to reduce disparities and impacts of disease and ill health, such as attempts to achieve the Millennium Development Goals [14, 31, 40], are in progress in many health friendly societies. Efforts to put in place sustainable initiatives is still in progress, resources and extensive financial mobilization is needed for effective implementation of programmes. The variation in health and health indicator analysis at the global and regional levels has a continuous influence on the health of the migratory population. There is an added challenge of financial cost towards the initiation of the sustainable control strategies of migrated displaced population. It has been shown that in the early studies, most of the health issues linked to migratory health were initiated at the national level. In recent times this health initiatives programmes has been achieved through immigration health actions, as a vital aspects of some local health programmes put in place. The importance of effective migratory health service needs to be put in place in most regions due to defined issues linked to displaced population [1, 13, 29, and 47]. The evolution of travel and migration has reduced the effectiveness of many national, point-of-arrival activities. New patterns of population mobility needs to reconsider the practicality and viability of border-health inspection for exclusion or containment strategies [42],.In most nations where large immigration medical programs are effective, there is a maintenance of specific screening or intervention programs for targeted diseases such as tuberculosis, syphilis and HIV/AIDS. Studies have also shown that in some situations a more effective screening outcomes could be obtained through interventions focused on disease control efforts in source nations rather than reliance on arrival screening alone [21, 28].

Studies on anxiety, depression and post-traumatic stress disorder (PTSD) in asylum-seekers are known to be linked to pre-migration trauma and post-migration stress. The number of documented mental health issues of refugees has increased in recent times, but there is a gap in the studies focusing specifically on the factors associated with psychiatric distress in asylum-seekers who have not been given residency status [11, 17, and 33]. Such studies associated anxiety scores with female gender, poverty, and conflict with immigration officials, while loneliness and boredom were linked with both anxiety and depression. A diagnosis of PTSD has also been linked with greater exposure to pre-migration trauma, delays in processing refugee applications, difficulties in dealing with immigration officials, obstacles to employment, racial discrimination, and loneliness and boredom of asylum seekers who find it difficult to *socio-culturally cross fertilize,* due to language barriers [24].

4. Conclusions

The global issue of migratory health has stimulated much interest in the public health sector in most developed and developing nation to the extent that policies towards addressing the problems is on the agenda of public health debates and putting in place strategy policy plan by stakeholders and states decision makers. There is a need to address migration problems at national and international levels especially as there are increasing displaced population under war, civil disorder, disease outbreak, political instability, natural disaster, *credit crunch,* or in search of better life and migration by the displaced population in developing countries. Population under refugee status needs a more advanced psychosocial service and procedures for dealing with asylum-seekers to reduce the high levels of stress and psychiatric symptoms in those who have been previously traumatized. Government in developing countries with displaced immigrant population and those in areas with intensive grazer migration, there is the need for the ministry of health and health actors to develop a system of global and national disease management in crisis.

The epidemiological issues that is linked to migration at the global and regional level have been shown to result from the movement of population flows across regional boundaries and frontiers and variation in disease prevalence outcome. The increasing trends of various types of migratory population has led to the gaps in health indicators. The changes in the trends of migration has also cause a rapid change in the implementation of health policy for the existing health programmes to meet up with these new challenges. The new action plan to deal with the new trends of migration has resulted in an increasing globalization that has a direct impact on health programmes and the indicators that is necessary for disease epidemics mapping.

The health effect of epidemics resulting from the mass displacement of migrants haa been demonstrated by the level of infectious disease health information that is available in the developing regions and there is also interest to develop information on non-infectious diseases in immigration receiving nations. The global health disparities and disease epidemics and prevalence will continue to exist in the national health programs and policies in migrant receiving nations and will continue to be challenged by illness and disease arising beyond their frontiers. A more holistic approach at the global and national level is needed to address migration of population irrespective of the circumstance predisposing the population to such migration, and strategic policy towards controlling migratory health issues within the framework of globalization.

Acknowledgements

The authors would like to thank the European & Developing Countries Clinical Trials Partnership (EDCTP) for the grant funding that enable us to realize part of this project. Furthermore we would also like to acknowledge the financial support of the Ministry of Higher Education (MINESUP) of Cameroon for the special presidential financial Research support of lecturers.

Author details

Charles Fokunang[1,2*], Estella Tembe-Fokunang[1], Zacharia Sando[1],
Marceline Ngounoue Djuidje[3], Barbara Atogho Tiedeu[3], Frederick Kechia[1], Jerome Ateudjieu[4],
Valentin Ndikum[1], Raymond Langsi[2], Dobgima Fomnboh[2], Joseph Fokam[1], Luc Gwum[1],
Obama Abena[1], Tazoacha Asongani[1], Vincent Pryde Titanji[6] and Lazare Kaptue[5,7]

*Address all correspondence to: charlesfokunang@yahoo.co.uk

1 Faculty of Medicine and Biomedical Sciences, University of Yaoundé, Cameroon

2 The University of Bamenda, Cameroon

3 Faculty of Science, University of Yaounde, Cameroon

4 The University of Dschang, Cameroon

5 The Universite des Montagnes,West Region, Cameroon

6 The University of Buea, Cameroon

7 Cameroon National Ethics Committee for Research in Humans (CNERH), Cameroon

References

[1] Khan MA, Islam S, Arif M, ul Haq Z. Transmission model of hepatitis B virus with the migration effect Biomed Res Int. 2013; 2013:150681. doi: 10.1155/2013/150681.

[2] Schär F, Trostdorf U, Giardina F, Khieu V, Muth S, Marti H, Vounatsou P, Odermatt P Strongyloides stercoralis. Global distribution and risk factors: PLoS Negl Trop Dis. 2013 11; 7-17.

[3] Harvey K, Esposito DH, Han P, Kozarsky P, Freedman DO, Plier DA, Sotir MJ. Surveillance for travel-related disease--GeoSentinel Surveillance System, United States, 1997-2011.Centers for Disease Control and Prevention (CDC).

[4] Zou G, Wei X, Witter S, Yin J, Walley J, Liu S, Yang H, Chen J, Tian G, Mei J.Incremental cost-effectiveness of improving treatment results among migrant tuberculosis patients in Shanghai.. Int J Tuberc Lung Dis. 2013 17:8-15.

[5] Montanaro M, Colombatti R, Pugliese M, Migliozzi C, Zani F, Guerzoni ME, Manoli S, Manara R, Meneghetti G, Rampazzo P, Cavalleri F, Giordan M, Paolucci P, Basso G, Palazzi G, Sainati L.Intellectual function evaluation of first generation immigrant children with sickle cell disease: the role of language and sociodemographic factors. Ital J Pediatr. 2013; 39:36-46..

[6] Lavender CJ, Globan M, Kelly H, Brown LK, Sievers A, Fyfe JA, Lauer T, Leslie DE.Epidemiology and control of tuberculosis in Victoria, a low-burden state in south-eastern Australia, 2005-2010. Int J Tuberc Lung Dis. 2013; 17(6):752-758.

[7] Maltezou HC, Tsolia M, Polymerou I, Theodoridou M. Paediatric malaria in Greece in the era of global population mobility. Travel Med Infect Dis. 2013; 11(3):178-180.

[8] Salinas Botrán A, Ramos Rincón JM, de Górgolas Hernández-Mora M Cardiovascular disease: a view from global health perspective. Med Clin (Barc). 2013 7; 141(5): 210-216.

[9] Bell TR, Molinari NM, Blumensaadt S, Selent MU, Arbisi M, Shah N, Christiansen D, Philen R, Puesta B, Jones J, Lee D, Vang A, Cohen NJ.Impact of port of entry referrals on initiation of follow-up evaluations for immigrants with suspected tuberculosis: Illinois.J Immigr Minor Health. 2013; 15(4):673-679.

[10] Selent M, de Rochars VM, Stanek D, Bensyl D, Martin B, Cohen NJ, Kozarsky P, Blackmore C, Bell TR, Marano N, Arguin PM.Malaria prevention knowledge, attitudes, and practices (KAP) among international flying pilots and flight attendants of a US commercial airline. J Travel Med. 2012; 19(6):366-372.

[11] Taylor AB, Kurbatova EV, Cegielski JP Prevalence of anti-tuberculosis drug resistance in foreign-born tuberculosis cases in the U.S. and in their countries of origin..PLoS One. 2012; 7:11-19.

[12] Ramos JM, Ponce Y, Gallegos I, Flóres-Chávez M, Cañavate C, Gutiérrez F. Trypanosoma cruzi infection in Elche (Spain): comparison of the seroprevalence in immigrants from Paraguay and Bolivia.Pathog Glob Health. 2012; 106 (2):102-106.

[13] Oviedo M, Muñoz MP, Carmona G, Borrás E, Batalla J, Soldevila N, Domínguez A.The impact of immigration and vaccination in reducing the incidence of hepatitis B in Catalonia (Spain). BMC Public Health. 2012, 12(1):614.

[14] Siriwardhana C, Stewart R. Forced migration and mental health: prolonged internal displacement, return migration and resilience.. Int Health. 2013;5(1):19-23

[15] Bayoh MN, Akhwale W, Ombok M, Sang D, Engoki SC, Koros D, Walker ED, Williams HA, Burke H, Armstrong GL, Cetron MS, Weinberg M, Breiman R, Hamel MJ. Malaria in Kakuma refugee camp, Turkana, Kenya: facilitation of Anopheles arabiensis vector populations by installed water distribution and catchment systems..Malar J. 2011 4; 105-:149.

[16] Buonomo B, Lacitignola D. Analysis of a tuberculosis model with a case study in Uganda.. J Biol Dyn. 2010; 4(6):571-593.

[17] Centers for Disease Control and Prevention (CDC).Rapid establishment of an internally displaced person's disease surveillance system after an earthquake --- Haiti, 2010..MMWR Morb Mortal Wkly Rep. 2010 6; 59(30):939-945.

[18] Westerhaus M. Linking anthropological analysis and epidemiological evidence: formulating a narrative of HIV transmission in Acholiland of Northern Uganda. SAHARA J. 2007, 4(2):590-605.

[19] Brian D Gushulak1 and Douglas W MacPherson. The basic principles of migration health: Population mobility and gaps in disease prevalence.*Emerging Themes in Epidemiology2006*, 3:3-12

[20] Gensini GF, Yacoub MH, Conti AA: The concept of quarantine in history: from plague to SARS. *J Infect* 2004, 49:257-261.

[21] International Organization for Migration WHO.Migration Medicine: First International Conference on the Health Needs of Refugees, Migrant Workers, other Uprooted People and Long Term Traveler's. In *Seminar Report* IOM, Geneva; 1990.

[22] Centers for Disease Control and Prevention: Technical Instructions for the Medical Examination of Aliens revised 2002. *Atlanta, Georgia* [http://www.cdc.gov/ncidod/dq/panel.htm]. (Accessed July 2014).

[23] McKay L, Macintyre S, Ellaway A: Migration and Health: A Review of the International Literature. Medical Research Council Social and Public Health Sciences Unit. Occasional Paper # 12. January 2003. University of Glasgow, Glasgow; 2003.

[24] Markel H, Stern AM: The foreignness of germs: the persistent association of immigrants and disease in American society. *Milbank Q* 2002, 80:757-788.

[25] Centers for Disease Control and Prevention: Recommendations for prevention and control of tuberculosis among foreign born persons. Report of the Working Group on Tuberculosis among Foreign-Born Persons. Centers for Disease Control and Prevention. *MMWR Recomm Rep* 1998, 47(RR-16):1-29.

[26] Taylor R, King K, Vodicka P, Hall J, Evans D: Screening for leprosy in immigrants – a decision analysis model. *Lepr Rev* 2003, 74:240-248.

[27] Stauffer WM, Kamat D, Walker PF: Screening of international immigrants, refugees, and adoptees. *Prim Care* 2002, 29:879-905.

[28] Uitewaal PJ, Manna DR, Bruijnzeels MA, Hoes AW, Thomas S: Prevalence of type 2 diabetes mellitus, other cardiovascular risk factors, and cardiovascular disease in Turkish and Moroccan immigrants in North West Europe: a systematic review. *Prev Med* 2004, 39:1068-1076.

[29] Feng W, Ren P, Shaokang Z, Anan S: Reproductive Health Status, Knowledge, and Access to Health Care Among Female Migrants in Shanghai, China. *J Biosoc Sci* 2005, 37:603-622.

[30] Bhugra D: Migration and mental health. *Acta Psychiatr Scand* 2004, 109:243-258.

[31] Acevedo-Garcia D, Pan J, Jun HJ, Osypuk TL, Emmons KM: The effect of immigrant generation on smoking. *Soc Sci Med* 2005, 61:1223-1242.

[32]   Adams KM, Gardiner LD, Assefi N: Healthcare challenges from the developing world: post-immigration refugee medicine. *BMJ* 2004, 328:1548-1552.

[33]   Dawson AJ, Sundquist J, Johansson SE: The influence of ethnicity and length of time since immigration on physical activity. *Ethn Health* 2005, 10:293-309.

[34]   El-Ghannam AR: The global problems of child malnutrition and mortality in different world regions. *J Health Soc Policy* 2003, 16:1-26.

[35]   Boadi KO, Kuitunen M: Environment, wealth, inequality and the burden of disease in the Accra metropolitan area, Ghana. *Int J Environ Health Res* 2005, 15:193-206.

[36]   Kullgren JT: Restrictions on undocumented immigrants' access to health services: the public health implications of welfare reform. *Am J Public Health* 2003, 93:1630-1633?

[37]   Bischoff A, Tonnerre C, Eytan A, and Bernstein M, Loutan L: Addressing language barriers to health care, a survey of medical services in Switzerland. *Soz Praventivmed* 1999, 44:248-256.

[38]   Eshiett MU, Parry EH: Migrants and health: a cultural dilemma.*Clin Med* 2003, 3:229-231.

[39]   Gushulak BD, MacPherson DW: Health issues associated with the smuggling and trafficking of migrants. *J Immigr Health* 2000 2:67-78.

[40]   Burnett A, Peel M: Asylum seekers and refugees in Britain. The health of survivors of torture and organized violence. *BMJ* 2001, 322:606-609.

[41]   US State Department: Trafficking in Persons Report. Washington.[http://www.state.gov/g/tip/rls/tiprpt/2005]. (accessed April 8,2014)

[42]   International Organization for Migration: Migration Trends in Eastern Europe and Central Asia: 2001–2002 Review. *The Organization, Geneva* 2002.

[43]   Wong W, Tambis JA, Hernandez MT, Chaw JK, Klausner JD: Prevalence of sexually transmitted diseases among Latino immigrant day laborers in an urban setting – San Francisco. *SexTransm Dis* 2003, 30:661-613.

[44]   Viani RM, Bromberg K: Pediatric imported malaria in New York: delayed diagnosis. *Clin Pediatr (Phila)* 1999, 38:333-337.

[45]   MANU Ibrahim Nformi1, BIME Mary-Juliet2, FON Dorothy Engwali2, Ajaga NJI. Effects of farmer-grazer conflicts on rural development: a socio-economic analysis. Scholarly Journal of Agricultural Science Vol. 4(3), pp. 113-120 March, 2014

[46]   Robinson, J. and Clifford A. (1977). Conflict management in community groups. Urbana University of Illinois. Cooperative Extension services. pp. 100-120.

[47]   Hornby, A.S. (1995). Oxford Advanced Learners Dictionary of Current English, 5th Edition. Oxford University Press, New York

Disasters and Public Heath — An Updated Review of the Role of Infectious Disease in the Post-Disaster Environment

David M. Claborn and Christie Oestreich

Additional information is available at the end of the chapter

http://dx.doi.org/10.5772/59123

1. Introduction

Both natural and man-made disasters affect the public health of impacted populations. This simple truth has been recognized for many years and several reviews and treatments of this topic have been written to provide perspective on how to prepare and respond to the impacts of disaster. One of the most complete of these treatments is the 1997 book edited by Erik Noji titled "The Public Health Consequences of Disasters." This comprehensive book compiled many of the lessons learned from disasters and conflicts that occurred in the latter part of the 20th century and then constructed some essential theory for public health workers who must contend with the post-disaster environment. Since the publication of that book, several noteworthy disasters have struck in various parts of the world: the Fukushima tsunami and subsequent nuclear power plant disaster, the Haiti earthquake of 2010, Hurricane Katrina, the Kashmir earthquake of 2005, Hurricane Sandy, the Indonesian tsunami, and many others. These and other disasters have added more insight into the field of public health as applied to preparedness for and response to disasters. More nuanced understanding has become available for how infectious diseases and mental health issues impact affected populations in the post-disaster environment. This chapter will attempt to update some of the information gained from these disasters.

2. Generalizations about Public Health and Disasters during the 20th Century

The rarity, unpredictability and suddenness of disaster occurrence historically led to a degree of neglect regarding the study of public health consequences of those disasters [1]. However,

---

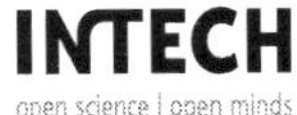

the sheer magnitude of the number of people affected by disasters eventually demanded a systematic analysis of public health issues. The number of people killed, injured, or displaced by disasters was estimated to be 311 million in 1991, a tripling of the population since 1980. This increase was due to multiple factors including population growth, but was also due to denser urban populations, especially along coastal areas, and to a large migration of populations from rural areas to the urban setting. Further complicating issues was an increasing reliance on a sophisticated, but vulnerable, infrastructure to provide power, transportation, and daily essentials to the densely packed urban populations. All of these factors contributed to increases in the amount of damage caused by natural and man-made disasters. Concurrent with this reliance on an increasingly vulnerable infrastructure was an increase in the number of complex humanitarian emergencies, a special category of emergency defined as humanitarian crises in which there is a breakdown of authority as a result of internal or external conflict [2]. The complex humanitarian emergency by definition requires an international response that is beyond the capability of any ongoing country program. All, of these factors led to the realization that a systematic study of public health and disasters was warranted.

One consistent finding from these studies was that displaced populations were particularly vulnerable to disease and other impacts of disaster. Population movements after disasters may move people into regions where health services cannot provide adequate support, with the result being increased morbidity and mortality [1]. Increases in infectious disease have also been noted in these displaced populations, often due to increasingly unsanitary conditions and the lack of potable water. Epidemics of infectious disease after rapid onset disasters are considered uncommon, but this is not the case for complex humanitarian emergencies [3]. In Africa, there have been epidemics of shigellosis, hepatitis and meningitis directly associated with complex emergencies. Displaced populations have also experienced outbreaks of cholera, bacillary dysentery, measles, malaria, schistosomiasis, and leishmaniasis. For example, a significant epidemic of leishmaniasis in southern Sudan was associated with a population that was displaced by civil war [4].

The assumption that epidemics inevitably follow disasters has been described as one of several myths about disasters [1]. Other erroneous assumptions include perceptions that medical volunteers of all medical backgrounds are necessary, all types of international assistance are needed immediately, disasters elicit criminal human behavior, affected populations are too shocked to help themselves, moving affected persons into temporary settlements is desirable, food supplements are always required, and that clothing is always needed to support the affected population. These and other myths may misdirect efforts or lead to a large degree of inefficiency during relief operations. For instance, one of the most frequently donated items is used clothing, most of which is not needed. Unnecessary supplies clog up the logistics and supply system, preventing the rapid arrival of truly necessary supplies. Piles of extraneous clothing and other unnecessary supplies often have to be burned simply to obtain necessary warehouse space.

Myths aside, several consistent recommendations regarding the practice of public health after disasters have been described. Perhaps the most important of these is the requirement for potable water. A sufficient amount of water is the most important commodity for a recovering population. This was most graphically demonstrated when a cholera epidemic occurred amongst the Rwandan refugees inside Zaire in 1994. The estimated death toll was more than 50,000 people [1]. Second to the provision of adequate food and water is the need for shelter, especially for displaced populations. However, communal shelters can present special problems, especially with regard to infectious disease and at times, security. In communal shelters it is particularly important to institute surveillance for diarrheal illnesses, upper respiratory infections and vaccine-preventable diseases. In 1997, a group of non-governmental organizations and the Red Cross movement collaborated on a project to identify minimum standards for disaster assistance in the fields of water supply, sanitation, nutrition, shelter and health services. This process eventually led to the publication of the first Sphere handbook in 2000. This book, which has been used extensively to guide disaster relief and humanitarian assistance in many situations, is currently in the third edition and is free for download at sphereproject.org [5].

3. Disasters and public health in the early 21st century

As mentioned earlier, one of the basic understandings concerning public health in post-disaster environments is that rapid onset disasters rarely lead to epidemics of infectious disease, especially among the healthy. As with almost all assumptions involving biology, there are exceptions to this rule and some have occurred in the 21st century. Post-disaster communicable diseases have been categorized into four groups: (1) those due to contaminated water, (2) respiratory infections (3) vector-borne diseases and (4) infections due to wounds and injuries [6]. The top five causes of death due to infectious disease after disasters are diarrhea, acute respiratory infections, measles, severe malnutrition and, in regions where it occurs, malaria. Between 1999 and 2008, over 7,100 natural disasters occurred causing approximately 1,243,000 deaths. Most of these deaths, especially those linked to communicable disease, occurred in Asia. However, increases in infectious disease rates after disasters also occurred in developed countries. For instance, the rates of West Nile virus neuroinvasive disease, one form of which is a paralytic disease reminiscent of polio, increased more than two-fold after Hurricane Katrina in portions of Louisiana and Mississippi that were affected by that storm [7]. Re-searchers speculated that the increased number of cases was due to increased human exposure to vector mosquitoes caused by the necessity of living in damaged houses without proper windows or screens. There was also an increase in the mosquito population due to increases in larval habitat as a result of the storm. In that instance, there was a sharp decrease in cases of the disease soon after aerial application of insecticides, suggesting that such vector-borne diseases are subject to effective control.

Another example of a post-disaster outbreak is provided by a fatal fungal disease that appeared after the 2011 tornado in Joplin, Missouri. The storm itself directly caused approximately 160 deaths, but in the aftermath, an outbreak of necrotizing cutaneous mucormycosis occurred, with thirteen confirmed cases. Five of the cases were fatal. Each of the cases had suffered from significant deep-penetrating trauma during the tornado and thus were examples of "infections following wounds and injuries." At least some of the victims were already in poor health prior to the storm; however, deaths were attributed to the infection.

Such fungal infections are not unique to the United States. Invasive fungal infections have been detected following eight different disasters including hurricanes, tsunami, an earthquake, a dust storm and a volcano. Other skin diseases are relatively common after disasters and have especially been associated with floods [9]. Prolonged immersion leads to keratinocyte damage and inflammation even without a typical immune cascade response [10]. This inflammation is often followed by a bacterial or fungal infections of the skin. Skin diseases as a result of flood exposure, can be categorized into four groups: inflammatory skin disease or irritant dermatitis, skin infections (usually bacterial or fungal), traumatic skin conditions, and miscellaneous. The latter includes insect bite reactions and psycho-emotion aggravation of existing primary skin diseases. The 2004 Indian Ocean tsunami led to many fungal skin infections, but also to several non-skin associated conditions. In one, an anesthetic was contaminated with a fungus, leading to infection of several delivering mothers receiving spinal anesthesia [9].

Although perhaps not as deadly as the example just mentioned and not caused by infectious disease, adverse birth outcomes have been repeatedly and consistently documented after disasters. Increases in rates of hypertension, anemia, pregnancy loss, birth defects, low birth weight, pre-term birth, intra-uterine growth restriction and decreases in head circumference have been attributed to trauma or exposures during or after disasters [11]. Also of importance to women's health, after Hurricane Katrina there was a documented increase in the rate of intimate partner abuse among displaced women, nearly three times that of pre-storm rates.

Due to the terrorist attacks of 2001 in the USA and subsequent attacks in Spain and London, public health agencies have had to assess what roles they must plan in preparing and responding to violent attacks on the civilian population, especially those associated with terrorism. Though this threat was not really new, the scope of the disasters mentioned above clearly required a public health response beyond that most agencies were capable of providing at the time. One significant challenge associated with terrorism is that terrorism's impacts go beyond the very obvious ones of illness and injury to cause significant increases in rates of anxiety and other psychological reactions. It is not surprising that the terrorists' actions cause such issues given that the goal is often to bring attention to the terrorists' causes through violence and terror. Such actions, by definition, are aimed at the mental well-being of populations. As professionals concerned with population health, the public health community often must become involved in disaster response following terrorist attacks and other violent events. Unfortunately, the success that developed countries have had in controlling disease may have led to a degree of complacency. In many ways, the public health infrastructure had somewhat deteriorated by the early years of the 21st century, leaving populations vulnerable to the repercussions of terrorism and other disasters. Laurie Garret discussed this issue at length in her book "Betrayal of Trust: The Collapse of Global Public Health" which was published just one year prior to the 2001 terrorist attacks. The threat of bioterrorism in particular suggested a need for improved epidemiology and disease surveillance, as well as more public health laboratories. Specific vaccines and anti-toxins were also needed, and several authors noted a need for improvements in mental health care capacity [18].

At the same time, the public health community expressed a concern that increased attention on responses to terrorism might take needed resources away from struggling but needed public health programs. The increasing likelihood that public health workers might have to work closely with law enforcement following bioterrorism events also raised fears that the public's trust in the public health community might be compromised. Nevertheless, the public health community demonstrated a needed capacity to respond to the needs of impacted populations after the attacks of September 11, 2001 [19]. Initial actions to assess health care availability and threats to those facilities were soon followed by environmental health sampling and public health education on re-entry and clean-up techniques for returning residents. Long-term efforts were initiated to establish surveillance programs on workers injuries and health. Also, environmental health actions after the building collapse were performed to ensure food and water quality, as well as adequate rodent and vector control.

Bioterrorism preparedness took on added importance after the anthrax attacks of 2001. There had been several hoaxes using powders to mimic an anthrax weapon previously, but the 2001 attacks were real and they utilized a weapons-grade formulation of the agent. The attacks led to 18 definite cases of anthrax disease, of which five were fatal. The attacks also contaminated portions of the mail delivery system, apparently causing infections in non-targeted persons far from the initial attacks. The anthrax attacks demonstrated the vulnerability of American society to bioterrorism and they stimulated much discussion about the need for a comprehensive bioterrorism plan. Discussions focused on the need for rapid detection and diagnosis, improved investigations and therapy, and effective communication. This latter was considered to be one of the larger extant problems due to unidentified lines of authority between the public health and law enforcement communities.

In the USA, the establishment of the Department of Homeland Security was a direct action to address many of the vulnerabilities to terrorism; however, officials noted that terrorism was still a rare event and that infrastructure built to address only the threat of terrorism would probably be unused for years at a time. The "all-hazards" concept of planning and response to disasters and threats to the homeland was developed to allow public health, public safety, law enforcement and other organizations with disaster response capabilities to be used on a variety of hazards whether related to terrorism or not. The concept stated that assets appropriate for a bioterrorist attack would also be appropriate for detecting and addressing other threats, such as natural outbreaks of a highly infectious disease (ex. avian influenza). In recent years, many investments in public health infrastructure have been related to the "all-hazards" approach that includes a homeland security focus.

4. The Haiti earthquake as an exception to many of the rules

Disaster events sometimes serve as turning points with regard to how organizations think about preparedness and response. For instance, the San Francisco earthquake of 1906 changed the way public assets, especially the military, were used in disaster relief efforts [12]. Hurricane Katrina and the 9-11 attacks caused responders to focus on improved communication in post-disaster response [13]. The 2010 earthquake in Haiti may serve as another of those turning points, particularly with regard to the risk of infectious disease in the post-disaster environment. Public health authorities have maintained that outbreaks of infectious disease are rare after many disasters, including earthquakes. Experience with many previous such disasters supported this claim, but post-earthquake Haiti proved to be an exception---with caveats.

The 7.0-magnitude earthquake struck the island nation on January 12, 2010 just west of the capital city of Port-au-Prince. Government estimates placed the number of dead at 217,000, with many more injured or rendered homeless. The recovery process has been long and incomplete. Reports of some infectious diseases, like malaria, did go up in the native population, though the degree to which increased surveillance played a part in those increases is unclear.

Several countries provided substantial aid to the stricken population and many relief workers, including UN peacekeepers, arrived to provide a variety of essential services, from engineering to medicine. This was the population in which the rate of infectious disease was specifically noted. There were documented outbreaks of dengue and *Plasmodium falciparum* malaria amongst international travelers, as well as acute diarrhea and upper respiratory infections. The latter was specifically noted to occur at higher rates in post-earthquake travelers than in the population of pre-earthquake travelers [14]. In one group of American missionaries, 25% were infected with the dengue virus [15].

The above-mentioned diseases, however, had been endemic to Haiti for many years. After the earthquake, a new disease emerged, one that had not occurred on the island previously. That disease was cholera. The first cases of cholera in Haiti were detected in October 2010. Within two months, cases were occurring throughout much of the island. By mid-December, the daily death rate was estimated to be 100. By 2012, over half a million people had suspected infections and over 7,000 had died [16]. The earthquake-damaged infrastructures for providing water and other necessities exacerbated the disease situation, but a real mystery developed as to where the causative organism, *Vibrio cholarae*, had originated. Haiti had no real history of cholera outbreaks and had even avoided the 1991 pandemic [17]. Initial conjectures were that *V. cholerae* is a normal but dormant part of many coastal waters and that an event that causes significant disruption to the environment, such as an earthquake, can stimulate an outbreak of the disease [16]. Others thought that humans must have brought the agent from another endemic region and this appeared to be corroborated by sanitation issues occurring at a United Nation camp in which soldiers from endemic regions were encamped. Some even linked the initial outbreak to one event in which a septic tank was dumped directly into a tributary of the Artibonite River. Microbial studies provided strong evidence that the bacterium was a recent import from the region of Northern India or Nepal. The obvious conclusion was that the Nepalese UN peacekeepers were the source of the agent and the epidemic.

Through late 2012, 604,634 cases of cholera had been reported by the government, along with 329,697 hospitalizations and 7,436 deaths. Though still too high, the relatively low death rate reflects a remarkable success given that untreated cholera may result in nearly 50% death rates in affected populations. International workers were also infected and sickened.

Thus, the perception that infectious disease outbreaks are not common after earthquakes was not accurate for the Haitian situation. Of course, Haiti presents a variety of complicating factors that affected the post-earthquake disease risk. Haiti is a tropical island with the accompanying risk of tropical diseases; malaria and dengue, though not strictly tropical, are certainly more common in tropical regions. Also, Haiti is the poorest country in the Western Hemisphere. Many diseases, including cholera, have long been associated with poverty, so it is not that surprising that these diseases emerged in post-earthquake Haiti. Nevertheless, Haiti demonstrates that there are exceptions to most rules. It is still true that large outbreaks are rare after earthquakes and some other disasters, especially if those disasters occur in developed countries. That conclusion is not as easily accepted in developing countries, especially those in tropical regions.

5. Conclusion

The disasters mentioned here and others have added knowledge and insight to provide a better understanding of the preparation needed to prevent adverse outcomes in the post-disaster environment. With the increase in the number of people affected by disasters, whether being killed, injured, sickened or displaced, a need for a public health response was warranted in each instance.

There have been many myths and assumptions stating the needs of persons after disasters; these have often proved false and have actually caused confusion and great wastage. Numerous disasters have demonstrated that the main need after disasters is potable water, often followed by food and shelter. In addition, the most at-risk population for adverse health outcomes is that of persons who have been displaced in the post-disaster environment. The health outcomes of these disasters can include the rapid spread of infectious diseases. Although uncommon after disasters, they do occur on occasion. The highest risk of infectious diseases exists outside the developed world; however, recent events have shown several instances of infectious diseases after disasters in developed countries as well, including West Nile virus after Hurricane Katerina and a fungal infection that appeared after the Joplin Tornado. Other outcomes that have come to be of concern are adverse birth outcomes and mental health issues. In addition, with the recent surge in terrorist actions, public health has had to develop the ability to respond to these events as well.

Preparedness for disasters is essential for a fast and effective response, but an important question that plagues public health is to what degree funding is allocated for these programs. It is important to avoid reducing funding for already struggling but necessary programs. The challenge public health professionals must address is the need to find a balance between allocating the proper funds to ensure essential preparedness programs are prepared for future disasters while not hindering other critically important public health programs.

Author details

David M. Claborn and Christie Oestreich

*Address all correspondence to: davidclaborn@missouristate.edu

Master of Public Health Program, Missouri State University, USA

References

[1] Noji EK., editor. The Public Health Consequences of Disasters. New York, NY: Oxford University Press; 1997.

[2] Chan JL, Theodosis C. Public-Private Partnerships During Emergencies. In: Kapur GB, Smith KP. (ed.) Emergency Public Health. Sudbury, MA: Jones and Bartlett Publishing; 2011.

[3] Toole MJ. Communicable diseases and disease control. In: The Public Health Consequences of Disasters. New York, NY: Oxford University Press; 1997.

[4] Claborn, DM. Conflict leishmaniasis In: Leishmaniasis-Trends in Epidemiology Diagnosis and Treatment. London: InTech Publishers; 2014.

[5] The Sphere Project: Humanitarian Charter and Minimum Standards in Humanitarian Response. Bourbon-on-Dunsmore, Rugby, United Kingdom: Practical Action Publishing, Schumacher Centre for Technology and development:2011. Sphereproject.org. (downloaded Aug 22, 2014)

[6] Jafari N, Shahsanai A, Memarzadeh M, Loghmani A. Prevention of communicable diseases after disaster: A review. J Res Med Sci 2011 16(7):956-962.

[7] Caillouet KA, Michaels SR, Xiong X, Foppa I, Wesson DM. Increase in West Nile neuroinvasive disease after Hurricane Katrina. Emerg Infect Dis 14(5):804-807.

[8] Fanfair RN, Benedict K, Bos J, Bennett SD, Lo YC, Adbanjo T, Etienne K, Deak E, Derado G, Shieh WJ, Drew C, Zaki S, Sugerman D, Gade L, Thompson EH, Sutton DA, Engelthaler DM, Schupp JM, Brandt ME, Harris JR, Lockhart SR, Turabelidze G, Park BJ. Necrotizing cutaneous mucormycosis after a tornado in Joplin Missouri in 2011. N Engl J Med 2012 367(23):2214-25.

[9] Benedict K, Park BJ. Invasive fungal infections after natural disasters. Emerg Infect Dis 2014 20(3):349-355.

[10] Tempark T, Lueangarun S, Chatproedprai S, Wananukul S. Flood-related skin diseases: a literature review. Int J Dermatology 2013 52(10):1168-1176.

[11] Zotti ME, Williams AM. Reproductive health assessment after disaster: Introduction to the RHAD toolkit. J Women's Health 2011 20(8):1123-1126.

[12] Foster GM. The Demands of Humanity: Army Medical Disaster Relief. Washington, D.C.: Center for Military History, U.S. Army; 1983.

[13] Degutis LC, Babcock-Dunning L. Risk communication and media relations in Health Care Emergency Management: Principles and Practice. Sudbury, MA: Jones and Bartlett Learning; 2011.

[14] Esposito DH, Han PV, Lozarsky PE, Walker PF, Gkrani-Klotsas E, Barnett ED, Libman M, McCarthey AE, Field V, Connor BA, Schwartz E, MacDonald S, Sotir MJ, GeoSentinel Surveillance Network. Characteristics and spectrum of disease among ill returned travelers from Pre-and Post-Earthquake Haiti: The GeoSentinel Experience. Am J Trop Med Hy 2012 86(1):23-28.

[15] Sharp TM, Pillai P, Hunsperger E, Santiago GA, Anderson T, Vap T, Collinson J, Fuss FG, Safranek TJ, Sotir MJ, Jentes ES, Munoz-Jordan JL, Arguello DF. A cluster of dengue cases in American missionaries returning from Haiti, 2010. Am J Trop Med Hyg 2012 86(1):16-22.

[16] Frerichs RR, Keim PS, Barrais R, Piarroux R. Nepalese origin of cholera epidemic in Haiti. Clin Microbio Infect 2012 18(6):E158-E163.

[17] Barzilay EJ, Schaad N, Magloire R, Mung KS, Boncy J, Dahourou GA, Mintz ED, Steenland MW, Vertefeuille JF, Tappero JW. Cholera surveillance during the Haiti epidemic-The first two years. N Engl J Med 2013 368(7):599-609.

[18] Levy BS, Sidel V. Challenges that terrorism poses to public health. In: Levy BS, Sideal VW. (ed.) Terrorism and Public Health: A Balanced Approach to Strengthen Systems and Protecting People. New York, New York: Oxford University Press; 2003. p3-18.

[19] Holtz TH, Leighton J, Balter S, Weiss D, Blank S, Weisfuse I. The public health response to the World Trade Center disaster. In: Levy BS, Sideal VW. (ed.) Terrorism and Public Health: A Balanced Approach to Strengthen Systems and Protecting People. New York, New York: Oxford University Press; 2003. P19-48.

Chapter 13

Health Risk Management and Mass Media — Newspaper Reports on BSE in South Korea

Satomi Noguchi and Hajime Sato

Additional information is available at the end of the chapter

http://dx.doi.org/10.5772/59080

1. Introduction

Risk management has become a dominant concern in public policy. In particular, health risks require delicate handling because of the scientific uncertainty surrounding them. In addition to performing a technical assessment of risk, an analysis of the social implications associated with health risks is indispensable. That is, one must consider that a society's coping with risk management leads to an understanding and strategy of each country. Furthermore, consideration of various stakeholders, such as professionals, citizens, and mass media, and how they are positioned is also a key issue in risk communication. Among these stakeholders, mass media are the most important source of information for most people and thus they influence how people understand particular health risks [1]. Specifically, news reports help shape the public definition of health risks and risk-related events, and politicians often interpret such reports as examples of public opinion [2]. Thus, news reports can set the public agenda, prime audiences to ascribe differing degrees of salience to available information, and provide frames for understanding risk events [3]. Therefore, examination of media reports on health risks will help in understanding how health risks emerge and are managed in society.

Bovine spongiform encephalitis (BSE) is a cattle disease that first emerged in the UK in 1985. BSE is caused by prion that is an infectious agent composed of protein in a misfolded form, and enter the food chain through the practice of feeding sheep remains to cattle. In 1996, when eating meat from infected cattle was associated with the human disease variant Creutzfeldt-Jakob disease (vCJD), the general public became extremely concerned about the safety of beef. The US Center for Disease Control and Prevention (CDC) announced that, by January 2007, 200 vCJD patients had been reported from 11 countries since the first patient was reported in 1996. The BSE crisis occurred mainly as a result of indefinite fears and categorization of BSE in the same light as other prion diseases even though the studies were still in process and no clear mechanism for developing and transferring BSE had been identified. In addition, it is

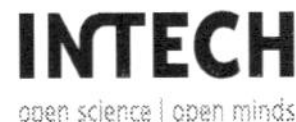

difficult to identify infected animals because biopsies are not possible and ordinary sterilization cannot eliminate the pathogen. A similar crisis also occurred in South Korea despite no BSE being reported in South Korea. According to the South Korea Centers for Disease Control and Prevention (KCDC), 5 CJD cases were reported in 2001, 9 in 2002, 19 in 2003, 13 in 2004, 15 in 2005, 19 in 2006, and 18 in 2007, while no vCJD was reported. In South Korea, a large percentage of consumed beef is imported from other countries, such as the US and Canada. When BSE was reported in those countries, the importation of their beef products was immediately suspended, and soon thereafter negotiations over the necessary risk control measures began between South Korea and its trade partners.

The aims of this chapter are to examine the visibility and faces of BSE issues as they appeared in newspaper articles in South Korea and to compare how the BSE issue was presented to the public during this period. We will first present a short history of the BSE issue and then examine related newspaper reports in South Korea. We will also illustrate the states of affairs and changes in policies and social awareness of BSE in South Korea. An analysis of the quantity and content of the newspaper articles will disclose how BSE incidents, the related health risks, and social effects were portrayed and what policy choices (e.g., aversion versus acceptance of risks, with regard to rationale) were considered appropriate. The results are discussed by comparison of US and Japanese cases, which we have previously explored [4]. The paper then discusses the roles the mass media played in appraising BSE-related safety standards and regulations and harmonizing them among countries. Additionally, implications for future health risk management are also considered.

1.1. Newspaper articles in South Korea

Three national dailies of South Korea, Dong-a, Chosun, and JoongAng, were selected for this study. At the time, these national dailies had the top three circulations in South Korea. According to the survey of 139 daily newspapers by the South Korea Audit Bureau of Circulation, which tracks the circulation of newspapers and magazines, domestic newspapers in South Korea had circulations of 1.84 million for Chosun Ilbo, 1.31 million for JoongAng Ilbo, and 1.29 million for Dong-a Ilbo from February through December 2010 [5]. The Chosun Ilbo was established in 1920 and is regarded as representing rightists, along with JoongAng Ilbo and Dong-a Ilbo. JoongAng Ilbo is a daily newspaper and a key product of JoongAng Media Network, which has 1,000 service centers in South Korea and additional branches in the US. The paper also publishes an English version, the JoongAng Daily, in alliance with the International Herald Tribune. The Dong-a Ilbo was founded in 1920 by Kim Sung-soo, who established Korea University during the Japanese occupation of Korea and later served as second vice president of South Korea in 1951.

1.2. History of BSE issue in South Korea

1.2.1. Period I: January 2002 through April 2003 and earlier

In June 1992, the first discussion of beef trade between South Korea and the US occurred, and the US claimed full opening for the beef trade [6]. On June 26, 1993, the countries agreed to postpone the full opening of the beef market until July 1997 [7]. In December 1995, the US initiated re-discussion of five items, including beef, and full opening for the beef trade was accepted with the condition of a tariff [8]. On March 26, 1996, due to the BSE problem, South Korea prohibited the importation of livestock products from countries in which BSE had occurred, including the UK and adjacent countries. In 1997, the government of South Korea modified the livestock infectious disease prevention law to cover BSE and scrapie. According to the Ministry of Strategy and Finance, the volume of beef imports increased constantly until May 1995 but after the BSE shock in the UK in 1996, beef imports began to drop (21% from May 1996 to May 1997). Then, by December 1997, imports had again increased and were 19% higher than imports in June 1997 [9].

In 2000, the Food Standards Agency (FSA) was established to evaluate food safety, to control hazardous food, and to exchange information about hazardous food. Being independent from government, the FSA made its own decisions, established its own strategy, and operated on a customer-oriented, open-door, independent, science-and evidence-oriented policy. In addition, the FSA performed its role in supporting local government's food safety tasks, evaluating food-related tasks and outcomes and supervising [10]. In February 2000, the government of South Korea established and ran the "Special Committee for Cow BSE" through the Ministry of Agriculture and Fisheries [11]. The government of South Korea banned importation of beef and related products from countries in which BSE has occurred since 1996. In addition, they also banned feeding meat or bone meal to ruminants such as cattle and sheep [12].

Starting in December 2000, the government gradually banned feeding ruminants meat or bone meal and leftover food; it also took action to prevent cross-contamination in cattle fodder. However, banning the feeding of meat and bone meal to ruminant animals in South Korea started much later than such bans in the UK and USA. Since BSE occurred in Japan, which is adjacent to South Korea, in September 2001 and since the US beef issue was considered one of four pre-conditions for the Free Trade Agreement (FTA) in 2006, the inspection and safety assurance system became a main concern. BSE was the main issue among parties who opposed the FTA: livestock farmers who worried about a decrease in beef prices, consumers who were concerned about a BSE outbreak, veterinarians, health professionals, and environmentalists. In 2003, a periodic audit by the Ministry of Health and Welfare and the Red Cross found that medicine made from the blood of patients who died of vCJD in the UK in 1998 was distributed and administered to 1,492 patients in South Korea, resulting in a hotly contested social issue [13].

1.2.2. Period II: May 2003 through August 2006

In December 2003, as BSE cases were confirmed in the US, the government of South Korea banned beef imported from the US. US beef's market share was 46% in the beef market of South Korea. Being relatively safer, demand for domestic beef was predicted to increase. However, due to customers' increasing concerns, demand for domestic beef also decreased significantly even though BSE had never occurred in South Korea. The decrease in beef consumption seemed to have originated from emotional factors such as fear and worry regarding BSE risk. As a result, even though BSE did not break out in South Korea, the information about BSE breaking out in the US resulted in a significant decrease in demand for domestic beef and thus prices for domestic beef as well.

1.2.3. Period III: September 2006 through October 2007

Importation of beef from the US resumed in 2006 with the condition that the beef must be from less-than-30-month-old cattle and be boneless. The mad cow disease outbreak in the US resulted in an increase in coverage; thus, importing US beef became a hot issue. On November 24, 2006, beef imports partially stopped because bone pieces were found in some imported beef [14]. However, on March 28, 2007, the South Korea and US governments entered "Korean-US technical agreements for livestock inspection," which stated that South Korea acknowledges the US livestock inspection system. On April 2, 2007, the South Korea and US governments reached a settlement in FTA negotiations [15]. On May 22, 2007, the World Organization for Animal Health (OIE) assessed the US as safely controlling for BSE [16]. This meant that the US could export any part of a cattle at any age without restriction if particular risky material was removed [17]. The OIE established guidelines for countries with less than a million cattle over the age of 24 months to perform tests on 20%~30% of them in seven years and countries with more than a million to test 450,000 head in seven years. Therefore, with about 40,000,000 head, the US performed tests per the second criterion and the percentage of tested individuals was less than 1%.

On August 2, 2007, spinal bones were found in beef from the US, and its importation was suspended [18]. At that time, the Grand National Party (Hannara), as the opposition party, strongly insisted on suspending imports [19]. However, after it became the ruling party, its members supported the resumption of imports and that created doubt in the public's mind. Despite the situation, restrictions on US beef imports were lifted on August 24, 2007 [20]. In 2007, the Ministry of Agriculture and Forestry reported to the government that the US was not conducting proper inspections, increasing vulnerability of South Korea to vCJD. This was disclosed by legislator Jang, Ki Kap (Democratic Labor Party) [21]. Some people believe this agreement was made in haste because it was settled just before the summit talks between South Korean President Lee and US President Bush.

1.2.4. Period IV: November 2007 through April 2008

In the beef negotiations in April 2008, South Korea and the US agreed to resume imports with drastic cuts in quarantine conditions [22]. Originally, South Korea was to open for importation of every part of a cattle under 30 months of age, excluding tonsils and the end part of the small intestine plus specified risk material (SRM) such as skull, brain, third ganglion, eye, backbone, and spinal cord, and every part of a cattle over the age of 30 months, excluding SRM. However, through additional negotiation, the parties agreed to remove SRM such as eye and brain from cattle under the age of 30 months. The government of South Korea announced that the agreement was in accordance with OIE criteria [23].

On April 29, 2008, MBC TV aired the first report regarding the risk associated with US beef in a program called *PD's Notebook*. The program resulted in great social shock and triggered a protest against US beef imports in South Korea [24]. In the program "Is US beef safe?" *PD's Notebook* insisted that 94% of South Koreans have BSE infectable genes and the possibility is 2 to 3 times higher than that of the British and Americans [25]. The program also quoted a US consumer association members' words: "People who eat US beef are like experimental animals." Many parody pictures became popular on the internet after airing of the *PD's Notebook's* video [26].

1.2.5. Period V: May 2008 through April 2009

Kookmin Ilbo (a newspaper) reported on May 2, 2008, that BSE transferable SRM would be brought into South Korea according to the Korea-US beef agreement. The paper introduced specialists' opinions stating that certain SRM (e.g., brain, spinal cord, eye, head bone, tongue, tip of small intestine) from cattle 30 months or older had to be removed. However, since quarantine authority had no way to confirm the history of beef, SRM could be brought in. The Ministry of Food, Agriculture, Forestry, and Fisheries explained that SMR from cattle 30 months or older would be completely removed in the slaughter and manufacturing process and dental examiners determined the age of cattle in the slaughter house under a veterinarian's supervision. Right after the agreement, the government of South Korea announced that consumers could buy and eat quality beef at low price and the choice was a matter for the consumer. The government did not respond to the argument, calling it a "ghost story" at first. The government did hold a press conference to announce that US beef is very safe on May 2, 2008 [27].

The contents of the agreement of May 5, 2008, were said not to reflect the people's opinion [28]. Many parties debated the issue and political parties, the press, and specialist groups amplified the debate. Since most BSE cases were found in cattle older than 30 months, countries throughout the world started to import only beef under 30 months but, by the agreement, South Korea also was to import beef over 30 months. The OIE recommended not importing seven parts, including the brain, skull, spinal cord, eye, and backbone, from cattle 30 months or older [29]. However, if under 30 months, only the tonsils and end part of the small intestine were to be excluded. South Korea requested an indication of age, but the US declined. The countries only agreed to indicate under 30 months for T-bone steak, which has backbone – one of the SRMs – for 180 days. For other SRMs, people of South Korea could only hope that the US respected the age guidelines [30]. The government of South Korea could not stop importing or impose a quarantine even though BSE had broken out in the US. Before that agreement, if the US quarantine system was suspected of having a significant problem, the government of South Korea could stop importing based on its own judgment [31]. However, under the hygiene conditions of the new agreement, the only requirement for the US was to conduct epidemiological research and report the results. For that reason, the government's beef negotiation of South Korea was criticized as abandoning the people's right to health and to quarantine.

On May 2-3, large demonstrations were held in front of the Chung-gea Square. Celebrities participated in the demonstrations or wrote comments on their mini internet home page criticizing President Lee and US beef imports [32]. President Lee's mini home page was filled with critical comments from netizens and this led to the home page being closed out. On May 5, 2008, the government started advertising at the bottom of the front page of the main newspapers. On May 6, the departments in charge started public announcements through the internet. Cheongwadae (the presidential residence), the Ministry for Food, Agriculture, Forestry, and Fisheries, and the Ministry of Health and Welfare posted articles such as "BSE, 10 questions and 10 answers" on their web sites and tried to put out the fire by advertising on the main internet portal sites [33]. On May 12, responding for the US federal official gazette easing the regulation for animal fodder, the government announced that there was a working-level error in the process of the agreement. On May 22, President Lee released a statement to the public [34]. Despite the government's explanation, the argument did not subside. From May 2 to May 6, candlelight rallies gathered 10,000 to 20,000 people. After that, demonstrations criticizing the agreement continued through the weekend. As the official notification date approached, starting May 18, 2008, the Alliance for President Lee's Impeachment held the rallies every day [35].

After May 5, 2008, debate regarding distortion of the agreement came up. The Ministry of Food, Agriculture, Forestry, and Fisheries had a history of declining private organizations' requests for disclosure of original agreements [36]. In addition, the ministry disclosed the information only after it learned that the English-language agreement was posted on the internet. People suspected that the government had hidden factors in translating the original [37]. Indeed, there were more than 20 delicate differences between the original agreement and the agreement in the official announcement of May 5, 2008, as discussed below.

Due to the continuing controversy, South Korea and the US passed an epistolary-style agreement on May 19, 2008. On May 22, 2008, the president released a public announcement indicating an apology for the US beef issue and urging the National Assembly to ratify the agreement [38]. In the public announcement, President Lee acknowledged the lack of effort to get the people's understanding and gather opinions. Despite the government's effort, the street demonstrations spread. From that time, the slogans went beyond the US beef issue and some participants started to turn to anti-government stances [39]. The police's hold-back became active accordingly. On May 29, 2008, Minister of Food, Agriculture, Forestry, and Fisheries Jung, Woon Chan disclosed the sanitary conditions for importing US beef and concluded from surveying 30 slaughter facilities in the US that there was no sanitary management problem such as SRM removal [40]. From June 5 to June 8, the people staged a 72-hour demonstration in Seoul Square, and some protesters stayed all night in tents [41]. On June 6, the first day of long non-working days, the number of participants was estimated at 56,000 by police, but 200,000 by the hosts [42]. On June 7, a candle rally was held in New York, criticizing the government of South Korea. On June 10, the participants numbered 100,000 (police estimate) or 500,000 (host estimate) and in Seoul, 1,000,000 (host estimate) [43].

On July 8, 2008, the government of South Korea began to indicate the country of origin on beef and rice based on the food sanitation law's articles 21 and 69. In December 2008, the products covered extended to pork, chicken, and kim chi [44]. From August 1 to September 5, 2008, the National Assembly's US beef investigation committee was initiated. The Grand National Party insisted that resuming imports of US beef had been agreed upon in the former government and the current government just signed on, while the opposition parties insisted that the negotiation was pushed ahead with haste just for the Korea-US summit talk. Minister Dong Suk, chief officer for agriculture and trade strategy, who led the negotiation, said that the beef negotiation was not South Korea's present to the US but rather it was a present from the US, and he asked for an apology from the opposition parties [45]. Starting on November 25, 2008, large retailers such as E-mart, Home Plus, and Lotte Mart started to sell US beef to customers

[46]. However, by June 2009, the sales proportion of US beef in large retailers had dropped significantly, to 1%, and US beef sales were being considered for elimination [47].

The BSE controversy in South Korea became a main social issue through the writings of netizens who transferred concerns and rumor with their opinions. According to JoongAng Daily's statistics, the issue was very active in internet communities such as the Daum Agora economy forum, free bulletin boards, politics forums and social forums, and many discussions, items of news, and opinions were exchanged. In addition, the issue was dealt with seriously in DC inside, Naver, Yahoo, and Hankyorea Hantoma [48]. Many internet media broadcast the candle rallies, and the videos spread through media such as YouTube, making internet media more influential than conventional news media [49,50]. People boycotted media such as Chosun, JoongAng, and Dong-a and posted a list of the companies that advertised in those newspapers so that netizens could pressure the companies by taking actions such as posting criticism on the companies' web sites. Meanwhile, a controversy about *PD's Notebook* became the trigger for candle rallies. The translator Jung, Ji Min's whistle-blowing caused the controversy to check whether the coverage was exaggerated. The PD personnel who planned and produced the program were arrested with warrants [51]. On June 17, 2009, the Seoul high court decided in favor of the plaintiff, partially in the case the Ministry of Food, Agriculture, Forestry, and Fisheries litigated against *PD's Notebook* claiming an objection and correction coverage. However, MBC *PD's Notebook* appealed to the Supreme Court [52]. On January 20, 2010, the Seoul central district court found that the PD personnel were not guilty [53]. On January 26, 2010, the court decided in favor of the defendant in the civil case of groups against *PD's Notebook,* ordering an apology and correction coverage, plus compensation for damages [54].

Restarting after the hardship, US beef sales did not reach even half of Australian beef sales in the second half of 2009, which is much less than the sales before the imports stopped [55]. The import increased when the quarantine resumed in June 2008 after the BSE shock, but before long, sales dropped. The remaining negative notions about US beef are regarded as the reason. One of the reasons for the distrust is that the disqualifying rate of US beef is the highest among all imported beef. According to the data Kang, Ki Kap, a member of the National Assembly, received from the Ministry of Food, Agriculture, Forestry, and Fisheries on August 13, 2009, the amount of US beef disqualified in the quarantine process reached 20 cases, 59 tons in the first half of 2009, which is 56.1% of the total of disqualified imported beef (105 tons) [56].

2. Study methods

2.1. Collecting and coding of articles

Our study targeted the period from January 2002 through April 2009, when BSE-infected cattle were discovered in the US and the import ban was introduced and later lifted in South Korea. Articles were searched and collected from the three mentioned papers, using the keywords BSE and mad cow disease. In addition, articles with related keywords, such as vCJD, safety of beef (products), and ban on beef trade, were searched and checked individually to determine whether they reported or discussed BSE-related events; those that did were included for analysis. We categorized each article as follows: First, we focused our analysis on the number of articles, ignoring their word counts, placement, and font size. Second, all included articles were coded and counted for article content/frame. Here, a frame denotes a way of packaging and positioning an issue so that it conveys a certain meaning [57,58]. Coders in both countries used a coding system based on a framework similar to those previously employed [59,60]. Issues framed elements for coding and were derived from the preliminary qualitative interpretation of articles/policy documents, comprising geographic focus (South Korea, US, and other countries) and topic categories (BSE incidents, biomedical effects and risks to humans, vCJD, effects on commerce and related policies, agricultural effects and related policies, and effects on international trade and related policies). As there could be multiple categories for each article, more than one frame category could be coded per article. Third, the tone or slant (i.e., advocacy orientation) of the articles was analyzed in terms of their advocacy attributes. An article was assessed as positive when it argued for stronger safety measures/policies and negative when it contained arguments for weaker measures/policies. Articles were designated neutral if they did not clearly argue for either stronger or weaker policies, were ambiguous, or had relatively equal coverage of both orientations. Finally, the argumentative bases (policy discussion contexts) of articles, if any, were coded using the categories of health, economy, balance of different policy objectives, and (rational) acceptance of health risks. All the coding was done independently by two pre-trained coders, yielding a reliability rate of 83%, which was considered within the acceptance levels for study [61].

2.2. Statistical analysis

The overall study period was divided into five distinct sub-periods: period I (from January 2002 through April 2003, when BSE problems were reported in the UK through mass media), period II (from May 2003 through August 2006, when the first BSE cases were discovered in Canada and the US, and the import ban was imposed in South Korea), period III (from September 2006 through October 2007, when the trade ban was partly lifted), period IV (from November 2007 through April 2008, when the FTA was negotiated and adopted between South Korea and the US), and period V (from May 2008 through April 2009, when media of South Korea reported US beef risks, the candle protests took place, and afterward). Trends in the numbers, topics, and tones were analyzed over these sub-periods. After obtaining descriptive statistics (numbers, means, and standard deviations), adjacent periods in the given study period were compared. Relationships of advocacy orientation with rationale were examined using multi-nominal logistic regression analysis. In the model, a neutral orientation was chosen as the base outcome, and the coefficients (relative risk ratios) of the presence of each rationale for the article orientation (positive or negative) were estimated [62]. Statistical analyses were conducted using Stata/SE 12.1 for Windows (StataCorp LP, College Station, TX).

3. Results of newspaper reports in South Korea

Table 1 shows the monthly average number of newspaper articles with their geographic focus and topic categories on BSE of three dailies in South Korea. During the study period, the number of BSE-related newspaper articles prominently increased in period III when beef imports partially stopped because bone pieces were found in some US imported beef and in period V, in which liberalization of the beef market in South Korea became a political agenda, invoking a public protest movement (4.7, 4.4, 8.6, 4.1, 60.9, monthly average of articles per period, respectively). We also draw a scatter plot showing time series trend of weekly average number of newspaper articles in Figure 1.

	Period I Jan2002-Apr2003				Period II May2003-Aug2006				Period III Sep2006-Oct2007				Period IV Nov2007-Apr2008				Period V May2008-Apr2009			
	mean	±	sd	p	mean	±	sd	p	mean	±	sd	p	mean	±	sd	p	mean	±	sd	p
Number of articles[†]	4.7	±	9.5		4.4	±	6.2		8.6	±	5.6		4.1	±	5.9		60.9	±	82.1	**
Geographic focus (%)																				
Korea Topic	32.4	±	32.5		64.3	±	23.0	**	89.9	±	11.6	**	82.8	±	17.6		94.3	±	6.2	
US topic	10.8	±	19.6		10.1	±	15.6		6.2	±	7.7		11.0	±	16.9		1.5	±	1.9	
Other country's topic	56.9	±	38.9		25.5	±	22.2	***	4.1	±	10.5	*	5.6	±	13.6		2.7	±	3.0	
Topic categories (%)																				
Incidents	19.9	±	23.0		21.1	±	23.2		3.5	±	5.6	*	2.4	±	5.8		2.8	±	3.7	
Biomedical effects	18.9	±	20.5		16.8	±	19.0		17.6	±	12.6		20.0	±	18.3		12.1	±	9.0	
Commerce	27.9	±	22.5		44.3	±	22.7		55.4	±	13.3		31.8	±	17.2		29.9	±	10.8	
Agriculture	9.3	±	12.3		37.2	±	21.2	***	42.5	±	13.4		32.9	±	24.5		19.7	±	9.1	
Trade	15.4	±	20.1		48.6	±	26.2	***	73.1	±	14.8	**	73.4	±	15.8		19.1	±	12.6	***

Tests were performed for before period by Bonferroni method. *$p < 0.05$, **$p < 0.01$, ***$p < 0.001$

[†]The numbers are shown as monthly mean per paper.

Table 1. Numbers and Topics of BSE articles in South Korea

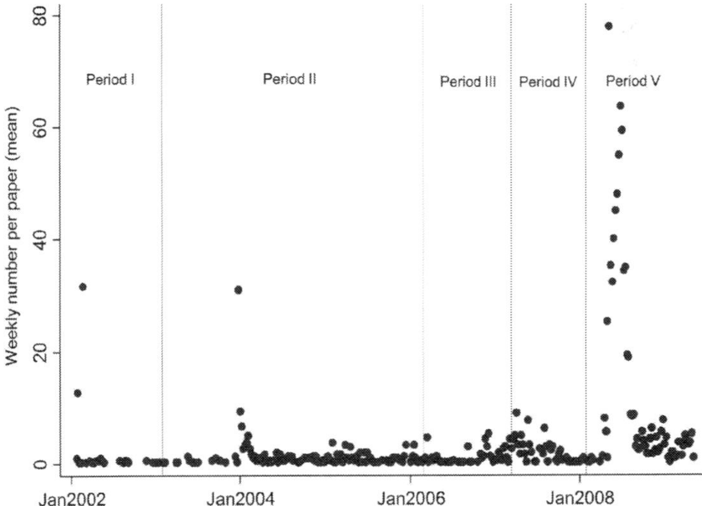

Figure 1. Number of newspaper articles in South Korea

Geographically, in the early phase in period I, more than half of the articles had a foreign focus (56.9%). This period covered the BSE problems reported in the UK through the mass media. In period II, articles with a domestic focus increased in accordance with negotiation of the US-Korea Free Trade Agreement. After this period, the numbers of articles with a domestic focus were high (period III, 89.9%; period IV, 82.8%; period V, 94.3%), while articles with a foreign focus were few. With regard to the topics reported, biomedical effects were reported constantly but with a small proportion throughout the study periods. However, the frequency of reports on trade issues changed remarkably over time. That is, from period III through period IV, trade issue coverage jumped up to a peak (73.1% and 73.4%, respectively) and sharply decreased in period V (19.1%). Articles containing arguments based on commerce and agriculture displayed similar trends but with different peaks in period III (e.g., commerce: 27.9%, 44.3%, 55.4%, 31.8%, and 29.9%, for periods I through V, respectively). These trends and contrasts of geographic focus and topic categories are also shown in Figures 2.

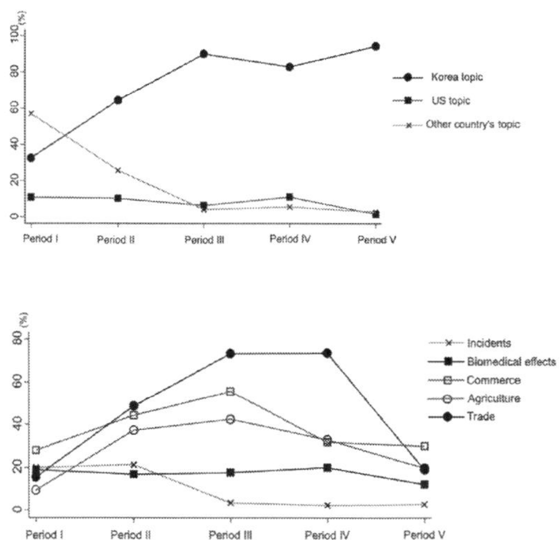

Figure 2. Geographic focus and Topic categories of newspaper articles in South Korea

The policy advocacy observed in newspaper articles in each period is shown in Table 2. Calls for stronger domestic policy peaked in period III (14.2%), which was after the beef trade ban was partly lifted, but in period IV, calls for weaker domestic policy gradually increased and became more visible (12.1%). In period V, when a trade issue became a conspicuous political agenda, calls for both stronger and weaker domestic policies appeared less frequently and none of them was dominant. Throughout the study period, the major rationale for policy advocacy was the economy (65.1%, 73.7%, 73.6%, 74.4%, 34.5%, for periods I through V, respectively). Gradually, advocacy articles based on health concerns decreased (e.g., from period I at 42.9% and period II at 39.5% to period IV at 29.5%) and the arguments for balance in different policy objectives increased (e.g., from period I at 6.0% and period II at 6.6% to period IV at 19.0%). In period V, arguments for rational acceptance of BSE risks became more visible compared to other periods, while the economy, health, and balance were less frequently argued. Graphical charts about policy advocacy and rational for policy advocacy are shown in Figures 3.

		Period I Jan2002-Apr2003				Period II May2003-Aug2006				Period III Sep2006-Oct2007				Period IV Nov2007-Apr2008				Period V May2008-Apr2009			
		mean	±	sd	p	mean	±	sd	p	mean	±	sd	p	mean	±	sd	p	mean	±	sd	p
Policy advocacy (%)																					
Domestic	Positive	6.5	±	8.2		6.6	±	7.4		14.2	±	5.2	**	4.5	±	6.5	*	3.0	±	3.1	
	Negative	0.0	±	0.0		0.6	±	1.6		2.4	±	1.9		12.1	±	18.9		3.5	±	2.9	
Foreign	Positive	1.8	±	4.8		1.7	±	3.6		1.1	±	2.2		0.0	±	0.0	**	0.2	±	0.4	
	Negative	0.0	±	0.0		4.0	±	5.3		9.9	±	7.2	**	5.3	±	6.6		0.9	±	1.3	
Rationale for policy advocacy (%)																					
Health		42.9	±	34.8		39.5	±	23.0		29.7	±	15.4		29.5	±	25.3		20.0	±	10.3	
Economy		65.1	±	32.7		73.7	±	20.8		73.6	±	14.5		74.4	±	22.4		34.5	±	11.7	**
Balance		6.0	±	14.6		6.6	±	10.1		23.6	±	14.1	***	19.0	±	11.5		10.9	±	7.4	
Acceptance		0.7	±	2.2		1.3	±	3.6		3.3	±	4.7		1.0	±	2.6		3.8	±	2.5	

Tests were performed for before period by Bonferroni method. *p < 0.05, **p < 0.01, ***p < 0.001

Table 2. Policy advocacy and its rationale for BSE articles in South Korea

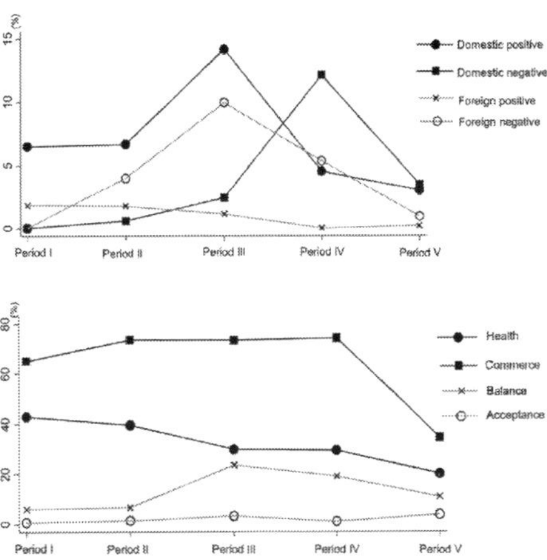

Figure 3. Policy advocacy and Rationale for policy advocacy of newspaper articles in South Korea

The results of the examination of individual articles using a multinomial logistic regression analysis are shown in Table 3. The citation of health concerns indicated a greater likelihood that a given article carried advocacy for a stronger domestic policy rather than no advocacy (RRR=2.62). A discussion of the economy indicated a 2.25 times greater likelihood of stronger domestic policy advocacy. The discussion on policy balance and risk acceptance is less associated with stronger advocacy (RRR=0.90, 0.61, respectively) and with weaker advocacy (RRR=7.24, 4.06, respectively). Additionally, health concerns was more associated with stronger foreign advocacy (RRR=4.06), and economic discussion was more associated with weaker foreign advocacy (RRR=1.92) with statistical significance, while other advocacy (balance, acceptance) were less associated with stronger/weaker foreign policies.

| | Domestic Policy | | | | | | | | Foreign Policy | | | | | | | |
| | Positive | | | | Negative | | | | Positive | | | | Negative | | | |
Variables	RRR	±	SD	p	RRR	±	SD	p	RRR	±	SD	p	RRR	±	SD	p
Health	2.62	±	0.28	***	1.55	±	0.24	**	4.06	±	1.43	***	1.27	±	0.20	
Economy	2.25	±	0.24	***	0.98	±	0.15		1.90	±	0.69		1.92	±	0.29	***
Balance	0.90	±	0.13		7.24	±	1.14	***	0.90	±	0.45		4.99	±	0.78	***
Acceptance	0.61	±	0.19		4.06	±	0.87	***	1.05	±	0.80		1.11	±	0.33	

Results of multinominal logistic regression analysis: Relative risk ratios (RRR) and their standard deviations for a given article to carry positive/negative advocacy (neutral orientation as baseline).
*p < 0.05, **p < 0.01, ***p < 0.001

Table 3. Relationship of advocacy orientation with rationale of South Korea newspaper articles

4. Discussion

In South Korea, the number of BSE-related newspaper articles increased with trade disputes and, throughout the study period, the major rationale for policy advocacy was the economy. In the early periods of our analysis, advocacy articles based on health concerns gradually decreased, and the arguments for a balance among different policy objectives increased. At the same time, calls for both stronger domestic policies and weaker domestic policies appeared less frequently and none of them was dominant. Calls for stronger domestic policy peaked immediately after the beef trade ban was lifted, but thereafter calls for weaker domestic policy gradually increased and became more visible. When a trade issue became a conspicuous political agenda, arguments for the rational acceptance of BSE risks became more visible, while the economy, health, and balance were less frequently argued. However, even when trade liberalization became a political agenda, newspapers of South Korea did not disproportionately call for stronger/weaker policies. The media did not focus on any single aspect as the base for their reporting and discussion, but rather argued for the rational acceptance of BSE risks.

4.1. Issue prominence and geographic focuses of newspaper reports on BSE

The framing of the issue, coupled with its visibility, helped set the agenda in the media and society. Characteristics of events/issues and the social configuration around them are the determinants of their social impact and associated news coverage. Therefore, tabulation of the domains of issue reporting reveals the social importance of each domain. Considering the dynamic nature of the relationships, media framing affects and reflects how people understand an issue and how society responds to the issue [63]. The case would be expected to be the same for BSE reporting, and media reports on health risks reflect the social implications of those risks and the configuration of social interests and powers in which they operate [64]. Discussion in the media of acceptance or aversion of health risks and what policy measures are desirable are also associated with these reports. The media are thus a key arena in which policy choices and responsibilities with regard to food system governance are negotiated [65]. With a focus on topic categories for articles, trade and agriculture topics drastically increased with Korean-US technical agreements for livestock inspection. Trade issues started to jump up in period II, when BSE cases were confirmed in the US in December 2003 and the government of South Korea banned importing beef from the US. In 2006, beef imports from US resumed with conditions (younger than 30-month-old cattle and boneless), but thereafter beef imports partially stopped because bone pieces were found in some parts of imported beef in November 2006. For South Korea, the BSE issue became an important international economic issue rather than a health issue for domestic consumers.

The number of BSE-related newspaper articles first increased when beef importation was partially suspended because bone pieces were found in some beef imported from the US in November 2006. On the other hand, period V could be treated as an atypical period because liberalization of the beef market in South Korea became a political agenda. Large demonstrations were held in front of the Chung-gea Square and media articles increased with the candle protests. Such visibility meant that the total number of articles increased about 15 times compared to the previous period. Under a social crisis such as the BSE issue, "social amplification" can be observed and Renn et al. conceptualized social amplification in their examination of risk-related social processes over time [66]. Events pertaining to hazards interact with psychological, social, institutional, and cultural processes, and they can increase or decrease the public's perception of risk and shape the public's behavior, which in turn can have secondary socio-economic and political consequences. When the initial influence of a risk dissipates and the secondary consequences grow, the risk is said to be socially amplified. However, Chung et al. noticed that risk amplification of media was not reported in South Korea [67]. They analyzed the role and framing of media with the BSE and H1N1 cases and reported that the effect of media was limited in the BSE issue. Rather, the media reduced the voice amplifying BSE risk while public unrest was building in South Korea. That is, the number of articles increased in period V, but those articles may simply have covered the candle protest and issued daily reports that the movement and contents were relatively rational. This is observed in South Korean newspapers that did not focus on any single aspect as the base for reporting and discussion, but rather argued for the rational acceptance of BSE risks.

4.2. Comparison with other countries: Cases of US and Japan

Acceptance of BSE-related risks was argued differently in each country, and those differences reflected and affected the public's perception of BSE issues, the related safety policies of the governments, and the configuration of social interests. Previously, we compared the newspaper reports on BSE-related events in major national dailies in Japan and the US around the period when BSE-infected cattle were discovered in the US and the import of US beef products was banned (between December 2002 and November 2006) and reported elsewhere [4]. After the discovery of BSE cattle in the US, articles of commerce and trade issues were dominant in

Japan, while the incidence of BSE, agriculture, and trade dominated in the US. From these results, the trend in South Korean newspapers about BSE was similar to the US rather than Japan because the BSE issue continued to be an issue of agriculture and trade in South Korea. BSE remained largely an issue of human health and trade, so news articles in the commerce category comprised a large part of the related articles in Japan. In the US, even after the detection of BSE in Canada and the US, confidence in the safety of beef products remained high. US newspapers carried significantly fewer articles on BSE than Japanese papers. This could be explained by the cattle-raising agricultural sector being relatively larger in the US and also the beef trade and commercial relationship between the two countries [68,69]. In many countries, a set of major frames provided by the preceding reports in the initial period of BSE dominated media reporting of the issue over time [70,71]. The differences evident in the media could serve as a vehicle for reappraising the existing policies as well as the possible international harmonization of risk management policies.

Beginning in the late 1990s, South Korea became a growing and important market for major beef exporters in the US. In 2003, beef imports accounted for nearly 75% of beef consumption of South Korea and South Korea was the third-largest market for US beef exports before the ban its government imposed after the first US BSE case was discovered. With regard to the trend in beef consumption in South Korea, in 2008, the quantity of US beef exports to South Korea decreased to about 57 thousand metric tons, about one quarter of its former total, and the slide continued to 2009. The falling value of the won and the candle protests evoked a negative attitude toward the government of South Korea and its agreement about US beef [72]. Beef exports to South Korea in 2010 totaled $518 million, about two-thirds of the record 2003 level. This shows that, in South Korea, although the news media were objective or rational, the reaction of people did not equal that of the media. That is, consumer behavior was typically characterized by panic or reaction to social crisis. A crisis is usually driven by a focus on particular events or one event that surprises people, limited time to develop a response, and threats to high-priority goals [73-75]. These focusing events highlight certain adverse conditions, increase public concern, trigger political mobilization, define the issues as serious, and propel them to a high priority on the political agenda [76,77].

4.3. Policy advocacy and international partnership for risk management

Closely related to aversion and acceptance of a risk is the media advocacy of policy, referring to judgmental statements on the policies already in place and/or calls for stronger or weaker alternatives. Such statements help shape public perceptions of what is left to be done and who is responsible. Therefore, the slant of newspaper articles (advocacy) can also be interpreted as the media's policy appraisal. Our study showed that calls for stronger domestic policy peaked when the beef trade ban was partly lifted (period III), but thereafter calls for weaker domestic policy gradually increased and became more visible (period IV). When a trade issue became a conspicuous political agenda (period V), calls for both stronger domestic policies and weaker domestic policies appeared less frequently and none of them was dominant. Throughout the study period, the major rationale for policy advocacy was the economy in South Korea. Gradually, advocacy articles based on health concerns decreased and arguments for a balance of different policy objectives increased. In period V, arguments for the rational acceptance of BSE risks became more visible, while the economy, health, and balance were argued less frequently. In summary, the media appraised domestic policy as positive based on health and economic viewpoints in South Korea.

The media play a pivotal role in setting goals, assigning responsibility, and assessing the efforts of governments [78]. For example, the public might be perfectly content with ongoing policies if people are persuaded to accept certain levels of risk or if they regard the policy efforts to be well in place and the incidents beyond the control capacity of the government. On the other hand, when the policy target is zero risk (i.e., the total elimination of risk), the discovery of BSE cattle can easily be interpreted as a policy failure, which might invoke calls for stronger (more effective) policies [4]. In the case of BSE, scientific uncertainty was always a key component of the environment in which the policies were made [79]. The handling of the uncertainty brought about by inconclusive scientific evidence has thus become an important aspect of policy management [80]. Furthermore, mishandling of health risks would undermine public trust in their governments. Therefore, the artificial introduction or the enlarged threat of such risks might be employed as a tool for political maneuvering. This aspect should be deliberately considered in the planning of public management for every government [81,82]. Although scientific information is shared among countries, information about the perception and management of risk is not. Policies are not always in concert and many remain to be internationally disputed, as exemplified by the South Korean import ban on US beef. Analyzing media reports helps in examining the process of policy making and offers an analytic framework for observing how issues are treated.

5. Conclusion and policy implication

We examined the visibility and faces of BSE-related issues in newspapers in South Korea. The media play a role in setting the agenda and assessing governmental efforts. Media reports on health risks and their management can serve as vehicles for the judgment of existing policies. The slant of newspaper articles can be interpreted as a call for stronger or weaker policy alternatives. Even when the trade liberalization became a political agenda, newspapers of South Korea did not disproportionately call for stronger/weaker policies. The media did not focus on any single aspect as the base for their reporting and discussion, but rather argued for the rational acceptance of BSE risks. Based on our findings, the utility of monitoring the mass media as an indicator of public policy appraisal is discussed, along with its use in planning health risk management. Health and safety regulations can be understood as expressions of a nation's political and social values; they are associated with the social configurations around the issue. Reports and discussions in the media reveal which policy measures are considered desirable by the public. Especially during trade disputes, which are sometimes triggered by the introduction of policies for health and safety purposes, the examination of media reports helps in reconsidering the existing domestic safety measures and facilitates international harmonization of health risk management, in addition to helping resolve trade conflicts.

Acknowledgements

This study was supported by the Grants-in-Aid for Scientific Research "Risk communications in mass media during heath crises: An international comparative study (2012-2014)," granted by Japan Society for the Promotion of Science to Hajime Sato.

Author details

Satomi Noguchi and Hajime Sato*

*Address all correspondence to: hsato@niph.go.jp

Department of Health Policy and Technology Assessment, National Institute of Public Health, Japan

References

[1] Goodell R. The role of the mass media in scientific controversy. In: Engelhardt HT & Caplan AL, editors. Scientific controversies: case studies in the resolution and closure of disputes in science and technology. Cambridge: Cambridge University Press; 1987.

[2] Kleinschmit D, Krott M. The Media in Forestry: Government, Governance and Social Visibility. In: Sikor T, editor. Public and Private in Natural Resource Governance: A False Dichotomy? London: Earthscan; 2008.

[3] Kim S, Scheufele DA, Shanahan J. Think About it This Way: Attribute Agenda-Setting Function of the Press and the Public's Evaluation of a Local Issue. Journalism and Mass Communication Quarterly. 2002; 79: 7-25. http://dx.doi.org/10.1177/107769900207900102

[4] Sato H, Campbell RG. Newspaper Reports on BSE around the Time of the Japan-US Trade Conflicts: Content Analysis of Japanese and US Dailies from 2002 to 2006. Advances in Journalism and Communication. 2014; 2: 20-34.

[5] ABC Journal. Firstly published the report on the circulation of daily newspapers. 2010; 85: 1-3.

[6] Daily record of negotiation. JoongAng Ilbo. 2 April 2007.

[7] Seoul Shinmun. UR negotiation agenda for agricultural products passed. 15 December 1993.

[8] Seoul Shinmun. US and Canada are imposing trade pressure. 8 December 1995.

[9]   Ministry of Strategy and Finance in Korea. The Analysis in Economical Effect of Beef Market Opening Expansion. May 2008.

[10] Shin K. SDI policy Report: Strategy for food safety of Seoul (21st edition). Seoul: Seoul Development Institute; 2008.

[11] Chosun Ilbo. Government organized 'special committee for cow BSE.' 6 February 2001.

[12] Chosun Ilbo. Rigid enforcement of illegal imports for blocking BSE. 10 February 2001.

[13] Dong-a Ilbo. UK exported blood infected BSE to 11 countries. 5 February 2001.

[14] Chosun Ilbo. US beef got rejected again, outlook on deepening trade conflicts. 1 December 2006.

[15] JoongAng Ilbo. Dongseok Min "US understood our stance on beef inspection." 2 April 2007.

[16] Kyunghyang Shinmun. OIE judged US as 'safely controlling country for BSE.' 23 May 2007.

[17] Dong-a Ilbo. Rising possibilities to import US 'beef with bones.' 23 May 2007.

[18] Kyunghyang Shinmun. Halt all inspections for US beef, resuming rib imports is not guaranteed. 2 August 2007.

[19] Chosun Ilbo. Korea "should prohibit to import US beef when necessary." 3 August 2007.

[20] JoongAng Ilbo. Release of halting US beef inspections, resumed imports. 24 August 2007.

[21] Joonang Ilbo. Restart US beef inspections in Yongin. 27 August 2007.

[22] Chosun Ilbo. Korea-US resumes beef negotiation tomorrow. 10 April 2008.

[23] Dong-a Ilbo. US "Eliminate restrictions on cattle age and parts." 14 April 2008.

[24] JoongAng Ilbo. 'PD's Note' report on US beef shocked the audience. 30 April 2008.

[25] Dong-a Ilbo. Amplified 'controversy about BSE', battles in politicians. 2 May 2008.

[26] JoongAng Ilbo. Increasing campaigns to obtain signatures for impeaching the president Lee, leaders are faced with ordeal as well. 2 May 2008.

[27] JoongAng Ilbo. President Lee bowed three times in the statement. 2 May 2008.

[28] JoongAng Ilbo. Revealed Korea-US beef agreement, main issues. 5 May 2008.

[29] Dong-a Ilbo. Korea-US beef agreement is stricter than OIE hygiene standards. 19 May 2008.

[30] Seoul Shinmun. Government "Possible to request for revision about hygiene conditions." 7 May 2008.

[31] Kyunghyang Shinmun. Additional discussion on US beef without the key points, 'Renegotiation is the only solution.' 20 May 2008.

[32] Chosun Ilbo. 'Hard time of President Lee', Netizens against 'US beef imports' attacked his homepage. 1 May 2008.

[33] Seoul Shinmun. Cheongwadae 'founding a capital solution' to block the ghost story. 7 May 2008.

[34] Chosun Ilbo. Same with US conditions about imported beef. 3 May 2008.

[35] JoongAng Ilbo. All-night demonstration occupying downtown roads in Seoul, from start to forceful dispersal. 25 May 2008.

[36] JoongAng Ilbo. Minister of Agriculture letting US beef shocks progress. 12 May 2008.

[37] Chosun Ilbo. Supplement negotiation about beef, Government should put heart and soul to resolve misunderstandings. 20 May 2008.

[38] Chosun Ilbo. President Myung-bak Lee's a statement to the nation. 22 May 2008.

[39] Dong-a Ilbo. Candle rally collided with police at dawn. 27 May 2008.

[40] Chosun Ilbo. Announced US beef import and hygiene regulations. 29 May 2008.

[41] Dong-a Ilbo. Continued the rally '72 hours nation action' for two day long. 6 June 2008.

[42] Chosun Ilbo. Candle rally spreads to US, rally in the center of New York. 5 June 2008.

[43] Dong-a Ilbo. 6.10 candle rally massively held throughout the nation. 10 June 2008.

[44] Kyunghyang Shinmun. Park, Byungryul. Indicating a place-of-origin for pork, chicken and kimchi from 22nd. 21 December 2008.

[45] JoongAng Ilbo. Woonchun Jung and Dongsuk Min's 'outspoken' comments. 1 August 2008.

[46] JoongAng Ilbo. Park, Hyunyoung and Im, Mijin. Big markets start to sale US beef tomorrow. 26 November 2008.

[47] Dong-a Ilbo. US beef has completely defeated Korea and Australia beef since last year. 26 November 2009.

[48] JoongAng Ilbo. Lee, Nari. 'Internet rumor' about BSE. 2 June 2008.

[49] Salman A, Ibrahim F, Hj.Abdullah MY, Mustaffa N, Mahbob MH. The impact of new media on traditional mainstream mass media. The Innovation Journal: The Public Sector Innovation Journal. 2011; 16(3): article 7. http://www.innovation.cc/scholarly-style/ali_samman_new+media_impac116v3i7a.pdf